A Multidisciplinary Approach to Managing Ehlers-Danlos (Type III) – Hypermobility Syndrome

Working with the Chronic Complex Patient

Isobel Knight

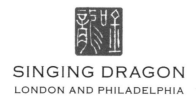

SINGING DRAGON
LONDON AND PHILADELPHIA

Permission has been given by all of the contributors for their material
to appear in the book.
Figure 5.1: Maslow's Hierarchy of Needs has been printed with kind permission from www.
maslowshierarchyofneeds.net.
The material on the Breighton Score and Brighton Criteria on pp.328-329 has been reproduced with
kind permission from the Hypermobility Syndrome Association.
Table A1 has been printed with kind permission from EDS-UK.

First published in 2013
by Singing Dragon
an imprint of Jessica Kingsley Publishers
73 Collier Street
London N1 9BE, UK
and
400 Market Street, Suite 400
Philadelphia, PA 19106, USA

www.singingdragon.com

Library of Congress Cataloging in Publication Data
Knight, Isobel, 1974-
A multi-disciplinary approach to managing Ehlers-Danlos (type III)--hypermobility syndrome : working
with the chronic complex patient / Isobel Knight ; foreword by Rodney Grahame.
p. ; cm.
Multi-disciplinary approach to managing EDSIII
Multi-disciplinary approach to managing EDS3
Includes bibliographical references and index.
ISBN 978-1-84819-080-1 (alk. paper)
I. Title. II. Title: Multi-disciplinary approach to managing EDSIII. III. Title: Multi-disciplinary approach
to managing EDS3.
[DNLM: 1. Ehlers-Danlos Syndrome--therapy--Personal Narratives. 2. Chronic Disease--psychology-
-Personal Narratives. 3. Chronic Disease--rehabilitation--Personal Narratives. 4. Patient Care Team--
Personal Narratives. 5. Professional-Patient Relations--Personal Narratives. WR 218]

616.7'7--dc23
2012051121

British Library Cataloguing in Publication Data
A CIP catalogue record for this book is available from the British Library

ISBN 978 1 84819 080 1
eISBN 978 0 85701 055 1

Printed and bound in Great Britain

*This book is simply dedicated to my mother,
Theresa Knight, my sister, Fiona Evans,
and my nephew, Thomas Evans.*

When my beloved father died, I was ten years old. My mum had to raise my sister and I entirely on her own, which she managed amazingly. She continues to be a hugely positive influence in my life – I have always admired her energy and determination in the face of difficulty.

My sister, Fiona, is also truly inspirational and has been a very constant and positive support throughout everything – tremendous in the face of her own personal challenges. I admire her very much – not least for the amazing job she is doing in raising my lovely nephew, Thomas.

Thank you both for all your unconditional support throughout my life, and particularly over the past few difficult months. It will always be remembered.

With much love,

Isobel

A Note on Terminology

Since this book was written, the numbering system for classifying the types of Ehlers-Danlos syndrome has been replaced by a classification that uses descriptive names. For example the term EDS-III has been replaced by the term EDS-Hypermobility Type (EDS-HT). It is not wrong to use the numbering terms, just that the named classification is the most up to date. So, in this book, EDS-III can be taken to mean EDS-HT.

To complicate matters many experts in the field consider Joint Hypermobility Syndrome-JHS/EDSIII and EDS-HT to be the same thing. They will use the terms interchangeably. The most important thing to appreciate about this is that whichever term is used the investigations, management, and advice are exactly the same for both JHS and EDS-HT. Also, currently there is no genetic test that can identify either condition or separate them.

Therefore, JHS and EDS-HT appear to describe the same condition albeit their classification originally derived from different clinical perspectives.

Dr Alan Hakim MA FRCP
October 2019

Contents

Foreword

Isobel Knight has already demonstrated her undoubted literary talents in her widely acclaimed book entitled A Guide to Living with Hypermobility Syndrome: Bending without Breaking (2011). This, her first book on this topic, approached the subject at several levels simultaneously: it provided an informative and reliable description of the syndrome, and also explained what it is like to experience it from the inside. Never before has anyone documented with such clarity and detail what living with JHS is really like. It certainly made its mark and became a bestseller. Then why (I hear you ask?) has Isobel gone to the trouble of producing a second book on the same topic less than two years later? Well, of course, it is highly significant that she has designed a new name for the syndrome – the 'Ehlers-Danlos (type III) hypermobility syndrome' (EDS3HMS) – thereby recognising the increasingly wide acceptance of the notion that hypermobility is EDS, and vice versa.

The new volume is very different from the first. It is longer and goes much deeper into the nature of the underlying condition and into Isobel's reaction to the changing phases of her condition. At times it becomes more erudite; at others more down-to-earth and user-friendly. What we have is a more analytical account of her journey through life thus far. And what a turbulent journey it has been! She is joined at various points by invited contributors whose expertise and contributions enrich the substance of the book and broaden its appeal. They include Alan Hakim, Howard Bird, Rosemary Keer, Andrew Lucas, Jane Simmonds and John Wilks.

Paradoxically, despite major advances in our understanding of hypermobility syndrome as a whole, as documented in this book, there has never been a more difficult time for patients to access much-needed treatment. It remains a major challenge for patients to seek out doctors or therapists who have accumulated sufficient knowledge and experience to help them. In consequence many patients wait in vain

9

for help and for many, it never comes! Effective treatment is available for the fortunate few. It should be available to all who need it. In the UK where we do have an (albeit diminishing) handful of dedicated centres, the service they offer is woefully inadequate to satisfy the national need. But this is not just a UK problem. It is a world-wide one. No other disease in the history of modern medicine has been neglected in such a way. It is a topsy-turvy world where patients often know more about a condition than their doctors! Patients left to their own devices show amazing resourcefulness in many different ways. Some (in fact, many) discover untapped poetic skills and utilise them to describe their condition and their feelings. Others dedicate their time (and some, their lives) to building up and sustaining magnificent self-help groups like the HMSA and EDS UK. For others, like Isobel Knight, drawing on their own life-long experience for the benefit of others helps them to make their own journey through EDS3HMS a less daunting, less frightening and less lonely experience . Such is the real value of this book. And, of course, it also makes for salutary reading for medical professionals.

Professor Rodney Grahame CBE MD FRCP FACP FRSA
Honorary Consultant Rheumatologist,
University College Hospitals, London
Honorary Professor, Division of Medicine.
University College London
Affiliate Professor, School of Medicine,
University of Washington, Seattle WA, USA
February 2013

Acknowledgements

There are a great many people to thank who have been tremendously supportive to me in the writing of this book, particularly in the final months.

I would like to thank Donna Wicks, who is the senior medical liaison officer of the Hypermobility Syndrome Association (HMSA), for giving me the courage to continue with this book in the face of difficulty. I am so grateful to you for all your personal support and for all the windows of opportunity that you have opened for me. You are an amazing person, and always so positive. Others have much to learn from you.

Professor Howard Bird has continued to be unstintingly kind and supportive to me, both as my physician, but also in contributing to this book. I am highly privileged to work with you, and have enjoyed our other writing and lecturing work.

Dr Alan Hakim has been unfailingly supportive to me, and I am extremely fortunate to have his invaluable clinical input, as the chief medical officer for the HMSA. Thank you so much for your work and time.

Dr Jane Simmonds has so kindly written some invaluable advice on cardiovascular fitness and endurance in Chapter 40 of the book. Jane has been extremely supportive to me throughout, and I will get on and write some case studies and journal articles, I promise!

I am extremely grateful to have had the input of Rosemary Keer who has so generously taken the time to explain some of the really difficult aspects of treating EDSIII patients – particularly in terms of strength gains and the problems with muscular patterning.

Dr Andrew Lucas has written a wonderful contribution to the psychological aspects of treating the chronic complex patient from a wealth of experience, and this is totally invaluable in this particular book. I very much enjoyed meeting you and felt reassured that I was generally 'normal' in the spectrum presented in this patient group.

I am immensely grateful to John Wilks who is a Bowen instructor and author and has written an incredibly detailed academic explanation of the Bowen technique, working on fascia and connective tissues and work with EDSIII patients. I think his writing about birth and birth trauma will be particularly eye-opening for many medical practitioners.

I would like to thank the physiotherapist who treated me for almost four years and for treating me for as long as she was able to, and the physiotherapist who has continued my care to ensure I maintain my condition optimally.

I am grateful to both Jessica Moolenaar (leading Pilates Foundation teacher trainer) and Maggy Burrowes (Feldenkrais) for so kindly and generously contributing to the book.

I would particularly like to thank Lisa Clark, my editor at Jessica Kingsley Publishers (Singing Dragon), who has been a huge support, and I know that this book has required a lot more work for her than my last book. Thank you!

I would like to thank Professor Rodney Grahame for so kindly writing a Foreword for this book and for times we have met and discussed EDSIII – for example during Hypermobility Club Meetings.

I cannot sign off without thanking the patients I have come across via Facebook and the HMSA online forum who provide such inspiration and support. I know that there are many areas I have not written about that you wanted me to (sorry!) – but I hope you will feel I have done *some* justice to this incredibly complicated condition, and other indirectly related medical conditions.

Last, but by no means least, thank you to my friends and family who have supported me so unconditionally with this particular book.

Preface

A Hypermobile body is like a credit card, it gives you immense satisfaction and happiness when it functions properly, when you overdo things it can be painful for months and when it reaches its limit you simply have to recuperate and start again.

Marie Chapman

This ingenious quote comes from a fellow EDSIII patient via my Facebook forum. Marie has so succinctly explained the benefits of a functioning hypermobile body, but also the pitfalls when it so clearly malfunctions and the patient has to (almost) go back to square one.

At the time of writing this it is 22 June 2012 on a cold, windy Friday afternoon, and I am in hospital. I have generally been in good health in recent months and getting fitter and fitter. I came to hospital for a bladder operation (see Part II: Physiology) and whilst here have suffered complications post-surgery and contracted three separate infections. I feel weaker than I have felt in a long time, but mentally determined. One of the doctors says it is a good job I had 'good reserves' and was 'fit' upon arrival because if my EDSIII had been unmanaged I could have been in a much worse state. He is not wrong. I know when I leave hospital (over a week later than expected) I will be weaker than I have been in a while. I will have to pace my activity, take rests and slowly re-start my previously excellent exercise regime. It will be frustrating, but I will have to pay back my credit card balance (as Marie puts it) until I reach my previous point of good health. This will be frustrating, but far from uncommon in this type of situation. It takes EDSIII patients longer than non-hypermobiles to gain muscle strength, but they also de-condition much faster (Simmonds and Keer 2007). Herein lies the problem or the conundrum faced by so many EDSIII patients who find themselves often going around in circles – trying to gain strength when they can, until they hit the next fatigue or illness and then they return to square one (or near there). I know that I will reach my former (post-surgical) fitness level and recover faster than at any other point in my life so far – mainly because my musculoskeletal system (at least) is functioning so much better. Where rehabilitation has taken place recovery should more swiftly follow. It could be argued that even non-hypermobile people take time to recover after surgery, and that is of course true – but it is the musculoskeletal system that is perhaps anecdotally slower to respond in many hypermobile/EDSIII patients, and also wound healing owing to stretchier and more fragile skin (Tinkle 2010).

After a few days 'bed-bound' I am in more pain, I feel more stiff and achy and I certainly feel much weaker than normal. Since exercise is so crucial to managing all of these symptoms, the delay in return to normal exercise will hinder my return to normal activity as I will need to work even harder to rehabilitate and reverse the resultant muscle atrophy, which is worst in the first five to seven days during inactivity, particularly the crucial endurance muscles (Keer 2003; Simmonds 2003). I see my physio about two weeks after leaving hospital and he says it will take me a further six to twelve weeks to regain my former pre-operative fitness. I find this both incredulous and upsetting, although wonder why I am so surprised.

Ehlers-Danlos syndromes are part of a range of genetically inherited connective tissue disorders (see Appendix 1). For the purpose of this book I am referring to the hypermobility type of Ehlers-Danlos also known as type III (EDSIII). This particular subtype is considered by many experts in the field to be the same as joint hypermobility syndrome (JHS). JHS is diagnosed using the Beighton Score, a nine-point scoring system, and the Brighton Criteria, which are designed to capture the multisystemic aspect of a connective tissue disorder. For further details please see Appendix 1 and other books which go into much greater detail.[1] Here the term EDSIII in my book should be considered the same as the hypermobility type of EDS and JHS. EDSIII overlaps with chronic pain disorders and fibromyalgia/chronic fatigue symptoms. Both these conditions are mentioned in this book, although more from a patient/symptomatic point of view. Further medical detail can be found in Hakim, Keer and Grahame (2010).

In order to get the best out of this book, I would like to suggest that the Introduction and Chapters 1 to 4 are core reading, after which the reader is free to choose which sections (e.g. physiology) or chapters are of most interest and importance to them, although I hope that you might read the whole book!

---

1   See Beighton, Grahame and Bird (2012); Hakim, *et al.* (2010); Keer and Grahame (2003).

Introduction

Researching a personal topic issue offers transformative potential for self and others. [In the first author's case] she has discovered personal attributes such as determination, courage and strength and has come to see how individuals, regardless of the specific circumstances, can share their humanity with others at a deep and fundamental level. Knowing that others have trodden a similar path is potentially liberating and relieves the burden of isolation and loneliness that many people suffer when keeping silent about the past. Experiences that have been seen as crises can become transformed into turning points or life lessons that enable the individual to move on to the future with both courage and renewed strength. Sharing the common bond of personal experience might ultimately serve to transform the lives of the participants, other researchers and the broader community.

Foster, McAllister and O'Brien 2005, pp.8–9

The quotation comes from an article about autoethnography in mental health nursing and offers the most succinct and elegant expression about the ultimate aims of this book.

In my first book *A Guide to Living with Hypermobility Syndrome: Bending without Breaking* (2011), I wrote with the patient in mind and set out to describe hypermobility syndrome (HMS) and the process of diagnosis. I explained my own story partly in autobiographical terms whilst looking at the lives of others with HMS. There were chapters about childhood, adolescence and then pain management. I started to address the story of managing and surviving with HMS in the most general of terms, whilst going into more detail through my experiences as a dancer. There were chapters about managing hormones and pregnancy, the psychological aspects of living with a chronic condition and then a chapter outlining overall management approaches including physiotherapy and other complementary therapies. *A Guide to Living with Hypermobility Syndrome* provided an introduction to what seems to be one of the first books of its kind aimed specifically at patients. Whilst writing that book I was still very much in the middle of my own therapeutic journey and so I stuck to referencing treatments and drugs and approaches whilst at times giving the reader a brief insight into my own treatment story.

This new book goes into my treatment in far greater detail and is therefore aimed primarily at the medical profession, whilst patients (and, I hope, professionals alike) will find the information inspirational, informative and thought-provoking. Some of what is discussed and described in this book will be new and therefore anecdotal. Whilst the book will go into what is traditionally done in the medical management of the hypermobility type of Ehlers-Danlos (type III) (EDSIII), the treatment plan, such as it was, will partly follow what I experienced during medical treatment. This book will not cover all aspects of EDSIII, and aspects such as diagnosis are only briefly mentioned. The book is likely to raise more questions than it can hope to answer. It is documenting what was done in a treatment context that went far beyond rehabilitating the presenting complaint (as described in the first book) of an injured right calf.

The general conclusion of this book is that it might be possible to rehabilitate a patient with a chronic complex pain disorder such as EDSIII, but it takes a huge amount of time and commitment from both patient and treating practitioners. There is a generally happy ending, the diagnosis now less important than the management of the symptoms. I am now managing more than I could have possibly ever dreamed of and have returned to completely normal physical exercise, which is very much the recommended treatment management of EDSIII, although I still experience and have both pain and flare ups.

The book falls naturally into four main parts: on 'the body and the self', physiology, psychology, and exercise and rehabilitation, including complementary medicine. What is perhaps revolutionary about this book is using the analogies of Maslow's Hierarchy of Needs to explain just how out of kilter the EDSIII (chronic, complex) patient is compared to normal physiological homeostasis and how critical this is to address. The psychology in working with this patient group is exceptionally important and so, in the psychology section, there are detailed discussions on the topic of the therapeutic relationship and, on the side of the patient, conditions such as self-harm and how these further complicate working with this patient group, and what sort of external support medical practitioners need when working with the complex patient.

I have chosen to write this book in an autoethnographical style, and so the account is interwoven with blog entries, memoirs, poems and 'my general life story'. At other times I write as an academic researcher and also as a Bowen therapist, the result ultimately being a rich cacophony of different voices, including the voices of other leading medical experts including Jane Simmonds, Rosemary Keer, Howard Bird, Alan Hakim, Andrew Lucas and John Wilks, with contributions from Pilates teacher trainer Jessica Moolenaar and Feldenkrais teacher Maggy Burrowes. Since I documented about 18 months' worth of physiotherapy sessions, there are also a wealth of transcripts to draw upon to further explain my treatment and how other medical professionals could also learn from ultimate triumphs and pitfalls.

I hope this book will encourage others to really think outside the box when approached by the most challenging of patients presenting with chronic complex medical conditions. There are practical tools for other readers to use, such as my subjective graphs and tables. The part on 'exercise and rehabilitation' serves to provide examples of the exercises that I was given during physiotherapy, but it is not my intention that this is followed as an explicit guide since every patient you see is likely to require a slightly different approach even though some exercises are invariably core to the group – for example pelvic tilt.

This book also raises questions of the difficulties when this particular patient group presents at A&E and the potential problems when some medical measures in this group fall outside medical testing. The book is expected to generate and attract wide debate, and the intention is to open the minds of all medical professionals who work with the complex patient who is suffering a chronic condition such as fibromyalgia, EDSIII and chronic pain, as well as other conditions which are perhaps pertinent to the author, though not linked to EDSIII, such as endometriosis. It is therefore important to point out that because of my personal and autoethnographical approach, I am discussing my experiences and how they link and interact together, again not because everyone diagnosed with EDSIII will have the same symptoms and conditions, but to discuss how EDSIII might interact with or impact other related conditions, such as endometriosis.

PART I

THE BODY AND THE SELF

CHAPTER 1

The body and the self in illness and health

An autoethnographical approach

My new urologist is taking my history. He asks me what I do. I tell him I have started my doctorate, a qualitative study of chronic kidney failure, transplantation and recovery. He pauses and lifts his pen from my life's story.

'What qualifies you to do that?' he asks.

'I lived it,' I reply.

Richards 2008, p.1717

Autoethnography might be defined as a genre of writing that connects the personal experience to the cultural and places the self within a social context (Reed-Danahay from Holt 2003). Autoethnography is usually written in the first person and involves writing from one's own experiences for academic purposes (Richards 2008). The autoethnographer will use their personal experiences as primary data, but will carefully link them into a wider cultural and social context (Chang 2008). Autoethnographical writing is particularly suited to more emotive or private subjects, such as health or medically related topics where researchers can investigate intimate information in detail (Chang 2008). We seldom choose our topics accidentally – our reasons for researching them are often personal: 'No one ever knows what I have been through unless I tell them' (Richards 2008, p.1718).

The advantages of autoethnographical research is that it is written in personally engaging ways that are often more accessible than academic writing (Chang 2008). Autoethnographical writing might help the researcher understand themselves and others and accordingly transform the reader's and other lives in the process. It might further encourage the reader to engage and reflect more actively on the material they are reading (Chang 2008). In the case of a medical condition, the expert is not necessarily the clinician, but the person experiencing the illness or condition (Richards 2008). In this case, autoethnographical writing offers the patient, who is usually in a position of less power than their medical doctor, a unique but powerful voice in 'telling the story'. This is particularly important because patients are often assumed to have far less knowledge than their doctors and devalued in what they might know about their medical condition. The patient 'lives' in their body but is seldom consulted about it. Writing autoethnographically gives a voice to the person actually experiencing the illness or medical condition, who is often rendered invisible (Richards 2008).

In autoethnographical research, it is important to balance engagement with personal experience with consideration of such experience in wider frames of research and understanding. This involves several challenges to avoid limiting the usefulness of such work by over-focus on introspection (Grbich 2007; Holt 2003). Chang warns that the autoethnographer is in danger of self-exposure if they do not adequately reflect back on analysis and cultural interpretation and reply on excessive narrative accounts (Chang 2008). Chang further cautions on personal memory, which can be selective and 'shaped', and so there is a potential for bias – memory is not always accurate (Chang 2008). Furthermore, confidentiality is still critical, even in autoethnographical writing, since the lives of others will be embellished via links to other stories and from true cultural representation. It is essential that the ethics of the usage of others' stories are also protected (Chang 2008; Holt 2003). There are also risks in the way in which other academics value autoethnographical writing, and the autoethnographical writer is still more apt for rejection in certain academic spheres (Holt 2003). However, if the autoethnographical writer ensures that their writing is culturally and socially representative, that they follow the rigours of academic research in the usage of others' stories in an ethical way and avoid mere over-indulgence, the results of autoethnographical writing are highly advantageous in gaining social and cultural insight into a personalised area, such as illness (Chang 2008; Grbich 2007; Holt 2003; Richards 2008).

I have chosen to write autoethnographically about my experiences of living with the inherited connective tissue disorder Ehlers-Danlos (type III) – hypermobility syndrome, or EDSIII (see Appendix 1 for diagnosis criteria), and other chronic conditions (endometriosis). The autoethnographical writing forms the 'tree' structure of this book. I am the trunk and overall shape of the tree. The branches of the tree are the social and cultural realities, which check back to the roots of the tree and ensure that my story accurately represents the many complex (and, at times, conflicting) aspects of the life of a person with EDSIII, and therefore speaks to the challenges, strategies, experiences and successes of the wider community of EDSIII patients/individuals. Richards writes, and I agree, that

> [the] lived experience of illness and disability is perhaps their ultimate truth and is a truth that can seem inaccessible to outsiders. This should not, however, prevent researchers from trying to reach it... I shall have to do that. I am still becoming myself.
>
> *Richards 2008, p.1726*

The body, illness and disability

Scambler (1997) describes illness as external and as a product of life. He further describes health as an absence of illness; a reserve of health, determined by constitution and temperament; and a positive state of wellbeing or equilibrium (p.35). The way in which we accept, value or experience our bodies is an important concept in terms of how we subsequently manage a decline in health. To that end, Shilling writes that 'we all have bodies but we are not all able to see, hear, feel or speak and move about independently. Having a body is constraining as well as enabling' (1993, p.23). Some attempts have been made to describe the 'body as a machine', which Shilling and others have questioned by implying the body is radically 'other' to the self. However, it is possible for individuals to use this construction – it is 'their' machine that can be maintained and looked after by diet, exercise and health check-ups (Shilling 1993, p.37). The 'machine' might be enhanced by performance, as in sport and performing arts, but the machine might also break down, thus questioning bodily wellbeing (Shilling 1993). Additionally, not all disabilities and illnesses are apparent to observers and not all disabilities are perceived to be disabilities by those who have them (Richards 2008). This is a particularly important point in a condition such as EDSIII where the patient frequently appears outwardly well (Grahame 2009), which can be deceptive to both the medical professionals working with this patient cohort, and their friends and family.

Freund looks at how people's experiences of health and illness are shaped with reference to social relations and subjective experiences (Shilling 1993). Freund defines bodily wellbeing in two ways. One is in a physiological context where the body must be regulated – for example, in terms of temperature, blood pressure, hormone levels and in balance. Freund's second premise for bodily wellbeing relates to having control over the intimate relationship of body and mind, which he might refer to as 'being in touch with the body' – for example, in monitoring pain (Shilling 1993, p.115). If one is in touch with their body, then they know when to eat, when they are cold or hot and how to respond to their bodily needs. Some people lose touch with their bodies and cause them harm – for example, an anorexic in denying their body nourishment. Such an example might explain how bodily wellbeing is related to social existence (the anorexic perceives themselves as 'fat'), and an emotional mode of being (Lawrence from Shilling 1993). Emotion is fundamental to human life and our social interactions with other human beings (Shilling 1993). For instance, being injured can affect both our bodily wellbeing and the way in which we behave emotionally (we cannot perhaps do something) and therefore our social interaction. Our bodily wellbeing might therefore impact upon both our social and economic tenure and the way in which we are valued. For example, difficulties with employment, reduced career prospects, social isolation from friends and family and loss of independence are some of the problems encountered by some patients managing a chronic medical condition such as EDSIII (Locker 1997; Shilling 1993).

Living with chronic illness

People do not often die from chronic conditions. Instead, people mostly 'live with' their chronic conditions (Locker 1997). Therefore, it is less often the cause of death, even if to the patient themselves the chronic condition can, at times, feel disastrous. According to research in the British population by the Royal College of Physicians, 1/5 have a chronic condition (Locker 1997). More recent research obtained by the Department of Health website and by the British Pain Society suggests that this figure might be closer to one in three of the population living in chronic pain (Price *et al.* 2012). A chronic illness might be defined as a long-term condition that has a profound influence on the patient (Locker 1997). However, it might be the way in which the person with the medical condition, 'the patient', chooses to interpret and define the role, in which their medical condition impedes or otherwise affects their life. They might not wish to be labelled as a patient at all, but as a 'person', primarily and foremost, in their own right. For all people with chronic medical conditions, it is the value that they place on their medical condition (or otherwise) that is likely to impact upon their attitude towards the condition and the way in which they live their life. For example, for some people, their medical condition has a profound effect upon their lives, and for others, who perhaps cope differently, the condition holds less magnitude in their life. However, every person is individual and unique, and the patients who are *not* seen as 'copers' cannot, in any way, be blamed for this, since everybody manages pain and symptoms differently. Charmaz (1987), as cited in Locker (1997), writes, and I agree, that 'chronically sick people are involved in a constant struggle to lead valued lives and maintain definitions of self which are positive and worthwhile…the loss of the self is a powerful form of suffering experienced by the chronically ill' (p.86).

To qualify this further, Lucy,[1] has type 1 diabetes, which would qualify as a chronic medical condition; however, she very rarely talks about her diabetes and appears to manage her insulin injections and blood tests and gets on with her life in a full and holistic way without it impeding her life. I am sure she doesn't always 'feel' well, yet she seldom complains about her body and how she 'feels', and yet I also have chronic medical conditions that are substantially less life threatening, but the symptoms and pain I have endured have impeded the quality of my life, although my fierce determination and stubbornness have put me in good stead to usually appear as a 'coper'. I complain a lot more about my medical problems than Lucy does, which does not mean that Lucy has a better or easier time, but does that make me weaker and more of a hypochondriac than Lucy? Some would argue that it does, yet my conditions are not always well managed with pain control and some of the symptoms I experience make me feel more unwell – particularly fatigue – and it is really impossible for me to do very much when I am very fatigued, even when I really want to 'do something' – for instance, write this book, or go to work. It might be that Lucy, who has had support for her condition and been well managed with it since she was young, places

---

1   Pseudo-name.

much less emphasis on her medical condition, whilst I have the very opposite experience and am only now getting the support I have so badly required in order that the condition has less of a hold and an importance in my life. I don't want it to be 'important' at all, but it just takes over, regardless. However, a delay in diagnosis of this condition (EDSIII) is far from uncommon, as might be seen from the Rare Diseases Report, which makes *the following significant points*:

- significant delays in diagnosis
- patients being misdiagnosed (often multiple times)
- patients 'rattling around the system' having to visit multiple specialists before receiving an accurate diagnosis
- difficulties in accessing information and support
- fragmented and poorly coordinated care
- patients and families having to attend multiple hospital appointments, often at a long distance from home
- a lack of effective treatments
- inconsistencies in access to medicines.

Hypermobility Syndrome Association (HMSA) 2011, p.13.

Throughout the book, several themes from this report will emerge and will be only too familiar to some readers. Recent HMSA research suggests that in 56 per cent or more of patients surveyed it takes over ten years to get a diagnosis (Hakim 2012). In addition, some doctors have difficulty in accepting this lesser known condition. Indeed, there are very few centres of expertise that even treat EDS as a condition: namely Glasgow Royal Infirmary, the Royal National Orthopaedic Hospital and University College Hospital (see Appendix 3). It would appear that there is clearly a disappointing lack of awareness amongst some medical professionals, as per a 2011 conference on EDS:

A rheumatologist's perspective over four decades by Professor Rodney Grahame

What do rheumatologists think of HMS?

- A majority believe it exists (only 7% don't believe).
- 51 per cent believe HMS is not a real disease (39% believe it is a real disease).
- 79 per cent believe that HMS is not a genetic disorder (10% believe it is a genetic disorder).

- 84 per cent believe that HMS does not affect the rest of the body aside from the joint.

- 57 per cent don't know if HMS is the same as EDS Type 3 (7% believe EDS and HMS are the same and 35% believe they are different).

- 50 per cent believe HMS has a significant impact on the patient's life.

- 72 per cent believe HMS has a minimal impact on the burden of society's rheumatological diseases.

EDS/HMS is the new rheumatological disability!

- Severely physically disabled.

- Musculoskeletal system largely intact.

- Chronic pain inhibits movement.

- All sorts of dysfunctions throughout the body occur. There is not one medical specialty that is not affected by this.

- Mostly young, highly motivated people affected, cut down in their prime.

- Often told that it is all in the mind.

- Feel dispirited, abandoned, angry.

> *Nadia Bodkin's interpretation of lectures given at the 2011 EDNF Learning Conference: www.edsers.com/ 2011_Conference_Notes.html. Kind permission has been given to include this extract from www.EDSers.com.*

These final bullet points resonate throughout my entire story – EDSIII *is* a newer rheumatological disability.

I have now met with many people with EDSIII and have been struck by the severity of their incapacitation, especially those who have ended up in wheelchairs. Even for those who don't, there is no doubt that this a cruel and poorly recognised condition, with a huge lack of resourcing and centres of expertise. Treatment is a postcode lottery and improved recognition and treatment management and resourcing are crucial.

Chapter 2 tells my story and where I came from.

CHAPTER 2

Isobel's story

I probably always knew I was hypermobile, certainly since the age of 13 when my ballet teacher mentioned I had 'swayback' knees. I didn't appreciate the value of my hypermobility until I learned a great deal more very recently. There is no doubt that hypermobility is a real asset as a dancer and I am increasingly grateful to it as I get older and start to lose some of my natural flexibility. Having hips that laterally rotate with ease makes ballet so much more possible, and my hyperextended knees are very useful when it comes to aesthetically pleasing lines and extensions. From the point of view of a dancer and not a patient, I am thrilled to be hypermobile. However, I would consider myself as a patient with EDSIII when it comes to a myriad of other bodily symptoms and injuries.

In February 2008 I suffered a grade 2 tear of my right medial gastrocnemius during the allegro or jumping section of a classical ballet class. I was doing assemblés, a step where the dancer jumps off one foot and lands on two. I heard a tearing sound and fell to the floor. I went to A&E where I was assessed and issued with crutches and told to follow PRICE principles. I was asked to attend the acute physiotherapy clinic the next day. I was told I would probably not be dancing again for at least six weeks, which seemed psychologically unbearable given my only recent return to dancing following a nine-year injury gap. I recall feeling incredibly depressed and that almost overrode the pain I was experiencing.

The physiotherapist who saw me the following day suggested that I start to take some weight on the leg when I felt comfortable to do so and that it was best if I tried to walk as normally as possible, that is not on tip-toe as I wanted to do, as she suggested this would store up trouble later and make it harder to walk normally. She commented upon the difference in my calf temperatures and said to seek help if this further changed over time. Soleus and Achilles tendon were assessed as normal. The physiotherapist then referred me for further physiotherapy at my local sports centre, which was an NHS Primary Care Trust (PCT) physiotherapy centre.

The next physiotherapist who saw me made further assessments of my legs and noted the considerable difference in calf muscle bulk, which I had not really thought about before. At this time my left calf measured 43cm, whilst the right was 39cm. He gave me some stretches to do hanging off steps and then suggested that I did parallel rises on the right leg when I felt ready to try them. At this point I was still using crutches a little bit (one week after the initial incident). Being a Bowen therapist, I had also done some Bowen work on my calf on a daily basis to support the soft-tissue injury. The Bowen technique is a gentle form of soft-tissue therapy that originated in Australia and involves small 'rolling-type' moves across muscle and tendon fibres, primarily working at the fascial-tissue level, and generating an integrated healing response. It appeared to be 'speeding' the healing process, which the physiotherapist commented upon when he saw me one week later and I no longer needed the crutches. I was also able to show that I could take weight on the leg and was doing my exercises. By the third week, the physiotherapist wanted to do some deep-tissue work on my calf. I was wary about this because my calves had always been rather sensitive and I had barely allowed Bowen therapists to touch them, given that Bowen *is* gentle. The physiotherapist did try, but I screamed blue murder and so he backed off. I understand his rationale for trying; he wanted to try and break down scar tissue, but in my case it was futile. Given that he couldn't work 'hands on' with me and had given me exercises and that time was now needed to complete healing, I asked if I could return to ballet classes, and since I was being discharged, the physiotherapist thought there was no reason why not, although he sensibly advised against demi-pointe work and doing any allegro.

When I did return to ballet classes the following week, with insight it was probably much too soon for me to be dancing again and I was severely limited in what I could manage in class. My drive to return to class was highly psychological and a need for an endorphin rush, as since my accident I had become quite depressed. I kept on trying to dance, but even with my apparent body knowledge, I couldn't understand why I just wasn't really able to dance as I could before, and I was frustrated and still in pain. After several more weeks with the calf still not recovering, and not really managing any demi-pointe work or allegro, I decided to seek the advice of a private physiotherapist with an expertise in working with dancers. My motivations for doing this were that I didn't believe that a 'standard' NHS musculoskeletal physiotherapist would understand my specific needs as a dancer, and perhaps because I hoped that their knowledge base would resolve my problem more rapidly.

It is of significance to note that my expectation from seeing a dance expert would be that she would resolve my calf problem within about five or six sessions and that I would then be able to return to allegro and ballet dancing. When I first met my physio, I was rather dismayed to realise that my gluteals, hamstrings and adductors were apparently extremely weak, that I was over-rotating my lateral turnout (a very common fault in ballet dancers) and that I was sitting in on the right hip, and that led to a weakness on the whole of the right lower limb. My physio gave me some exercises to strengthen the gluteals and abdominals to give me some initial stability – although I was completely oblivious of the extent of my weakness, my systemic hypermobility and my instability. At this stage I had no idea of what I would be embarking on – I merely thought that doing the exercises that my physio recommended would resolve my problem and I would be back to dancing in a very short time. I requested that my physio inform my ballet teacher about her findings, and she commented that I underused my right hip in extension and that I was weak in abduction, leading me to sit in on my right hip, and that there was a weakness throughout the right lower limb. My physio also suggested that because of weakness in my right turnout muscles I would also be underutilising my available lateral turnout range, which led to overuse of excessive lateral rotation and the knee, and increased use of the medial calf. She further commented that the left hip looked better, but the quadriceps were overused and turnout of the left hip also underused. In April 2008 my physio suggested that I reduce the degree of turnout I had whilst strengthening all weakened areas until sufficient control was gained.

I must step back at this point to reflect on my previous experiences of physiotherapy, which had frequently been unsuccessful for the various soft-tissue injuries I had sustained, and in particular for any attempted management of chronic lower back pain, where I had been episodic since I was 17 years old. Therefore, my motivation to seek help from a physiotherapist was almost rather strange, since by then I had relied on Bowen solely as my treatment method since 1999. However, the

Bowen technique does not work for muscular re-education (and motor repatterning) or strengthening, and in the end I knew that I needed to approach my calf problem in a different way. The calf episode wasn't merely restricted to the initial trauma I had endured in February 2008, but in fact a catalogue of minor calf tears throughout my adolescent years. I had just put up with this and with being unable to walk easily first thing in the morning as 'normal' and accepted it.

My first experiences of physiotherapy began weeks after my eighteenth birthday when my lumbar spine and sacral area had been painful for a few weeks. I had done a ballet exam just prior to my birthday and my teacher felt that I might have overdone things at the time. I had particular pain doing arabesques and had pain local to L4/5 where I have a hinge at that level of my spine. The physiotherapists attached to my GP said that my problems were related to my sacroiliac joint, and I had six sessions of physiotherapy that seemed to help somewhat; although my back still hurt a little I carried on dancing, because I enjoyed it – my hypermobility being a real asset in this respect. As time went on the pain became more insidious, and an area that started off the size of a drawing pin gradually spread in diameter and in intensity over time. In addition to back pain that was becoming a chronic and unrelenting feature of my life, I was having increasing difficulties with dysmenorrhoea, and this caused increasing problems for me as a student teacher and when I was working as a student in the holidays. By the time I was in my fourth year of my BA course, I had seen an osteopath for several sessions, which were unsuccessful in addressing the back pain, and I was sent for an X-ray to rule out spondylothesis. I also saw a gynaecologist who 'seriously' suggested I should consider having a baby and that I should try a different brand of oral contraceptive to help with the dysmenorrhoea. I was also referred for more physiotherapy at my local hospital. The physiotherapist who saw me gave me abdominal exercises, which I did, and also taped up my lumbar spine to give me support. This was helpful and gave me relief from pain, but I only had a few sessions of physiotherapy and was then discharged. I doubt that I kept up with the abdominal exercises for long and my back still hurt – although I was still dancing a little. I recall his comments that my back was 'horrendous', which still sticks in my mind, and that it was probably not going to ever really change very much in the future.

In 1997 I graduated from university and left to work in London as an examinations administrator for a dance examination board. I did not go into teaching, but I can now see this would have been impossible given that I could hardly stand for long periods of time and primary school teaching in particular is very physical. I had been in constant pain by the time of my final teaching practice. I think that I realised I could not have coped with this, coupled with severe dysmenorrhoea. In 1998 I was also diagnosed with endometriosis, which explained why I was experiencing such severe menstrual pain.

By 2001 it was becoming increasingly difficult for me to work owing to the back pain and endometriosis. I ended up leaving one job and then having six months off work before I re-started working part-time. I had many medical investigations in 2001, including an MRI scan of my lumbar spine. The MRI showed that I had a posterior disc bulge at L4/5 and disc degeneration. I was reviewed by a gastroenterologist as I was experiencing abdominal pain, which was partially explained as irritable bowel syndrome (IBS) as well as being related to having endometriosis. I was also referred for pain management and was given acupuncture for my back pain, which did not benefit me for that, but did help me feel less nauseous at times. I also tried using a TENS machine, which did benefit me somewhat, so I obtained my own machine, for use at home. I often had the TENS machine on a very high setting and still the relentless pain came through. I was finally put on Gabapentin and Dosulepin for pain management and asked to do as much exercise as possible, but was given no information about how to start the exercise regime and precisely what to do. I suffered a very bad reaction to Dosulepin, suffering from severe tachycardia, and ended up on a very high dose of Gabapentin with no change or improvement to my pain. This was eventually terminated by a pain management consultant at a different hospital in 2003.

In 2003 I moved to Cambridge with my partner at the time. I stopped the swimming and Pilates and substituted walking for cycling, the way that one gets about in Cambridge. I was still in pain, although my endometriosis was managed by artificial and temporary cessation of menstruation by GNRH analogue subcutaneous Zoladex injections with add-back Tibolone HRT for bone density, something that the Zoladex can impede. This was helping tremendously, although my back still hurt. I was given the option to try having lumbar steroid epidural injections for my back pain, which did appear to help, and that coupled with more Bowen therapy seemed to improve things. I imagine that not having the additional factor of incredibly painful menstruation also helped. I stopped any form of exercise and for a brief while I was 'fairly' stable and enthused in my new occupation as a Bowen therapist. I was offered, but declined, another well-paid part-time job as a volunteer manager, but declined this (wrongly) as I thought I could manage to be completely self-employed. Unfortunately, the clinic I was working in, which was doing very well, closed down and I never managed to do very well at the other clinics I was in. My partner and I bought a house together and this, coupled with doing less work and perhaps a myriad of other issues, led to both the demise of my relationship and the depths of depression and to me taking a minor overdose in August 2005. At this point I knew that if I did not leave the relationship and return to London I would 'die' completely. It was not the fault of my partner, it was just that I was in the wrong relationship for me.

The year 2006 ended up being very pivotal for me. I returned to London early in the year and, although I was still practising as a Bowen therapist in a London clinic, I needed other work. I was then not paid for the work I did which, coupled with being in more pain again with endometriosis and back pain, led me to having a spell on benefits so that I could 'recover' more easily. In the summer of 2006 I had several hospital admissions for the management of severe endometriosis pain and I was then sent to attend a four-week residential pain management course at a leading central London hospital. One of the first things I learned was that 'pain does not always equal damage'. That expression has stayed with me ever since and has allowed me at times to make a crucial judgement as to whether my pain is indeed dangerous or part of the complexities of my chronic pain syndromes. It doesn't mean that my pain is any less irksome, it is just that I do need to see a doctor for it (see Knight 2011, Chapter 6).

Part of the rationale of the physiotherapy at the pain management course was that the physiotherapists did not perform manual therapy. Instead we had to do a generic programme of daily stretches and 'circuit' exercises where we all learned the repertoire of exercises and were then given our own starting points for the exercises, which we then used pacing strategies for. One of the reasons that the physiotherapists did no manual work on any of the patients attending the course is that they had realised that many of us had developed a heightened sensitivity to touch, presumably linked to amplified pain responses. For me this explained other things – such as why I could no longer tolerate massage or deep-tissue work, since it was just too painful for me to experience. It was probably also a significant reason why I had taken so well to Bowen as it is very much gentler soft-tissue work. However, even touch that is so gentle as to be barely palpating the body can cause me pain. I can only just about tolerate palpating my own calf muscles, let alone anybody else making contact with me. It is for this reason I believe the physiotherapists at the course I attended did not conduct manual work with us.

By the time I got to see my physio I had seen many different medical practitioners and hadn't necessarily had particularly successful or long-term outcomes from previous physiotherapy sessions. I don't know why I expected my physio to be any different, but because she was a dance expert I thought she might just understand how to solve the problem in a different way. I recall giving my physio my injury history to date and had brought an A4 sheet of paper with a catalogue of different incidents. I had no idea whether the back and calf could indeed be related – but I wasn't interested in my physio working on my back and I think I was politely firm with her that my back was stable at the time and that she didn't need to have anything to do with that. At the same time, I wasn't keen on her palpating my calf as the NHS physiotherapist assessing my calf had made me scream – so I have no recollection of what I let my physio do on my very first appointment, but from her point of view it must have been highly observational and listening. My physio gave me some exercises to do, which I was really pleased about because it provided me with some control of my 'problems' and a sense of personal responsibility about what I could do for myself. I left the session happy, with a plan of exercises and things to avoid doing in class – for example forcing my lateral turnout.

Treatment and work began with my physio. I brought the following documentation to my first physiotherapy session in April 2008.

Notes for my physiotherapist: April 2008

- Partially tore R gastro medially during allegro section of a ballet class on 10.2.08. Took two weeks off dancing only – Bowen helped with the immediate healing (physio had said 4–6 weeks) but did remedial calf exercises to bulk muscle, as R side has less muscle than L. Have done exercises since. No further tears, but took a while to fully regain confidence.

- Last week L calf medially very, very sore – only strained muscle but this general pattern of re-injury is causing me great frustration and limiting progress in demi-pointe work and allegro.

- Spiral fracture of R tibia age seven from falling downstairs – in plaster for six weeks, walked like a duck for a year afterwards. No physio.

- L ankle sprain – age 11 running down a hill.

- Disc prolapse at L4/5 and disc degeneration. Diagnosed in 2001 by MRI – injury was probably sustained many years earlier – difficult to know. Lumbar epidural injections and Bowen resolved a chronic pain situation, coupled with pilates. I re-started ballet in September 2006 following a six year injury break.

- Both legs swayback, particularly the R which has significantly more hyperextension. Arms are also swayback. Quads are over-developed and abductors (inner thighs) weak, though been working on them. Abs weak, though working on this through pilates and losing weight. Muscles in the soles of the feet – weak, although good flexion and extension. High instep. Lower back very mobile. Lordotic posture – although this is under control. Lateral turnout very good, particularly standing on the L, which is my much stronger 'supporting' side.

- In general, whilst Bowen is being very effective for me in treating the acute or soft-tissue injuries to the calf when they occur, this is not a good enough long-term solution and is not treating the cause. It is becoming increasingly unnerving for me to dance safely with my gastrocs sometimes being so sore and vulnerable.

Isobel Knight, 13.4.2008

My physiotherapist picked up on the real complexity of my case and the possibility of EDSIII, and this was (partly) how I came to see Professor Howard Bird.

CHAPTER 3

Visit to consultant rheumatologist

Professor Howard Bird

Professor Howard Bird's report

Isobel has invited me to contribute to her book as someone she considers to be her 'over arching physician'. This is an extremely generous accolade in that my main contribution has been to see her just once (though on that occasion in detail) on 15 August 2009, a little before my retirement from the NHS. Although I have seen her both professionally and socially since then (notably at the launch of her first book), I do not have a full set of notes from these meetings and some of the information has been sent by e-mail. I will, therefore, restrict my comments to our first appointment together.

Ironically, she came to Leeds to see me not in my capacity as a rheumatologist with an interest in inherited disorders of connective tissue but having identified me from the British Association of Performing Arts Medicine practitioners register as a physician specialising in performing artists since, at that time, she was working at Trinity Laban Conservatoire of Music and Dance in London, where she had previously obtained a masters degree in dance science. I was, therefore, able to give her an appointment longer than that normally offered by the NHS.

Her blog detailed her recent complicated medical and dancing history, and the main reason for attending was slow healing of an injury at the right calf. I obviously took a hypermobility history as well as a dance history, the former perhaps more relevant to this book.

Helpfully, she brought with her a list of symptoms. It was clear that while some of these related to her hypermobility, others certainly did not, although for some, this was a fine balance of opinion.

Typical of hypermobility were her late walking, possibly her poor coordination when she was younger, her chronic low back pain from a disc prolapse (L4/5) at the age of 18 years and her temporomandibular joint problems from the age of 28 years. Clicking of the right hip, the neck and both knees and discomfort at the right elbow were typical of hypermobility as well, as was the asthma, which is often associated, though could have arisen from other causes. Hypermobile patients are subject to overuse syndromes, which might have accounted for her tiredness. In turn, the constant pain of the calf might also have been attributed to hypermobility, providing more serious causes of calf pain were excluded.

There was clearly significant history of endometriosis, present for over ten years. This is not a result of hypermobility but can aggravate symptoms from any hypermobility previously present. For this, she was taking Zoladex and tibolone and she had also had surgery for her endometriosis on four occasions.

Injuries in the previous history that were compatible with hypermobility included a spiral fracture of the right tibia at the age of seven years, a fracture of the left arm at the age of 11 years, a sprain of the left ankle at the age of 12 years and a grade 2 tear of the medial gastrocnemius at the age of 33 years.

Features that I felt, on balance, were not associated with hypermobility were the slow learning and anxious disposition (the main psychological syndrome associated with hypermobility is panic attacks), though poor handwriting, because of her inadequate pen control, might also have contributed. Poor concentration and poor short-term memory are not associated, though might be more convincingly associated with the psychiatric symptoms that she conceded, including a history of depression with mood swings (which had been adequately treated in the past) and self-harm. In turn, there was a suspicion that the 'disconnection of the body at all times' and the feeling of 'being out of control' with 'distraction' and 'agitation' were psychological, not associated with the joint laxity.

The dance history was that she did ballet from the age of 6 to 9 years, returning to it between 14 and 23 years and again at the age of 32 years. I felt the joints were probably loose before she started dancing. She had not practised in other styles of dance.

Her mother is alive, and was thought not to be hypermobile, but the maternal grandmother had had successive surgical procedures for dislocating shoulders. Her father died at the age of 40 years from a myocardial infarction and probably subluxed his knees. There was an impression, therefore, of a hypermobile trait inherited from both sides of the family.

She was trained in teaching and practising the Bowen technique, which occupied her two to three days a week. Otherwise she was at this time a full-time student at Trinity Laban and also worked as a volunteer manager for a charity.

On examination, her hypermobility was quite localised. It was not present at the hands or wrists nor particularly at the feet or ankles. It was most marked at the shoulders, almost as marked at the hips and marked at both knees, though the right knee hyperextended significantly more than the left. I felt there was no significant twist or scoliosis in the spine, although X-ray might reveal a minor deformity. If it did not, the difference between the two knees probably reflected previous local injury at the right knee.

There was no clinical evidence of Marfan syndrome or osteogenesis imperfect and, at a time when most authorities considered that EDS type III could be separated from benign joint familial hypermobility on clinical grounds, I favoured the latter diagnosis rather than the former.

There were local problems at the left calf, which was swollen compared to the right, though she did not have clinical signs to suggest a venous thrombosis, though this clearly had to be excluded, not least because of her gynaecological history.

Because of her asthma and her irritable bowel syndrome, which is sometimes linked to hypermobility, I gave her information leaflets for both of these problems. There had to be a strong suspicion that many of her musculoskeletal symptoms were mediated at her hyperlax joints through the influence of hormones because of her endometriosis. Most patients with endometriosis experience wild hormonal swings. Whilst oestrogens tend to stabilise the collagen in joints, progestogens invariably make it more lax; hence the loss of coordination around the time of menstruation in the normal menstrual cycle, which becomes even more pronounced with the wide hormonal swings that can occur in endometriosis.

Hypermobility can arise from various causes, and an understanding of these is perhaps much more important than simply counting the number of joints that are lax. My suspicion was that she has inherited a mild dysplasia at the hip and shoulder joints from her mother and a mild collagen abnormality, more widespread throughout the body, from her father.

The immediate need was to exclude serious pathology such as a venous thrombosis as a cause for the symptoms at the calf. I recommended that she visited her GP to make arrangements for this to be done in London.

Otherwise, management from a multidisciplinary team would clearly benefit the hypermobility, particularly with physiotherapy to strengthen the muscles around the lax joints (as an adjunct to the ballet training, which I suggested that she continue). However, the overwhelming impression was that the single most useful factor would be to seek gynaecological advice for treatment of the endometriosis, not necessarily by a hormonal route which might further aggravate the joints.

A later X-ray at Kings College, London, subsequently revealed a slight uncompensated C-shaped curve in the spine, which would have contributed to unequal clinical signs between the two knee joints.

Isobel illustrates the diagnostic and management difficulties when a patient with hypermobility syndrome, itself a multisystem disorder, has additional pathology, notably endometriosis and mild depression characterised by mood swings, both of which might aggravate symptoms of hypermobility and/or even cause symptoms mimicking hypermobility in their own right.

CHAPTER 4

Implications of diagnosis

Diagnosis

Diagnosis of EDSIII is made using the Beighton Score and Brighton Criteria, and these documents can be found in Appendix 1. There are plenty of other books with very detailed discussions about diagnostic criteria.[1]

What diagnosis meant for me as a patient

For me, finding out that I had HMS was initially quite a shock and I was initially quite upset about it. I knew I was generalised hypermobile from my teenage years when a ballet teacher had told me about my 'swayback knees' but I had no idea at all that my regular calf tears, my back pain, fatigue, poor sleep patterns, anxiety, depression, asthma, IBS, poor coordination, poor concentration and endometriosis might also be linked to having HMS. My physiotherapist was the first to suggest I had HMS and some months later this was officially confirmed by a consultant rheumatologist. I think that when I had a diagnosis I could start to put together all the pieces of the jigsaw that for me made the HMS. Once I was able to accept this I was able to look at where I went from there, and although I am a great deal more 'stable' than I was, it has taken about four years in real time to attain this level of control of my instable body. I think I would in fact add instable mind as well because now that my body feels stronger and more stable I feel calmer in my mind and have much less difficulty with mood swings than I did in the past.

From Knight 2011, pp.60–61

---

1   Beighton *et al.* (2012); Hakim *et al.* (2010); Keer and Grahame (2003); Knight (2011).

Picking up the pieces

Once I had a diagnosis I had to pick up the pieces both from my clinical history where I had so frequently been dismissed in the past, and in terms of a treatment journey which I embarked on in April 2008 (a little before official diagnosis) and which was to involve a considerable number of different medical specialities and departments. Hypermobility syndrome is a multisystemic condition (Grahame 2009) and as such it means that numerous experts have been involved in my care at the helm of any resultant treatment. Of course, ultimately there lies a responsibility with the patient themselves to manage their condition, but it is a great challenge, and many patients fall by the wayside through no fault of their own, but often due to lack of holistic support. I am, without doubt, one of the luckier ones. I have been fortunate to have obtained medical treatment from the leaders in their field. In temperament I am incredibly determined, which has no doubt helped me – but what about all those equally other 'determined' people who also so urgently require the same level of care and treatment? What is happening to them?

I cannot conclude this chapter without mentioning politics. Patients like myself place a huge and costly demand upon the NHS. Resources and expertise are scarce and, in the current economic climate, further cuts seem inevitable and waiting times are likely to increase. There are centres of expertise in the care of patients with EDSIII – for example, the Glasgow Infirmary, the Royal National Orthopaedic Hospital in London, University College Hospital, London and the (private) Hospital of St John and St Elizabeth which has a Hypermobility Unit (see Appendix 3), but this is woefully inadequate for the numbers of patients who are so badly affected. Research would tend to suggest that approximately 10–30 per cent of males and 20–40 per cent of females are hypermobile (Hakim and Grahame 2003). Only the most severely affected end up requiring regular hospital treatment, and research shows that EDSIII has overlaps with other medical conditions such as fibromyalgia (FM), chronic fatigue and pain, and a myriad of other bodily problems. This book seeks to explore in great detail the sheer complexity of the condition, whilst describing the investigations and treatments I went through in my journey through the system (both bodily and the NHS!), and is supplemented by my own experience as a patient, as an academic researcher and as a Bowen therapist. I am extremely fortunate to have an outstanding team of leading medical authors in their field to explain more academically and clinically the rationale behind treatment and some of the underlying pathologies of a truly chronic, complex medical condition and its management. I hope that the book will provide a useful resource for all medical practitioners and interested patients.

PART II
PHYSIOLOGY

CHAPTER 5

Maslow's Hierarchy of Needs and homeostasis

Being in my body is like being at a fairground without the fun!

Isobel Knight, Facebook, 11.7.2012

This part explores the sheer physiological complexity of living with a multisystemic, chronic, complex condition such as EDSIII. The use of Maslow's Hierarchy of Needs provides an excellent framework to explore the lack of homeostasis in EDSIII and how basic physiological needs may be unmet. I describe my own experiences in relation to different bodily systems and academic writing. Dr Alan Hakim explains in technical and medical detail what is going on physiologically in Chapter 6.

Maslow's Hierarchy of Needs

Although I very much consider my hypermobility to be an enormous asset in terms of classical ballet,[1] my quality of life was otherwise poor, and it made me consider the Maslow Hierarchy of Needs (see Figure 5.1), which I recalled from my teacher-training days. The starting points for motivation, Maslow writes, are the 'physiological drives' (1970, p.35). It then struck me how very crucial the red or bottom-line biological and physiological needs are to primal survival, and most of them were not working very well in my body. Maslow defines physiological needs as paramount. He writes that

in the human being who is missing everything in life in an extreme fashion, it is more likely that the major motivation

---

1   See Knight (2011), Chapter 10.

would be the physiological needs rather than any others. A person who is lacking food, safety, love and esteem would most probably hunger for food more strongly than anything else. (Maslow 1970, p.37)

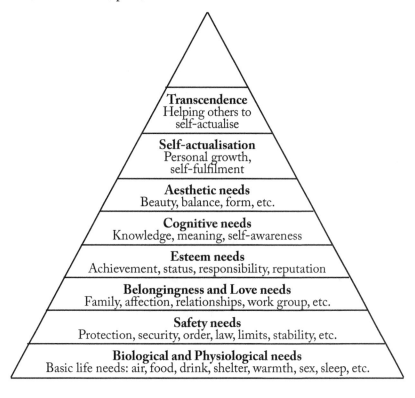

Transcendence
Helping others to
self-actualise

Self-actualisation
Personal growth,
self-fulfilment

Aesthetic needs
Beauty, balance, form, etc.

Cognitive needs
Knowledge, meaning, self-awareness

Esteem needs
Achievement, status, responsibility, reputation

Belongingness and Love needs
Family, affection, relationships, work group, etc.

Safety needs
Protection, security, order, law, limits, stability, etc.

Biological and Physiological needs
Basic life needs: air, food, drink, shelter, warmth, sex, sleep, etc.

FIGURE 5.1: MASLOW'S HIERARCHY OF NEEDS
Source: from www. maslowshierarchyofneeds.net, with kind permission

Homeostasis

I lacked any sort of homeostasis. Montpetit (2012) writes that, 'French Physiologist Claude Bernard was the first to define a state of internal dynamic equilibrium that is achieved unconsciously and constantly in the body (heart breathing, temperature) as homeostasis' (p.17). Maslow defines homeostasis as:

the body's automatic efforts to maintain a constant, normal state of the blood stream... [However,] not all physiological needs are homeostatic. That sexual desire, sleepiness, sheer activity and exercise, and maternal behaviour in animals are homeostatic has not yet been demonstrated.

Maslow 1970, pp.35–36

Breathing/respiration

Although I was generally breathing well, and not breathing apically, but diaphragmatically and correctly, I did at times have problems with asthma if allergic to something or as a result of a cold or infection. Asthma has been partly linked to EDSIII on account of the collagenous tissues found in the lungs which are also subject to laxity like other collagenous tissues in the body (Morgan *et al.* 2007).

Breathing is essential to life. If we stop breathing, we die! Breathing or respiration is about filling the body with nourishing oxygen and removing waste carbon dioxide. It is essential fuel to the body, and poor breathing leads to poor circulation and resultant complaints such as Reynaud's syndrome (Tinkle 2010), which is common for some EDSIII patients. The muscles are also affected, and research already shows that EDSIII patients have poor endurance or slow-twitch muscles (Simmonds and Keer 2007, 2008). If the muscles are not adequately fuelled with nourishing oxygen their performance becomes impaired, so breathing is crucial to everything. Endurance, in relation to cardiorespiratory and cardiovascular fitness, is discussed in Chapter 40.

Research is beginning to show how circulation and problems relating to disruption to the autonomic nervous system (ANS) or autonomic dysfunction are related to EDSIII, again because of tissue laxity (Bravo, Sanhueza and Hakim 2010). Any such disruption to circulation, temperature and heart-rate might be having an impact upon homeostasis, and both ANS disruption and a condition called postural orthostatic tachycardia are described in Chapter 6.

Autonomic dysfunction and postural orthostatic tachycardia syndrome (POTS)

Leading EDS consultant rheumatologist and HMSA chief medical officer Dr Alan Hakim explains the following about disruption to the autonomic nervous system (ANS).

AUTONOMIC DYSFUNCTION
Dr Alan Hakim

Introduction
The autonomic nervous system is a highly specialised network of nerves that regulate a number of important systems, automatically adjusting functions in the body and compensating for change. Activity is driven and controlled from structures in the brain stem and spinal cord over which we have very limited control. Highly intricate reflex reactions between organs and blood vessels of the body are constantly taking place without need for recourse to the brain.

The autonomic nervous system is made up of three parts: the sympathetic, parasympathetic and enteric nervous systems. Essentially, the sympathetic and parasympathetic systems work in opposition to each other, not in conflict but in balancing the various functions they control. For example, the sympathetic nervous system tends to speed up the heart, with the parasympathetic system slowing it down. The sympathetic system will slow down bowel activity and the parasympathetic nervous system will speed it up. When you are running for cover to avoid the rain your sympathetic system has switched on to give you energy and drive. The term 'fight or flight' is used to describe this activity. When you sit down in the evening and relax with your favourite drink your parasympathetic system switches on: 'rest and digest'.

The enteric nervous system is a network of nerves that looks after itself and regulates the various functions of the digestive system. Unlike the sympathetic and parasympathetic systems that use the chemical transmitters norepinephrine (noradrenaline) and acetylcholine to send signals along nerves and into organs, the enteric system also employs the chemicals dopamine, serotonin and nitric oxide. These chemicals are also found in the brain; so, manipulation of them by medications can affect a number of central nervous system functions and give rise to a variety of benefits and side-effects.

Given the intricacy of these systems and the fine balance they achieve it is perhaps not surprising that when they go wrong a person can suffer with quite considerable symptoms, many of which can be difficult for the individual to 'put their finger on'.

Although there is huge medical literature on the symptoms and clinical findings of autonomic 'dysfunction', it was not until the early 2000s that these problems were recognised as present in people who have joint hypermobility syndrome (JHS)/Ehlers-Danlos hypermobility type (EDS-HT). The work of Dr Gazit, based in Dr Jacobs' lab in Haifa, Israel, and published in 2003, was the first large study performed demonstrating the presence of symptoms and abnormalities of autonomic dysfunction in JHS (Gazit *et al.* 2003) Further work at University College Hospitals (UCH), London, found that up to 6 out of 10 patients with JHS describe some form of symptomatic autonomic disturbance (Hakim and Grahame 2004).

Symptoms

The most common concern is the sensation of feeling faint or even passing out. This happens most often when an individual changes position, such as sitting from lying, standing from sitting, etc. This is due to a drop in blood pressure and is called orthostatic hypotension. A similar problem often relating to change in posture is palpitations. Here, the heart beats much faster than normal and sometimes one can also experience shortness of breath and chest pain. Sometimes this can happen when resting and need not be related to change in posture.

A variation on orthostatic hypotension is the condition 'orthostatic intolerance'; this may be the most common of the vascular problems encountered in EDS. The condition occurs after a period of time standing. It may be obvious after only two to three minutes but can take ten minutes to appear.

Not all patients will describe heart and vascular symptoms. Some patients experience uncontrollable bowel symptoms, much like irritable bowel, with constipation, diarrhoea and abdominal pains. One also needs to be cautious in that bowel symptoms may arise for a number of reasons, not least due to hernias or a weak abdominal/pelvic floor due to tissue laxity, as well as medications such as pain killers. One should likewise be aware that the heart and vascular symptoms described might also be side effects of certain medications.

The UCH study showed that JHS/EDSIII patients with symptoms of autonomic disturbance are two to three times more likely to report fatigue and night sweats than those who have no vascular or bowel symptoms (Hakim and Grahame 2004). The fatigue reported by some patients is very similar to that reported in chronic fatigue syndrome (CFS). Interestingly, autonomic dysfunction is increasingly reported in CFS as well, suggesting considerable overlap between these conditions.

Mechanisms

When we sit at rest blood pools in large vessels in our legs and abdomen, the heart slows down and our breathing becomes shallow. The body, via the autonomic nervous system, keeps close check on the small volume of blood flowing through the heart and up to the brain. When we stand up the body has to react instantly to the fact that gravity is pulling all the blood away from the brain. Blood vessels in the neck sense changes in blood pressure and blood flow to the brain; these are called baroreceptors. A drop in blood pressure to the brain triggers the heart to pump harder and a little faster, and the leg and bowel blood vessels to constrict, forcing blood back to the heart. This generates a better blood pressure good enough to push blood into the brain.

When this mechanism goes wrong a person may experience 'postural' or 'orthostatic hypotension', feel dizzy and might even black out. Sometimes the heart also beats so quickly that one experiences palpitations. Here, the term 'postural orthostatic tachycardia syndrome' is used.

Study in this area suggests that some of the problem with the autonomic dysfunction in EDSIII lies in the stretchiness of peripheral veins. For example, in orthostatic intolerance the blood vessels no longer contract as well as they should and blood 'pools' in the leg veins. The legs swell and the blood pressure falls. But, how much these problems are due to combinations of changes in the chemical transmitters mentioned earlier, tissue laxity in the veins or even 'deconditioning' of blood vessels and muscles because of poor mobility is unknown. In individuals that do not respond to simple treatments sophisticated tests in an autonomic lab may be required to better understand the mechanism.

Clinical signs and tests

Cardiovascular signs can be recognised clinically by taking the blood pressure and feeling the pulse in the sitting and standing position. However, for a lot of patients the clinical signs can be very subtle even though the symptoms are strong (author's experience). Blood pressure and pulse monitoring for 24 hours wearing a machine that records the measurements whilst going about normal routine may also be helpful in making the diagnosis. More sophisticated tests require the facilities of an autonomic unit. There are several ways to stimulate the autonomic nervous system including tilting the body between upright and flat positions, using heat and cold to stimulate nerves, and even eating to stimulate the enteric system. Bowel investigations include upper and lower bowel endoscopy, stimulation tests and possible biopsy of bowel tissue.

Treatment

The three simplest ways to avoid many of the cardiovascular symptoms are:

1. Keep well hydrated and maintain salt intake. Drink two to three litres a day (preferably of water and 'isotonic' drinks), particularly on a hot day, and try to avoid caffeine and alcohol if these make symptoms worse. The colour of the urine is a good clue as to whether one is well hydrated. It should be a very pale straw yellow; anything darker suggests dehydration. It is important not to overload with water, and thus passing lots of urine that is very clear, as this can be harmful because it dilutes and reduces the normal salt balance in the blood.

2. Stand up more slowly and try to avoid having to stand in one position for too long. Just rocking back and forth lifting the ankles and working the calf muscles, whilst standing in a queue for example, can make all the difference.

3. If more unwell after heavy meals, cutting down the size of meals and trying to eat regularly through the day may also help.

Physical exercise might improve autonomic symptoms and fatigue by improving muscle conditioning. If one improves muscle quality in the legs and abdomen one should improve blood flow through the body and reduce the problem of venous pooling. Reducing venous pooling should lower the risk of orthostatic hypotension and orthostatic intolerance.

Medications

Several classes of medication might be used to help reduce symptoms, but it is important to note that their potential side effects might make other symptoms worse. It is for this reason that it is important to identify all the issues that may be present from the outset. Most require specialist input from either cardiology, neurology or gastroenterology.

Prescribed medications may be introduced to:

1. reduce the risk of palpitations by slowing down the heart. The most common group of drugs are the beta blockers. These, however, may make your blood pressure drop and increase pooling of blood in the legs that might make your symptoms worse

2. increase the blood pressure

3. control bowel function. These might include anti-sickness (anti-emetics), antacids and anti-spasmodics.

A patient describes her symptoms:

> One of my daughters has autonomic dysfunction and faints a lot with no warning. The cardiologist who diagnosed her just told her to step up her salt intake. It can happen at any time but does seem worse if she gets too hot.
>
> *EDS patient, Facebook*

Postural orthostatic tachycardia syndrome

Postural orthostatic tachycardia syndrome (POTS) occurs because of disturbances in the autonomic nervous system (ANS) resulting in changes in blood pressure and heart rate from lying or sitting to standing (Grubb 2008). As Hakim explained, patients might complain of the following symptoms: palpitations, fatigue, lightheadedness, problems with tolerating exercise, fatigue, dizziness, temperature changes, headache and mental clouding (Grubb 2008; Raj 2006). The condition predominantly affects women, 4:1 compared to men (Raj 2006). Bohora writes that

> orthostatic intolerance is, by definition, a change from supine to an upright position [which] causes an increase in heart rate of more than 30 beats per minute or to a heart rate greater than 120 beats per minute within 10 minutes of an upright position.
>
> *Bohora 2010, p.158*

Overactivity of the sympathetic nervous system results in the tachycardia and may affect other organs and include slow venous return and resultant changes in temperature (Bohora 2010). Unfortunately, the symptoms often closely mimic anxiety, which results in some patients being incorrectly diagnosed as having panic or anxiety attacks (Bohora 2010; Grubb 2008).

The cause of POTS is yet unknown but recommendations include improving fluid intakes and sodium intake – up to 200mEq/day (Raj 2006). Medications such as SSRIs, including Duloxetine, are suggested (Kanjwal *et al.* 2009). Increasing exercise is also beneficial, but it takes some time for patients to cope with dizziness and increased fatigue, so must be carefully paced (Grubb 2008). POTS might be explained in the EDSIII group owing to the increased tissue laxity in the connective tissue vasculature (Kanjwal *et al.* 2009). In addition to disturbances to the heart rate and blood pressure, other organs might also be involved, such as bladder and bowel, because of the overall effects on the ANS (Grubb 2008). There is little doubt that autonomic disturbance might count as physiological imbalance, and a lack of homeostasis, as per Maslow (see Chapter 5). My experiences of having POTS are described in the three following blog extracts:

> I was also having vascular responses and my blood pressure varied significantly during physiotherapy and then for an ongoing 24 hour period (although things did settle a bit). There was also a significant difference between the left and right side in terms of body temperature. The left side was cold and clammy compared to the right which was a normal, albeit cool!
>
> *Blog, 29.10.2010*

Today I feel 'out of my body' and I am experiencing both chest pain and then changes to heart rate level and nasty pressure in my head. It is all on the left side of my body. My temporomandibular joint (TMJ) hurts, I have a left-sided headache, and my hands are very different temperatures with my left hand being significantly colder than the right.

Blog, 17.7.2011

I don't know how or why I am still on a computer given my existing symptoms. I could be cut in half and in pain on the left-side of my body from the top of my head and down the whole of my left-side of body. I have extremely cold hands, but my legs are warm and normal temperature. I am 'locked' solid and as is if it is squeezed on the left side of my head and neck and into my TMJ and have been seeing 'stars' but not of the 'I'm a Celebrity get me out of here' kind.

Blog, 25.11.2011

POTS and physiotherapy experiment

During September 2010 and during a particular 'POTS' time, I decided to wear a BP/HR monitor for a 24-hour period to see what happened to my BP/HR during that time. The results can be seen in Figure 6.1. The results show a startling drop during physiotherapy when work was being done on my neck, thus having a very profound effect, including dramatic temperature changes during the session. At lunch time I felt like I was having palpitations. There was another significant dip in BP/HR after a hot bath at 10.50pm. The experiment was repeated again with very similar results two weeks later. Almost two years later I managed to have formal testing – there is an incredibly long wait for autonomic testing because of such high demand.

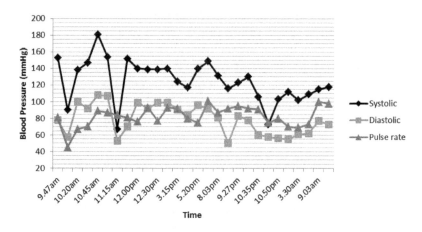

FIGURE 6.1: ISOBEL KNIGHT'S BLOOD PRESSURE/PULSE RATES 28.9.2010–29.9.2010

POTS testing and diagnosis

By the time I went for my own POTS testing, I had heard so many unpleasant things about it, I was thoroughly dreading it, and had postponed my assessment appointment several times because I was so worried about the implications of the 'tilt test' on my neck, but I really needn't have worried. The staff at the National Neurology Hospital were wonderful, and I blogged the following account of the entire two-day experience:

POTS testing: day 1

I finally had my long-awaited POTS assessment at the National Neurological Hospital in Queen's Square, London. I had been put on the list two years ago, but deferred my original assessment appointment because I was so worried about having the Tilt Table test at the time – although in fact nothing was done other than a blood pressure and symptom history – back in February. I had deferred because my physio and I had been concerned about the testing making my symptoms worse. Then would have been the time for these tests! As a result I feel that my symptoms are much less severe two years later, so am not sure how much benefit will be gained from the tests – other than my ability to contribute to their research and for me to document the experience now.

I woke in the morning with the symptoms of a cold and had a sore throat and cough all the previous night, so was not feeling well. I reported this to the nurse who met me on this pleasant and calm ward. It was strange being admitted to a ward where one is a day-patient. Nonetheless upon arrival my blood pressure was taken, and an MRSA swab as well as the usual clerical details – e.g. next of kin, allergies, wrist-band. I was then taken to the Autonomic Unit and entered a small laboratory where I spent the next four hours.

My 'scientist' was lovely and explained everything to me as it unfolded. He began with taking some notes about my symptoms and when they occurred and anything that made them worse. I was then asked to lie on the table (to become the 'tilt' table) and was hooked up to a blood pressure machine around my right arm and some base line readings were taken. Heart monitor pads were added to my chest and a heart monitor put around my middle left finger, which created a pulsing sensation (to the rhythm of my own heart). I had to have my hands warmed up as they were so cold – particularly to the left as is often the case. I was then left for a good ten minutes whilst several baseline readings of my Blood Pressure (BP) and Heart Rate (HR) were taken whilst I was horizontal. Then came the first of the testings...

I was asked to squeeze something as hard as possible and hold it there for several minutes to create a tornique. It was quite painful, and I just about managed to do it. All the while BP/HR readings were taken.

Next I was asked to do some mental arithmetic. I found this quite stressful at the start of the test, but got into it OK and then the maths became harder. Doubtless my HR/BP readings will bear out this stress!

After this I was asked to do some deep-breathing whilst readings were taken. This was fine.

The next test involved having two icepacks put onto my right hand, one under it and one on top of it. This was most unpleasant, and again I survived the experience.

Once I had recovered from this test I had to do a lot of shallow breathing – or hyperventilating. This did make me a bit dizzy/lightheaded.

After this I had to go to the bathroom before a few more baseline HR/BP readings were done, and then I was tilted abruptly (though not violently) to 60 degrees. I then had to spend a very long time in this position. I was taken well past the ten minutes – although I was having symptoms of HR and temperature change as well as feeling sick. I then had a cannula inserted and bloods were taken and my response to the stress measured. After I really could tolerate no more and was getting to stage of hypervenilation, I called it a day and requested the test to end (I think my tester wanted me to hang on a bit longer, but my back was killing me). I was then tipped back to horizontal, though this did not feel horizontal anymore – felt strange. Once a few more readings were done, whilst in horizontal, I was asked to stand still. A few minutes into the test Blood was taken from the back of my hand, rather than using a cannula, which I found strange, but it was another stressor designed to see how I would cope – which I did. After this came the exercise test!

The exercise test involved me lying supine on a bed where I was hooked up to another BP monitor and a few baseline readings were taken. I was then positioned into an exercise bike, whilst lying horizontal, which is hard to imagine, but was possible. I enjoyed this test the most of all. I had to cycle keeping the bike at a certain pace. The first level was easy, then pressure was increased to make the resistance harder and I had to cycle for a bit longer and then third level was harder still. I had no problems at all with this test and seemed to recover quickly.

The final part of the morning involved me being fitted with the portable BP/HR monitor and being given a diary to complete with various activities for the following 24 hours. I was told how to remove the monitor and what sorts of things to be doing in the different tests – e.g. some sitting, lying, walking, assessing myself before and after food. After this I was able to go to the ward and have my lunch before running off to work – and did a brisk walk there. It was very embarrassing having the machine on me at work as it was quite noisy and sounded like flatulance! Everyone was laughing. By this point in the afternoon, I was feeling increasingly poorly and was very definitely coming down with a cold.

I didn't get home from work until just after 8pm and did some more readings in different positions. Bed time was another issue altogether...!

POTS testing: day 2

I had left the Neurology Hospital with a 24-hour BP/HR monitor with a diary and instructions about how to use the monitor and the sorts of things to record in my diary. This started with me recording my BP 5 minutes before eating, then ten minutes after to see how food affects my BP. I then had a very brisk walk to work so these things were all recorded.

I did not sleep well that night. Aside from the fact I had a nasty cold the BP monitor was going off every hour, so was waking me up hourly as well!

In the morning I foolishly decided to run a few errands in the notoriously busy Oxford Street before going back to hospital. This was definitely a mistake – especially when feeling unwell.

I arrived into the lovely calm of the day ward and shown to another nice green chair in a room shared with others having intravenous medications – mainly for MS. I was then taken back to the Autonomic Unit for my final testing situation – the 'feeding' test.

I told my scientist of the day that I was not well, but we agreed I could proceed with the test, and I requested to be given a soya-milk complan drink as I was presently on a dairy-free diet.

The test started with a few base measurements starting on the tilt-table, in a horizontal position, after this I was tipped again to 60 degrees and left there for ten minutes. I did feel some fatigue and nausea, but not much else. My scientist then bought me back to horizontal and then fed me two plastic cups worth of the liquid meal I had to consume, whilst lying flat, and I had to drink the meal through a straw. It was strange doing this, but I managed to swallow the drink, which tasted quite pleasant. I then had to wait 45 minutes in order for the drink to be digested, but had to remain on the tilt table, horizontally. I was covered with a blanket and said I would probably fall asleep – although I was asked to 'preferably' remain awake to avoid my BP dropping, as would be the case if I slept.

Sleep, it seemed, did not feature in the agenda, particularly with a BP monitor going off every 5 minutes. My HR rocketed and I started to have palpitations. This went on, past the repeat of the ten minute tilt-test and actually went on for several hours after the test. This was not something I expected to happen, neither did my scientist. Although people sometimes do have palpitations (as per having POTS) they don't normally last too long. I had to be taken back to the ward and further monitored for a few more hours. My 'resting' heart rate ranged between 80–110 beats. As a precaution I was also given an ECG, but this was normal. I was also given more food in order to try and stabilise me. I did eventually feel better and got home at about 8pm. I should imagine the fact I had a bad cold and chest would have possibly had an effect on my tests and their outcome. However, I will definitely say that this 'Feeding Test' was nowhere near as bad as I had expected, even despite the outcome of my testing – which was unusual. Nobody should worry about this test or indeed any other POTS testing.

I get the results of my tests at the end of the month.

Everyone was absolutely lovely at hospital, and nobody should worry about having POTS testing – although some aspects of the testing are slightly unpleasant (as in my Day one experience) nothing lasts too long. You will be fine, and they will really look after you even if something strange does happen! At least it is not like being at A&E where nobody believes your symptoms or thinks you are making it up!

Blog, 26.9.2012

Results: formally diagnosed with POTS, management conservative.

POTS update: October 2012

Although I still get occasional POTS episodes, as my treatment progressed, particularly when I was able to commence cardiovascular exercise (see Chapter 40), I realised that my POTS symptoms have generally diminished over the past two years. The only time I have to be more careful is if I am squatting and coming up to standing (e.g. in a library or going shopping), when I do get dizzy. Otherwise dizziness, temperature changes and sudden changes to heart rate are all more 'homeostatic'. This certainly relates to the literature (Grubb 2008; Hakim's writing earlier in the chapter). As a result of my diagnosis, I continue to follow the recommendations of increasing my fluid levels, and slightly increasing my sodium levels, as well as conditioning exercise (Grubb 2008; Hakim in this chapter).

In this chapter Hakim also described how autonomic dysfunction affects digestion, which is discussed in Chapter 7.

CHAPTER 7

Digestion and bowel problems

Of all the symptoms I have endured, some of which have included very sensitive issues such as self-harming (skin-picking) and gynaecological problems (endometriosis), it has been the bowel-related problems that I have found the hardest to confront. I first remember having some problems with my bowels not long after I started at university, and in fact came home for the holidays. I just couldn't do a bowel movement, which was unlike me because I had always had regular bowel movements prior to that time. I remember speaking to my mum about it and I went to see my GP. I cannot remember what medication I was prescribed but suspect it was either a mild laxative or something that would have supported IBS. I took the tablets for a while and then things returned to normal.

A year or two later I started to experience problems with my upper GI tract and was suffering from terrible indigestion and acid reflux. I saw my GP and was prescribed Gaviscon and advised to stop smoking! I continued smoking, but the upper GI symptoms did go away, eventually.

When I did stop smoking (I only smoked for about five years) in 2001, I recall having problems with my bowels again. I think this isn't uncommon because many smokers I know tell me that smoking helps them to be able to go to the toilet, and caffeine is another helpful substance! I was referred to a gastroenterologist in 2001 because I had recently had a negative laparoscopy where at that time no endometriosis was found. I was otherwise asymptomatic in a GI capacity and only a vague diagnosis of IBS was suggested. All tests, including a barium meal, came back normal. A small haemorrhoid was found, but it was barely commented upon.

Several years later, my bowel habits changed completely and I started to pass what I now understand as 'overflow diarrhoea' several times a day, but not 'normal' bowel movements. Unfortunately, I started to accept this as a normal state of affairs, not even worrying about blood that I was finding. I was more than aware of skin-tags in my anus and just coped with this as best I could. Finally, when my rectal area became so painful and a long period of time had lapsed where I was not able to fully empty my bowels, I eventually decided that enough was enough and went to see my GP. My GP was very understanding, but said it was a great pity I had not been able to talk about this much sooner. He quickly referred me to a colorectal surgeon where I was diagnosed with an anal fissure. The first-line treatment for this was diltiazem ointment, which is meant to relax the anal sphincter muscles. The first surgeon who saw me said my colon was 'loaded' and I was put on fybogel, which I did not respond well to, and then a second surgeon told me I could take a senna laxative, which I have taken since. I was sent for other tests, which included a colon transit test, which involves having to take two tablets at the same time each day. Each capsule contains different shapes – for example crosses and circles. After taking a different set of shapes each day for three days, I had to return to hospital for a pelvic X-ray, the idea being to see where these shapes were within my digestive system. The X-ray showed there was some faecal matter remaining in my rectum, but otherwise the shapes had passed through my digestive system within a 'normal' transit time.

The next test I had was a colonoscopy. In order to prepare for this I had to take picolox, in order to completely clear my digestive system prior to the colonoscopy. I had the day off work and took one lot of this medication before waiting for it to pass through my system, which took a surprisingly short time.

I had my colonoscopy the following morning. I was dreading it – the being sedated. I don't think the sedation ever really worked on me at all. I was fully conscious the whole time. Normally doctors opt to carry out a colonoscopy with the patient lying on their left side, but I couldn't tolerate this and it was causing me more pain, so they carried out the procedure with me lying supine. The outcome of the colonoscopy was that I was diagnosed with mild diverticulosis in three separate areas of my left colon, which for me tallied beautifully with the pain I experienced in that area of my abdomen. One doctor said to me, anecdotally and informally, that it was just possible the diverticulosis was linked to EDSIII because of the high pressure that the bowel is put under, resulting in these pockets or diverticuli forming. However, despite this find, there was nothing more sinister, and treatment and management of the diverticulosis involves a high fibre diet, so there was a continued request for me to take fybogel, which I still hated.

In late August I was sent back to the colorectal surgeons again and seen by their most senior consultant – mainly given my clinical complexity – and he said that he would take over my care and perform the surgery to repair my anal fissure and skin-tagging. The surgery took place on 14 September 2011 and I had been dreading it because of a huge fear of anaesthesia. My fear of anaesthesia was not unfounded. I had had wisdom teeth removed under local anaesthesia in 1997 when I 'swore' I could still feel what was happening. As my research into EDSIII continued, I realised it probably wasn't my imagination since the effects of local anaesthesia are less potent in hypermobile patients (Beighton *et al.* 2012; Hakim *et al.* 2005). Of two of the four surgeries I had had involving general anaesthesia, two had not worked well initially as the anaesthetist had missed my veins completely and I just wasn't going under. Another surgery involved waiting over 12 hours following a pre-med, which had long since worn off and one where things seemed to be uneventful. I had a huge fear of being out of control and the fear of feeling pain whilst under anaesthetic. I was actually terrified of being put under and I requested Nicola, a close friend, to attend with me.

On the day of my actual surgery, I remember my name being called and Nicola came to go in with me, but was denied access. I hastily bid a retreat to the toilet and hid – mainly through fear. Shortly after, the staff asked me to come out of the bathroom and then said they would allow Nicola back in once I had signed my consent forms, etc. The anaesthetist was brilliant. She said she did this every day of the week, but for me it wasn't something I would be used to. She prescribed a dose of midazolam, which is a jelly-like texture and taken orally via a syringe. Nicola did some Bowen moves to calm me down and then, frankly, I don't remember anything else. I have no recollection at all of going to the theatre, although Nicola apparently kindly stayed with me whilst I was put under. The next thing I remember is waking up on the ward and being given coffee and biscuits – with a very sore backside!

My anus was repaired. For the first 24 hours after surgery I seemed amazingly fine, but I think this is often the case as the anaesthesia and other drugs give you a big high. However, a few days later, doing any sort of bowel movement caused unbearable pain. There were tears, and I recall breaking into a cold sweat on several occasions for about two weeks. Several things helped, including raising my feet on to books to use the lavatory and breathing. Lactalose solution did help a bit, but it was still taking about six attempts to evacuate my bowels, the most painful hours of the day being prior to 2pm. After that I could sit a bit more easily. It takes a whole four to six weeks for the area to be sufficiently recovered, which was just as well as I had been booked on to a cycle tour in Washington DC, and bicycle seats are not the kindest to one's behind at the best of times!

Amongst all of this, I had a flare-up of my neck pain and symptoms days after the surgery. I saw my physio for a treatment two days post-surgery, which was probably not advisable – but I had done it to aid my recovery. The following day I had some of my worst neurological and POTS symptoms. It was hard to say whether these had been caused by what my physio had done for me in treatment or from anaesthesia, and my neck being in an awkward position during surgery. I was seen by a local GP surgery which is an NHS walk-in centre. There was a very long wait, so I went back home to sleep before firstly being seen by a nurse who spotted my old familiar problem of having the possible start of a UTI. She asked one of the doctors to see me, who was quite unhappy with what was going on with me, did a referral letter for A&E and sent for an ambulance.

Yet again, I cannot really blame my local A&E department. Despite my myriad of symptoms, some disturbing (e.g. the neurological ones, change in pulse rate, temperature and dizziness), I was not near death (even if I felt it) and was not an 'accident' – so was I an emergency? Given that my vital signs were otherwise stable, probably not. The doctor who saw me was clearly quite 'pissed off' with me and asked me what medications I usually take for this kind of eventuality. I explained, and was forthwith given diazepam, codeine, anti-emetic medication and oramorph in more or less that order. The doctor said they were going to do nothing else for me and thus I was discharged in a bit of a daze to return home, so was it all worth it at all? Probably not, but how can I know or be sure that any of these severe neurological problems I get are not sinister?

Further bowel treatments and investigations
MRI proctogram
There is no doubt that I was very definitely not keen on having this test given the number of times I had postponed it, and for good reason. I had to be at hospital for 8.40am and had two nights in a

row of very bad sleep, and had needed codeine on the second night owing to pain, so thought this might be difficult for the test as I had been unable to do a bowel movement in the morning and dreaded the implications of this.

The radiology nurse was absolutely lovely and told me what would happen. I was asked to put on a hospital gown and told to remove any underwear and anything metal. The first thing that happened was that I was asked to lie on my left side and was given an enema to clear my rectum. She then sent me to sit in a cubical waiting area. It wasn't long before nature took its course and I needed to use the bathroom! I was left to wait for about 20 more minutes before then being brought to the MRI scanning area. I was put on to the MRI scanner and had to lie on my left side again so they could insert some jelly into my rectum before the scan of me evacuating the jelly. I was then asked to lie supine with my knees slightly apart in the scanner. The problem was, I was 'spasming' all over the place and just didn't have any control to keep my knees apart whilst lying flat. In the end they just told me to lie flat. The scanning started and then I was asked to eliminate the jelly. I tried very hard and was pushing until I was red in the face, but nothing would come out! The nurse then came back and asked me if I could try again lying with my knees bent up with sandbags on my feet to help me. The scan started and I was asked to push the jelly out, and this time I was successful. It was only clear jelly, but felt a bit embarrassing. The nurses were really good about preserving my dignity at all times and got me up. I was then able to get dressed and leave straight away.

I received a phone call from the doctor to say that the outcome of the MRI proctogram was that biofeedback training was entirely the right course of action for me.

Biofeedback

I was a little apprehensive in attending biofeedback training because of the part of the treatment that included having a balloon inserted in my back passage. However, I overcame my anxieties about this aspect of the treatment because I realised how valuable the treatment could be in terms of my bowel problems. I met Nurse V in late March. She couldn't have been kinder or more reassuring. The session began with a review of my MRI proctogram, which V explained showed that I was not using the right muscles to evacuate effectively and hence why I often needed to visit the toilet several times in order to completely clear my bowels. The muscles apparently required for effective evacuation are transverse abdominals and internal and external obliques. Despite all my efforts to develop these muscle groups in physiotherapy, my efforts were futile when it came to recruiting these muscles for the purposes of evacuation. Nurse V reiterated why biofeedback training would be helpful to me.

We had a discussion about my diet overall and this was barely commented upon in the end because my diet is generally good and contains plenty of roughage, fruit, vegetables and water. I explained that I was still taking senna laxatives, and Nurse V felt that I should be able to reduce these owing to the fact that my bowel movements were quite loose and that a slightly firmer stool would be easier to pass. We discussed the effects that other medications such as codeine would have on my bowels, and I explained how I was on minimal doses of these types of medications and fully understood their constipating effect.

After this we discussed posture on the toilet. I had never known that it would be much better if I slumped forwards and relaxed my forearms and belly. I had been sitting very upright before. I was also told not to take deep breaths and strain! It was difficult to consider letting my muscles relax whilst working out which ones I needed to access in order to improve my evacuation. This was where the balloon came into it!

I was asked to lower my undergarments and cover myself with a sheet and lie on my side with my knees bent. A tampon-like device was inserted (with lubricating jelly) into my rectum and I was asked to try and push it out. I couldn't. Herein lay the problem. Nurse V asked me to cough and palpate the muscles required. I did this. She then asked me to squeeze these very muscles (transverse abdominals and obliques). I did this a few times and was able to almost expel the balloon/tampon device. Having the device in situ really helped me to understand what I needed to do and which muscles I needed to engage for this to happen. It was quite hard work, but unfortunately all my experiences of learning to use new muscle groups have been the same – it is hard work and very fatiguing for me.

Nurse V explained how the squeezing of the muscle groups involved would act as a pump for the evacuation process and that combined with the relaxed slumped posture (no deep breaths) would eventually mean that I evacuated more efficiently and with fewer attempts. She told me this would take time and that the muscles would re-learn what was required, I would ultimately need to use the toilet fewer times and my bowel movements would also improve so I could reduce the use of laxatives. She said that I should allow proper time for taking bowel movements and also to wait until I needed to go 'quite urgently' because the more times I tried would encourage the gut muscles to activate and cause me to keep needing to go more.

ONE WEEK LATER

I felt very fatigued for two days after the biofeedback training session, but this has often been the case when I have been required to learn new movement patterns. My toilet posture is automatically better and the muscles are working better already and have more of a 'pumping action'. I am already evacuating more efficiently although still needing to do more than two or three attempts. I have already reduced my intake of laxatives from two to one and will start to cut this further to one tablet every other day. I am managing to wait until I more urgently need to evacuate and I hope that in time I will be able to reduce my attempts to evacuate. I am still a bit prone to holding my breath, but am mindful of this, and I hope to stop doing this and to be able to relax the other abdominal muscles I do not need to activate for the process of evacuation. Nurse V said this would all take time.

REVIEW UPDATE WITH NURSE V: MAY 2012

I had my review with Nurse V on 29 May 2012. I was a little disappointed that things seemed to have deteriorated, but upon discussion with her, we revised the bracing technique and decided I was still using too much effort and not relaxing in between 'bracing'. Nurse V reminded me to use my bracing technique and to 'pump' my waist muscles and then wait a few moments for nature to take its course before trying again. She reminded me not to take large inhalations in advance and to remain slouched and relaxed. She also suggested the use of glycerine suppositories for later on in the day, if I needed to complete my clearout. We booked a new appointment for late July and I left full of new resolve to sort out my bowels. A follow-up consultation with the gastroenterologist was also planned for August.

AUGUST 2012

I saw Nurse V again at the end of July. She decided to terminate my biofeedback training as it was not really resolving my problem. I was still unable to evacuate properly and inserting glycerine suppositories meant only passing the suppositories and not completely clearing my rectum. In addition, I had started to have a recurrence of anal fissure symptoms, meaning that it was becoming extremely painful to defecate, leading me to avoid doing so to avoid the pain. I realised upon discussion with Nurse V that this would then become a vicious cycle. Once there had been two separate episodes of deep anal pain again I made contact with my colorectal surgeon for a review and to seek advice from my gastroenterologist. However, I still believe that the biofeedback training had been helpful and said to Nurse V that I would continue working on the principles involved in the hope that my body would eventually get the message. She admired my positivity.

Gastroenterology update: October 2012

I saw my gastroenterologist for review and aside from having the symptoms of IBS, which is related to EDSIII, my symptoms of difficulties of evacuation were not considered particularly related to EDSIII, but are caused by difficulties in the muscular coordination of bowel evacuation. It was thought that this was also contributing to my anal fissure symptoms and was, in effect, becoming a bit of a vicious cycle. My gastroenterologist felt that that there was nothing more she could do for me, although we did discuss diet, which was something I was addressing, including a reduction of fermenting foods, such as wheat and gluten and high-sugar foods. Other than that, she felt it was going to have to be up to my colorectal surgeon to work out a longer-term management to address and target my symptoms.

Colorectal update

Unfortunately, once a patient has already had an anal fissure, the chances of this returning are apparently somewhat likely. I seem to be unlucky in this regard. It looks like I will require further surgery in the future, or at least give me more Botox injections in the area to relax the muscles involved. I may never be able to do more than simply manage my symptoms. They are just likely to return. As is so often the case with the symptoms connected to my EDSIII (or otherwise), there is seldom any 'cure' – we can only look at management.

Bowel and IBS problems

Research is now beginning to show links between EDSIII/HMS (fibromyalgia) and functional bowel-related problems such as IBS, heartburn and constipation (Beighton *et al.* 2012; Bird 2007; Farmer and Aziz 2010; Zarate *et al.* 2010). In the previous chapter the role of the ANS and autonomic dysfunction were described by Hakim.

Farmer and Aziz (2010, p.85) write that

clinical symptoms of dysautonomia such as poor sleep and syncopal episodes are common in functional gastrointestinal disorders, hypermobility syndrome and fibromyalgia. Particular patterns of dysautonomia, specifically dysregulation of sympathetic nervous system control of the cardiovascular system, have been described in patients with hypermobility syndrome and fibromyalgia.

Research also links poor sleep to conditions such as FM and IBS. In a study by Fass *et al.* (2000), of the 71 per cent of patients who had IBS, 55 per cent had problems with sleep and would wake with abdominal pain. Keefer *et al.* (2006) also report that lack of sleep also negatively affects gut motility when the gut is supposed to be at rest and in recovery.

Professor Howard Bird explains the following with reference to IBS, collagen and bowels.

Collagen and the bowels

[…]because the collagen that makes up the joint capsule that stabilises the joint resembles the collagen that lines the wall of the bowel, in patients where hypermobility is caused mainly, if not exclusively, by abnormal collagen structure, it makes very good sense to suggest that the bowel would be similarly involved. One helpful clue to determining whether a patient falls into this group is the bladder. If the bladder wall is comparably floppy and the bladder sphincter correspondingly weak, such patients will experience urgency in passing urine as well as stools.

Some X-ray studies have been done putting dye into the bowel, which suggests segments of the bowel with the loosest collagen might balloon out, allowing stools to collect in them and, in turn, these stretched sections of the bowel sometimes alternate with tighter structures, all of this tending to cause constipation unless, once all the floppy reservoirs are full, there is a constant overflow of stools, which may present as diarrhoea.

Email, 5.8.2012

Hernias and prolapse

Hernias and rectal (and uterine) prolapse are another finding in EDSIII patients owing to ligamentous laxity and resultant tissue weakness (Beighton *et al.* 2012; Farmer and Aziz 2010).

Symptoms

Tissue laxity being present in the bowel wall might explain why EDSIII patients experience symptoms which include bloating, nausea, reflux and constipation (Farmer and Aziz 2010). A study by Zarate *et al.* (2010) shows that connective tissue could be the link in unexplained gastrointestinal symptoms and in those with 'hypermobility syndrome' as opposed to hypermobility. Of the 17 with hypermobility syndrome, '81 per cent experienced abdominal pain, 57 per cent bloating, 57 per cent nausea, 48 per cent reflux symptoms, 43 per cent vomiting, 38 per cent constipation, and 14 per cent had diarrhoea.' Furthermore, a study by Mohammed *et al.* (2010), as cited in Beighton *et al.* (2012), shows links in terms of hypermobile patients with rectal evacuatory disorder (RED). Further research is now required to explore further links between connective tissue defect and intestinal motility (Beighton *et al.* 2012).

Management

It might seem an obvious oversight to consider the relevance of diet in terms of management of IBS or digestive symptoms, but even with my diet, which is 'reasonably good' and contains plenty of fruit and vegetables, meat protein and fish as well as plenty of water, this is still not enough in the management of gut problems at the helm of a connective tissue disorder. In a book about persistent fatigue, a symptom common to both EDSIII and FM patients, Montpetit (2012) suggests that a craving for chocolate might indicate a magnesium deficit, a craving for yeast foods or bread might imply candidias, and a strong interest in meat might imply an iron deficiency. In specific relation to IBS, Montpetit writes that:

> if you suffer from irritable bowel syndrome, you could very well require more food than the quantity that constitutes your normal intake, especially if you frequently have diarrhoea. If you suffer from food rather than respiratory intolerances, avoid the foods to which you are intolerant; this will help enormously.
>
> *2012, p.93*

In the light of Montpetit's research, a food diary might be a useful suggestion for some patients. From personal experience I have come to realise that eating too much wheat does seem to have an effect on my bloating symptoms, so I would not have bread, pizza and pasta all on the same day. Conversely, eating curry does not change or improve my ability to thoroughly empty my bowels! I have also sought advice from a nutritionist, and we are now looking to try a low-fermentation diet (so no wheat/gluten, dairy, and a low-sugar diet). It will be another attempt to manage (IBS) symptoms.

Medications do not seem to make a huge difference, as can be seen from my story of trying various medications for constipation and overflow diarrhoea. Other EDSIII patients made the following comments on Facebook:

Avoid all dairy, that seems to be my trigger.

Avoid eggs and too much fruit.

Sensible eating, no bread in the evening and few carbs, seems to help.

Avoid all dairy to stop the pain. Thinking about Fodmaps to stop the bloating though I can bloat without pain. Peaches and nectarines are my downfall here. I also take colofac and lactase enzymes as well as live culture probiotic capsules.

Aloe vera!!!!! Has changed my life. My IBS was crippling me until I started to drink the juice. One dose a day and my symptoms are totally managed. It is Amazing!

Buscupan and hot water bottle + years ago I kept a food diary to see what made things worse but I've been living with this for 25 years now so kind of know what to stay away from, still manage to eat stuff that make it worse at times.

Cut out caffeine in the end and that seemed to help, but still get days from hell.

Obstruction defecation and lower urinary tract dysfunction

Bird explained earlier in this chapter that in some patients, if their bladder sphincter is weak, they may need to pass urine urgently as they do for a bowel movement. A study by Manning *et al.* (2003) suggests that women who present with lower urinary tract dysfunction

(LUT) are more likely to have symptoms of obstruction defecation (owing to chronic straining) than controls. Furthermore, there was a relationship between childhood constipation and hypermobility syndrome. The study concludes that:

> Symptoms of obstructed defecation are associated with LUT dysfunction. The association may be explained by an increased prevalence of disordered bowel motility and uterovaginal prolapse among women presenting for LUT dysfunction. This in turn may be partly a result of an underlying congenital connective tissue disorder.
>
> *Manning et al. 2003, p.131*

The study shows how both bladder and bowel can be dually affected owing to tissue laxity, and in the next chapter we look at the bladder.

CHAPTER 8

Bladder

I have an extremely overactive bladder as does my 9 year old son who also has EDS. We don't do anything about it though, as we just deal with it and pee a lot.

EDS patient, Facebook

My mum can't go an hour without peeing. I can go for 8 hours, up to 18 hours sometimes (don't worry, I usually go every 4–5 hours) but if I need to go I need to go right then and there!

EDS patient, Facebook

I can't remember if I ever used to sleep through the night, but certainly from about the age of six I do recall regularly having to wake to use the bathroom. Over the years the amount of times I needed to use the bathroom increased to the extent that sometimes I would be waking in excess of six times a night, meaning that my sleep was highly disrupted. Mainly I think it was the bladder that would wake me up, although it is true that historically I often used to self-harm in the form of skin-picking, and I mainly did this at night. As with all of us from time to time, I would be kept awake after using the bathroom with a very busy head, to the extent I could then lose a further two hours of sleep. I frequently fell deeply asleep in the early hours of the morning, which made waking up extremely hard. I would often be asleep on my way to work and school and would feel 'jet-lagged'.

Sleep is so essential to growth and repair, as well as cognitive function and wellbeing, that it is of little surprise it counts as an essential item on the Maslow Hierarchy of Needs. Having not slept well for so long, I had come to see it as a normal state of affairs. I didn't expect this to change and coped as best I could in my brain-fogged, headachy, slow, little way. I had tried medications and an array of complementary therapies, of which Bowen, Shiatsu and Reiki had been helpful. I certainly didn't expect physiotherapy to have any impact upon sleep, or bladder for that matter, but it started to help following some discussions with my physio about both matters.

I recall discussing with my physio how, for example, car journeys were a complete nightmare for me and that within ten minutes of leaving the house I would need to use the bathroom. I remember being made to 'hold on' or would have to stop off in fields. The same was a problem in terms of long theatre or cinema shows, which I usually dreaded because I would always need the bathroom before the interval. The following extract was part of a discussion with my physio:

> The physio said: 'So you have not slept through the night since you were six? I can't believe that hasn't been addressed.' My response was that I was 'murder' on car journeys because I constantly needed the toilet. However, help had never been sought, and I had come to accept it.
>
> *Physiotherapy, 3.11.2010*

Following that session I started to have very occasional nights of sleeping through or needing to wake only once to use the bathroom. There were some other things that seemed to help. For example, I think that when my physio was working on C2/3 it seemed to affect both bladder and sleep. This might be explained by calming nerves in the autonomic nervous system. Working on the iliacus also seemed to improve the bladder, which could be explained by working on the sacral plexus and bladder innervation. Working on specific neural pathways combined with increased and improved postural core strength and control could explain why the bladder has improved. One thing that my physio did discuss with me was what happened during night-time micturition and that a hormone is released which slows production of urine and concentrates it. I remember when I was aware this had actually happened in me because I woke up, but my bladder did not feel full and I was able to go back to sleep. When I did wake later on to pass urine, the urine was much more concentrated and almost 'thick' compared to day-time urine. I had never experienced this before.

Six months after I started to get very odd nights of complete sleep, I started to get more than one night in a row and then several nights, so that by the time I went on holiday in June, it had become the norm for me to sleep right the way through. Unfortunately, being on holiday disrupted my sleep, which I was not expecting, but upon return from holiday, I was able to sleep through again. I cannot explain powerfully enough what an enormous impact this has had upon my quality of life and functioning. My bladder is subsequently better during the day time, almost becoming retentive! I feel much calmer in myself and my brain is clearer. I feel refreshed and energetic, and my brain function and memory are significantly improved.

I wrote the following reflective writing to my physio that was unsent:

> When I now move on two years to now and what has just been happening in terms of managing to sleep through the night without having to need to use the bathroom is an enormous deal to me. I have not slept through the night since being a very young child and didn't think that it was possible for me to manage. Ever. I didn't think I could get help for it and I didn't ask. I recall talking about it with you on one of our sessions in early November. It wasn't long after that that I managed to sleep through. This was revolutionary. I would like to suggest that it was possible for me to do that partly because we talked about it and you listened to me and showed genuine interest in why it hadn't been addressed before etc. You wondered why I should settle for this state of affairs and I suppose made me question this too.
>
> *Physiotherapy, 1.12.2010*

VCMG bladder test and bladder appointment

I met with Mr H in January 2012. Upon looking at my notes he quickly realised I was a much more complicated patient than he had anticipated. He realised he had to factor in my EDSIII and endometriosis which had been involved in the bladder and ureters. He offered me tablets for an overactive bladder, which I politely declined at this time owing to improvements in the numbers of times I needed to pass urine at night. I discussed the fact that my urine repeatedly tested positive for UTIs whenever I attended A&E, and indeed he found my sample to be infected on the date of examination. He decided to send this to the lab for bacterial growth which came back negative and for me to have a 'videocystometrogram' – VCMG bladder test – to look at bladder dynamics under pressure and via radiology.

My bladder ultimately required further investigation as it has never been 'right' – even though there were improvements during physiotherapy. However, following stress at work, needless to say this had a significant impact upon the behaviour of my autonomic nervous system (ANS) and therefore bladder, with some occasions of me needing to pass urine 15 times at night. By March 2012 my bladder became highly disruptive, yet again.

The account below describes what happened when I was sent for a VCMG bladder test:

I was due to have some VCMG Bladder investigations (under X-ray/video) done to measure bladder pressure on voiding – so I had to arrive with a full bladder and pressure was measured in a special toilet. The next part of the process was supposed to involve insertion of catheter in both bladder and rectum whilst fluid was introduced into the bladder and I had to say when I could first detect fluid in my bladder, to when it would feel full to slightly needing to go to really needing to go. Unfortunately I failed at the first hurdle when the doctor failed to insert the catheter. I was writhing in agony and had never known pain like it and promptly burst into tears. The doctor, who was very nice and said he did this all the time to children and had even done the procedure on himself, was most surprised, but said that this is all information in itself. He noted my history of endometriosis as well as EDSIII. He said he would report all this back to my consultant urologist Mr H. After this I needed to go to the bathroom and was in excruciating pain on passing urine and was bleeding. I was in terrible pain and crying – I think from shock as much as anything else. The staff were fantastic and so nice to me. They said to take paracetamol straight away and got me drinking lots of fluids. Then took some ibuprofen. I managed to go to the bathroom again and it was marginally less painful. The rest of my body particularly left abdominal, bladder area, adductor and back had gone into spasm and I was in a lot of pain. I was kept in the department a further hour before managing to leave. I felt exhausted, but then had to teach later in the day.

I am still in pain on emptying my bladder, but my bladder just isn't feeling very full, which is extraordinary given the amount of fluids I have consumed. My appetite has been poor for days and I am in quite a lot of pain, hence writing this at 2.30am. I have just taken some codeine now so will hope this helps.

It now appears I will most likely require a full examination of bladder and urethra etc under general anaesthetic in a procedure known as a cystoscopy (see Chapter 9). I am going to contact my consultant's secretary to see if my next appointment could be brought forwards. I definitely don't feel right or myself since having this done and will seek advice as needed in the morning, if need be. The fact I am managing to pass some urine is obviously a good sign, but the pain I experienced was totally out of proportion for this type of test and could indicate some kind of blockage. I am sure it will all get resolved and sorted eventually. Not a great day!

Diary, 16.4.2012

Update: August 2012

I was about to have another bladder-related autonomic dysfunction episode and finally decided to try the solifenacin (Vesicare) tablets that had been sitting in my cupboard for months. Solifenacin is a drug that is designed to help with an overactive bladder, as Hakim documents later on in this chapter. Unfortunately, it made my symptoms worse, including having one of my 'passing urine 15 times in just over an hour' episodes. I saw my urologist who, upon discussion of my increasing need to pass urine later in the day in plentiful quantity and several times per night, thinks that my bladder might be in a state of 'physiological confusion' (his words, not mine!). I am sure there will be a technical term for this, but Mr H did say that the problem would be easily solved with the correct medication. In order to determine a diagnosis, Mr H requested me to produce a diary for three days recording all fluid intakes and outputs. He also felt that there was no point in repeating the VCMG any longer as the fluid diary would provide sufficient information. He also wondered whether I am retaining urine, since upon measurement of my bladder capacity during my cystoscopy he maintained I had a bladder volume of 900ml. Bladder retention is possibly related to my EDSIII.

Fluid diary: outcome and ongoing treatment

I completed my fluid diary and Mr H has said that over the course of three days I never allowed my bladder to fill beyond 400mls before emptying it, meaning I am passing urine more than is necessary given a bladder capacity of 900mls. He noted no significant increase in output at night compared to the day, although it was evident I was getting up sometimes up to six times to micturate. The next part of the treatment requires bladder re-training, trying further medication and also Mr H has suggested fitting a neural implant (sacral nerve stimulation therapy), which will effectively stop my bladder telling my brain that it requires emptying under false pretences. I will also be trying to leave it longer and longer before I go and empty my bladder, whilst not making it uncomfortable or stressful for myself. If these outcomes fail, then further surgery becomes a possibility. However, conservative management is always preferable. Mr H said in an ideal world he would also like to re-attempt urodynamic testing, but so far this has been intolerable for me. It is something to be discussed in the future, pending my bladder re-training and neural implant.

EDSIII patients wrote the following on Facebook about their own bladder problems:

> I've had recurrent prolapses of the bladder and bowels, had more surgery than I care to mention, none of it works. I'm currently on Vesicare for minimalising the urinary incontinence, I must say though recently being diagnosed with severe depression they put me on anti-depressants and this in conjunction with the Vesicare has had a real effect on quality of my life its interacted and now my leaks are so much less!

> My bladder problems tend to be worse when my bowel problems are flaring up. My bladder becomes irritated and I need to go quite frequently and sometimes there is some incontinence while sneezing, rigorous movement and so on. Other times my bladder is so stretchy that it holds a great deal and I don't notice that I need to go. I get a fair few UTIs every year.

Dr Alan Hakim writes the following about the bladder and bladder investigations and treatments for patients with EDS, and it very much dovetails with my own experiences of both bladder treatment and management.

THE BLADDER
Dr Alan Hakim

Bladder dysfunction is common in the female general population and often manifests as 'urgency' (desperate need to pass urine), 'frequency' (having to pass urine on a number of occasions throughout the day) and 'nocturia' (needing to pass urine at night), with the risk of stress or overflow urinary incontinence and/or pelvic discomfort/pain.

The causes of urinary tract dysfunction may be functional and related to changes in the anatomy of the bladder and pelvis, neurological and affecting the autonomic control of the bladder, psychogenic (influenced by things like anxiety and pain), or as a consequence of infection, inflammation or cancer of the urinary tract. An 'over active bladder' (OAB) is common in both men and women and related to neuromuscular instability of the bladder wall and controlling sphincter muscles (Cardozo 2011).

Because these problems are common it can be difficult to determine whether they are a direct consequence of EDS. Nevertheless, it is important to note that the presence of EDS and the inherent potential for greater laxity of the pelvic floor might account for an individual developing urogenital problems and require additional thought during treatment.

The mechanical problems related to weakness in normal structures that support the bladder, vagina and pelvic floor, and anatomical issues such as pelvic wall prolapse, are concerns that intuitively might be expected to arise in patients with EDS. Anatomical abnormalities such as diverticula (pouches) in the bladder wall, rupture of the bladder, fistulas (abnormal connections between the bladder and other organs, e.g. the bowel) and prolapse have all been reported as complications in cases of EDS and urinary dysfunction.

The neurophysiology of bladder function specific to EDS is not an area that has been researched in detail. Its investigation and treatment is discussed below in general terms.

The common types of assessments and tests that might be undertaken to identify the nature and cause of urinary dysfunction are well described by Nager and Albo (2004). These include:

1. a visual examination for prolapse and other anatomical issues

2. urinalysis to exclude infection

3. a bladder diary, recording daily events – number, duration, volume, etc.

4. bladder filling and measurement of bladder pressures. This can be performed in clinic, gently filling the bladder after normal voiding of urine. It may be helpful in conjunction with a stress

test to see if the bladder leaks due to increased pressure, e.g. induced by coughing

5. cystometrogram or cystometry – these are the mainstay of urodynamic tests

6. measures of bladder emptying – e.g. volume of urine left after voiding

7. pressure-flow studies

8. video-urodynamics

9. tests of function and mobility of the urethra (the canal from the bladder and exterior).

These tests mostly require specialist expertise. Treatment will very much depend on assessing all the findings, whether physical or neurological or both.

In most cases conservative (non-surgical) treatments will apply. Lifestyle advice is an important aspect of treatment. Reducing fluid intake can help control urgency, frequency and nocturia. Reducing fluid intake may be difficult, however, in patients who are trying to control cardiovascular symptoms such as POTS and orthostatic hypotension. Caffeine and diet soft drinks have also been associated with a higher rate of urgency and frequency.

Pelvic floor muscle training may be effective in individuals with urgency incontinence. A therapist might also introduce a bladder re-education programme with biofeedback and bladder drill.

A wide variety of drug therapies are available in OAB. The most commonly used are agents such as oxybutynin, tolterodine or festerodine, propiverine, trospium, solifenacin and darifenacin. Several ways of giving these drugs has resulted in a more even concentration in the body, reducing peaks and the side-effects thereof. These include slow-release tablets, patches, gels and the intravaginal ring.

Desmopressin is a drug used to treat nocturia and nocturnal enuresis (bed-wetting). The major concern with desmopressin is that it can cause hyponatremia (low blood sodium), which can cause very serious neurological problems.

Although antidepressant drugs are sometimes used for the treatment of OAB, they are not licensed for this and there are no clinical trials with supportive evidence of their benefit.

New classes of drug, including calcium channel blocking agents, potassium channel opening drugs, beta agonists and neurokinin receptor antagonists, are under investigation.

Botulinum toxin injections to the bladder wall may offer an alternative, temporary, measure in women with intractable bladder muscle overactivity. Neuromodulation of the sacral nerves may also assist in specific cases.

Surgical interventions are beyond the scope of this review but the potential for complexity in EDS should be considered, including:

1. fragility and elasticity of tissues

2. tendency to bleed

3. delayed healing

4. abnormal scarring

5. resistance to local anaesthetics.

My bladder treatment is further described in Chapter 9, which is a stand-alone chapter on surgical and nursing implications for patients with EDSIII.

Surgical and nursing implications for EDSIII/chronic complex patients

Operations and treatment management for EDSIII/chronic complex patients

Having had about seven operations in my lifetime, it made me think about the implications for the EDSIII, complex 'chronic' patient. Having an operation is stressful for anyone, however minor the procedure and however fit the patient might be. When a patient has to worry about whether part of their body might dislocate during the procedure when they are under general anaesthetic (GA), or whether in fact the anaesthetic will even work, more of a problem with EDSIII patients with local anaesthesia (Hakim *et al.* 2005), and then factor in potentially slow healing times, and you can already gain a sense of mounting anxiety surrounding a surgical procedure.

Preparation and communication

I have learned to my cost that very careful preparation and impeccable communication are essential to the best possible outcome of any surgical procedure.

Prior to my most recent bladder surgery I tried very hard to be helpful to the pre-operative nurse by giving her a list of my regular medications, a list of medications I was allergic to and then some specific requests for the anaesthetist – for example, that I would very much like a pre-med and that they need to be very careful moving me about in surgery. Whilst I do not dislocate, I do have a disc prolapse and hinge in my spine which would certainly be aggravated, not to mention problems with my neck and temporomandibular joint (TMJ). I then asked if it would be possible for me to be admitted to the ward in advance of my operation rather than to the pre-operative ward so that I had a sense of where I would be returning to. I explained how very anxious I could become and that I could take to hiding in toilets and become very upset and distressed. This is very definitely out-of-character behaviour for me, but just down to general terror. The nurse looked at me and said that if they admitted everyone for that reason it would be impossible. However, having gained a sense of the complexity of my conditions, she agreed to email the consultant. My request paid off. Ten days later I heard from the consultant's PA who informed me that I would be admitted to the ward the day before the procedure. It got better than that.

I also discussed at the pre-operative assessment how very nervous I was about the removal of a catheter given my recent terrible experience at the VCMG testing (that had failed). I also explained how because of my EDSIII I might take longer to recover post-operatively and wanted to ensure I was properly alright and able to pass urine without crying before I left hospital. I therefore felt it would be sensible that they kept me in overnight. The PA also handled this for me and communicated this to the urology nurses. It turned out they were still working out when, after my surgery, they would be able to repeat the VCMG testing. They decided to keep me in for two more days post-surgery, and promised that I would not be discharged following the VCMG testing until I could pass urine without it being too excruciating. Finally, I managed to have a discussion about my chronic pain, heightened sensitivity and 'sensitised sensation', particularly in the pelvic area, and that this meant I might react more and experience more pain than other patients. It is not that I wouldn't be prepared for post-operative pain – but that my pain might be more amplified. I felt this was very important to communicate. The nurse I spoke to seemed to take this all on board and said they would find some creative ways to help me cope with passing urine following the catheter being removed upon completion of testing. Although I still felt anxious about the prospect of surgery, I did feel I had done everything in my power to communicate my needs in advance of my arrival to hospital and the nurse said she would ensure everyone was informed. It took several different conversations to achieve this, and developing a good relationship with the consultant's PA certainly helped! I also made it known how grateful I was to the PA and nurses who helped to coordinate all of this and sincerely thanked them.

Pre-operative

Having an operation is frightening. Most people are anxious about it. Some worry about pain, and some worry about the anaesthetic or waking up in the middle of the operation itself. Others don't like the concept of anaesthesia. EDSIII patients have more reason than others to be worried about anaesthesia – local rather than general – as lidocaine doesn't work as effectively in these patients. This is a particular risk with dental surgery. I am fairly terrified about the process of being put to sleep. This has become worse the more surgeries I have had. The first surgery I had was to reset a 'bent' arm bone when I was 11. The anaesthetic did not take effect and I did not fall asleep as expected. It turned out they had missed my vein. This same experience was repeated during one of my four laparoscopies. During another laparoscopy all the pre-theatre rooms were busy so I had to be wheeled into theatre and put to sleep there. I was very upset. On another occasion I was kept waiting pre-operatively for over 12 hours and pre-meds had long since worn off, and I was wheeled screaming down the corridor as I had been waiting for so long and completely lost my nerve. As soon as I got there I was rapidly gassed (to shut me up) – but this shouldn't have happened. When I was admitted to day surgery to repair my anal fissure I was told I was not allowed to have anyone with me and then locked myself in the toilets because I was so frightened. It took several people coaxing me before I would come out. After this they gave me midazolam and I remembered nothing more. On my most recent surgery, they didn't end up giving me midazolam, but 20mg of temazepam, which didn't have any sedation effect on me at all. Although I felt very anxious and had gone into a traumatic 'freeze' pose (lay still and motionless), I managed to cope as I was wheeled into a 'receiving bay' in the theatre before being wheeled into the anaesthetic room. In there, the anaesthetist was very reassuring and had been told all about me by her colleague. She inserted a cannula and then gave me an induction agent, after which time I knew no more about it until I woke up in the recovery room.

I didn't need to have experienced all that I did pre-operatively in the past. Some of these problems could have been avoided. I would urge anaesthetists and surgical staff to take on board the issues with anaesthesia and EDSIII patients because lidocaine and local anaesthesia can sometimes be ineffective (Hakim *et al.* 2005). The EDSIII and chronic complex patient will also experience heightened sensitivity to pain owing to changes in their central nervous system.

Anxiety is already known to be linked to EDSIII (Bulbena *et al.* 2004; Martin-Santos *et al.* 1998) and slow skin-healing (Russek 1999; Simpson 2006). Surgical staff need to be aware of the fragility of the joints in this patient group and the propensity for dislocation. Surgical staff also need to be more aware of reactions and changes in temperature and pulse rate in this group, particularly in those who have/experience POTS and autonomic symptoms (Grubb 2008; Raj 2006). EDSIII patients made the following comments and suggestions on Facebook:

> Be careful when you move me! My knee cap dislocated when I was moved from the hospital bed to operating table.

> Ask to walk to theatre or be wheeled and to get on operating table yourself, make sure you are very comfortable. It is a strange request, but best in long run. Be prepared for a possible reaction to anaesthesia, such as palpitations, pressure like feeling on chest including did ECG readings. Also you should never be a day case patient, always stay at least one night.

> I always warn them that anaesthesia wears off very quickly for me. I have woken up in the operating room (luckily just minutes after surgery was completed). I'm very small but it takes a lot to get and keep me under.

Post-surgery recovery and the chronic complex patient

When I had my latest surgery I experienced a huge surge of pain about 24 hours post-surgery resulting in the on-call doctor running to me. They weren't sure at that stage what was causing my pain. My pain escalated over the following day, and when I was sent for bladder testing it transpired that my suprapubic catheter had possibly caused a tiny puncture in my bladder. Putting a urethral catheter in situ would allow the suprapubic catheter hole to heal whilst checking the bladder was emptying properly and well. I wouldn't let the radiologist insert a catheter as I was in too much pain (and my abdomen was like a board). However, I was facing surgery if they didn't insert a catheter. After a lot of oramorph and bribery, the urologist inserted a catheter and the pain improved. I was glad they had found the source of my pain because it was beginning to look like I was going to be otherwise disbelieved.

Following this episode I then started to experience severe wrist pain and asked for my cannula to be removed – not soon enough as it turned out because it had become infected and I ended up having cellulitis. Although there is always the risk of infection for anybody post any surgical procedure, the skin is simply more fragile in the EDSIII population (Russek 1999; Simpson 2006) and so this resulted in a need for antibiotics for the 'hole' left in my bladder, and then my skin also became incredibly itchy and irritable from having to wear anti-coagulant stockings (TED stockings). The next day I started to feel incredibly sick and then had an episode of diarrhoea. Since there was a suspected outbreak of diarrhoea on the ward, I had to be moved to an isolation room and treated as 'infectious' until it turned out that I and the other five culprits were clear! However, it was another complication I had to endure and more bodily systems affected. Finally, my muscular strength really started to deteriorate, meaning I was struggling to manage to hold my catheter once it was over 500ml full, and I really started to 'hang' into my hypermobile joints. I couldn't walk far because of being in an isolated room and was struggling just to walk around that. My muscles hurt and my 'EDSIII' pain increased. Research has also shown that muscle tissues atrophy greatly in the first five to seven days during inactivity, particularly the endurance slow-twitch muscle fibres (Keer 2003; Simmonds 2003). Additionally, and interestingly, muscles also atrophy in response to pain and fear (Simmonds 2003). This meant that my musculoskeletal endurance might be really compromised when I left hospital and that I was going to have to pace my activity very carefully upon return.

I have actually had to request possible home-help for the first time during my life as an EDSIII patient, based on my immediate post-operative needs. I felt some guilt about this, but I had weakened so much I couldn't comprehend doing shopping or managing to get about very easily whilst I recovered. I also had the support of my family during my recovery.

Information for ward staff

Since there might be problems with blood pressure/pulse rates for some EDSIII patients, nursing staff should be aware that BP/HR levels might fluctuate more than 'normal' in these patients. Dizziness and lightheadedness can also be symptoms that relate to EDSIII/POTS (Grubb 2008; Raj 2006), and so nursing staff should be aware of this and allow more time in getting patients up and about, or when they first mobilise post-surgery. Mobility is a problem in general and people with EDSIII might take longer to get about, and so having the patient situated nearer to a bathroom might be a useful consideration in ward-planning.

Fatigue is a huge problem for patients with EDSIII, fibromyalgia and other chronic complex pain-related syndromes. With this in mind, they may be even more fatigued following the impact of surgery, the medication used both during and post-surgery and the 'general stress' of the situation overall. Additionally, some patients may lose their appetite during this time and so nursing staff shouldn't be unduly concerned if such patients are eating a little less. They will eat again as soon as they feel able to do so. An EDSIII patient on Facebook comments:

> Don't rush me. I will get washed and ready at my speed. Could I be moved to a bed nearer a toilet/shower or possibly ensuite room? Ask for physio and occupational advice while you [are] there, they [are] always on wards even if you [are] not in with a mobility issue. I am not an easy person to get blood from so please note it on my file. Sometimes fatigue takes my appetite away…do not shout at me… I will survive on yogurt/mousse till nausea clears!

Pain management is going to be a problem in those with already heightened sensitivity and chronic complex pain. They are already often taking high doses of painkillers, making targeting additional acute pain as a result of surgery all the more of a challenge. The stress of surgery is likely to exacerbate their 'usual' chronic pain. It may be that anaesthetists or related pain management consultants might need input in the management of this type of patient. However, the patient will usually know which drugs work best for them and might also have some of their own pain management strategies that they can put in place themselves – for example relaxation and imaging (Knight 2011).

EDSIII patients are prone to dislocations, so there needs to be great care when moving them – especially when they are in surgery or post-surgery. Additionally, it appears that the skin is more easily bruised and slower to heal in the EDSIII patient group (Russek 1999; Simpson 2006). It would therefore be especially important to be gentle in conducting blood tests, and perhaps using alternatives to plasters, or being aware of the skin fragility.

Since it is known that anxiety (more specifically panic attacks) is genetically linked to EDSIII (Bulbena *et al.* 2004; Martin-Santos *et al.* 1998), it may be worth noting that these patients require more time, patience and reassurance than perhaps others might. Just giving them time and space might be especially appreciated. If patients are upset it might be worth arranging for them to talk to someone (psychologist, counsellor) as well as perhaps informing their family, or making sure they have support from friends and family.

However, when the medical staff get it right – this is the difference:

This Wednesday I had surgery, my anaesthesiologist was amazing, knew about the EDS, I just ask [him] to be careful, and he promised to me [to] be very extra careful, even 'explain [to] me' that connective tissue is everywhere so promised to me [to] watch the surgeons don't hurt me too much, but they were prepared as well. I think the good thing is to ask your surgeon to prepare nurse staff about the special needs the EDS patients may have after surgery.

EDSIII patient, Facebook

CHAPTER 10

Hormonal aspects of hypermobility and living with endometriosis

We have seen in my case how the bladder and bowel are affected in patients with EDSIII and other related chronic conditions. Hormones also have a role in the homeostasis of patients. Professor Howard Bird has written about this.

HORMONAL ASPECTS OF HYPERMOBILITY
Professor Howard Bird

Some female patients with hypermobility have been disappointed when symptoms of which they are complaining to their doctor, nurse or friends are summarily, even chauvinistically, dismissed as 'hormonal'. There is actually a considerable amount of truth in this, though only occasionally will the person making this diagnosis have thought through all of the ramifications.

This section considers what types of hypermobility might be susceptible, what hormones might aggravate the symptoms and, when this is occurring, how things might be improved.

Hormones involved

A hormone is sometimes described as a 'chemical messenger' that is secreted from a gland, circulates through the bloodstream and, finally, reaches the organ at which it is directed where it exerts its effect. Although there are many types of hormones, all of different structures, two main groups are relevant to hypermobility.

First are the corticosteroids, which comprise three families. The first group, the mineralo-corticoids, alter minerals and fluids within the body and probably have no influence on hypermobility. The second group, sometimes referred to as metabolic steroids, are secreted from the adrenal gland and control the diurnal (or 24-hourly) variation in body function, which allows organs to rest during sleep but 'tones them up' during the day. This, in turn, may produce cyclical symptoms of pain and stiffness over a 24-hour period in joints, but this is normally only a minor problem. The third group comprises the sex hormones, which are divided into three types: androgens (mainly in males) and oestrogens and progestogens (mainly in females). The balance between oestrogens and progestogens, which is constantly changing, controls the 28-day menstrual cycle in the female in whom these hormones are almost absent prior to puberty and tail off after the menopause.

A further group of hormones relevant to hypermobility have a specific function in pregnancy. Relaxin is considered to relax the ligaments just prior to childbirth so the pelvis can open widely to allow the safe passage of the foetal head. Prolactin produces milk when the mother is breastfeeding and also has a relaxing effect on the joints. In addition, during pregnancy, oestrogens and progestogens climb in concentration, all of which accounts for the undoubted loosening of the joints in pregnancy. This normally remits soon after childbirth but may be prolonged if the mother is breastfeeding. Some research that we did several years ago suggested that this invariably made joints looser in a first pregnancy, made them slightly looser in a second pregnancy but gave no further additional loosening in third or subsequent pregnancies.

What types of hypermobility are affected?

In males, in whom hypermobility is often less pronounced than in females of the same age, cortisol may contribute to diurnal variation in symptoms as in females, but hormones related to pregnancy, clearly, are not produced. The predominant sex hormones in males are androgens, which probably have very little effect on collagen though may increase muscle bulk around the joints. In general this is likely to be helpful, with the increased muscle power more than outweighing any effect on the collagen structure.

In females, it is quite a different story. Although oestrogen tends to stabilise collagen, progestogens loosen it. Many hypermobile patients, though not all, notice a worsening in symptoms, more pain in the joints, clumsiness or a greater tendency to dislocate in the five days leading up to menstruation and in the few days after menstruation. This is exactly the time when the progesterone compounds far exceed the stabilising oestrogen compounds. This effect is most pronounced when the joint hypermobility is due mainly to collagen structure (the clue here is that all joints are almost equally lax throughout the body). Where the hypermobility is a marker of unusually shaped bony surfaces at the joint (typically these individuals have very pronounced hypermobility at only a small number of joints), the effect of hormones is much less pronounced.

Those females whose joints become worse at the time of menstruation often note that if the periods become irregular, for whatever reason, joints not only become worse but are worse for longer. This may be because in these patients progesterone is present in high concentrations at times when it would not normally be present.

Sometimes, irregularity of periods suggests gynaecological conditions such as a cyst on the ovary or a condition called endometriosis. In a few patients we have suspected this diagnosis on the basis of joint deterioration alone, even before symptoms have become severe enough to attract the attention of a gynaecologist!

Problems with contraceptives

A variety of hormonal contraceptives are available. Many are 'combined' contraceptives, either a mixture of oestrogen or a progestogen given at the same time or containing these two drugs sequentially, the progestogen after the oestrogen to mimic the normal female menstrual cycle. Others are entirely progestogen containing. Injected contraceptives (the most common is called Provera) are entirely progesterone, and recently intra-uterine devices that are impregnated with a reservoir of progesterone (e.g. the Mirena coil) have become popular.

When careful gynaecological and rheumatological histories are taken together, it is surprising how frequently hypermobility, which was only slightly worse at the time of normal unmodified menstruation, becomes significantly worse with certain contraceptive pills, especially those containing progesterone alone or with progesterone depo contraception preparations or mechanical devices impregnated with progesterone.

If you have hypermobile joints and have been taking hormones to modify menstruation or as contraceptives, you should discuss this further with your doctor, perhaps showing him/her this section, since doctors tend to be well versed in other side effects resulting from hormones, though not necessarily with the effect these have on your ligaments. Oestrogens, like progestogens, have their own side effects, one of the principal ones being a slight tendency to cause venous thrombosis, a feature much less frequently seen with progestogens. Therefore, a progestogen-only preparation may have been prescribed for good and well-intentioned reasons, even though the downside is it will have made the joints worse. In general, however, patients with hypermobility are safer avoiding injectable progesterone and progesterone-impregnated devices. They might also be better avoiding contraceptive pills that contain progesterone derivatives alone. However, if such a preparation was introduced deliberately in a patient for whom high oestrogen levels would be dangerous, it may be worth trying a different progesterone contraceptive. Newer progestogens (such as desogestrel) are derivatives of nor-ethisterone, which is more closely related to testosterone than the early progesterone analogues such as didrogesterone and medroxyprogesterone. There does seem to be individual variation in response within this group, so it may be worth trying one or two such hormones in turn.

The hormonal content of all contraceptives is clearly listed in the *British National Formulary*, allowing general practitioners a wide and informed choice.

If there are increased joint symptoms associated with menstrual irregularities in a patient not taking a contraceptive pill, it may also be worth trying an oestrogen-only preparation for a trial period in the first instance to see if this improves things. If it does, the choice of whether any slight risk in using such a preparation is worth taking for the significant improvement in the joints might ultimately be a decision for the patient, though should be taken in conjunction with the general practitioner, if necessary with expert gynaecological advice.

Similar arguments apply to hormone replacement therapy after the menopause. This normally involves a small amount of oestrogen to which a progestogen is added in women with an intact uterus. Since the oestrogen amount is very small (deliberately so in view of the slight increased risk of breast cancer when oestrogens are given to the elderly, as well as the risk of thrombosis), the amount of oestrogen is often not enough to provide a protective effect for the joints.

Hormones: gynaecological condition – endometriosis

Comments from EDS patients on Facebook include:

> Diagnosed with endo age 15!!! Since had three lap and cauterisation, injections, and then after having very debilitating symptoms causing a month in bed and anaemia – ablation – which so far has been best solution!! This is one of my worst problems with EDS!

> I have horrible inflammation around that time of the month and even more pain. Was told my symptoms can and even do replicate Endometriosis down to the flow issues. Then I do have fundal fibroids and cysts, but no tissue build up. My doctor even lets me use birth control to limit my cycle to four times a year. No actual reason for monthly menstruation if it is causing you pain, your body only needs it on occasion to stay healthy naturally actually. I also get PMSD worse than just cramps and craving it is really bad cramping, hormones going nuts, and going from screaming to crying in about no time. If given the choice I would probably do a chemical hysterectomy as I heard a regular one can make us have even more bladder issues with the opened space. I already have a very overactive bladder verging on incontinence.

In addition to problems with bowel, bladder, sleep, neck/temporomandibular joint (TMJ) and postural orthostatic instability, I also suffered from gynaecological conditions, namely endometriosis, which caused me significant pain and distress. It is essential to point out to the reader that so far there are no research links with EDSIII and endometriosis. A paper by McIntosh *et al.* (1995) suggests a 27 per cent prevalence of women with endometriosis in a study about gynaecological disorders involving 41 women with Ehlers-Danlos syndrome. Other gynaecological disorders included prolapse in 29 per cent which would link with EDS (Grahame and Keer 2010). However, the McIntosh study is very small, and further research would be required on a much larger scale to explore any correlations with endometriosis and EDSIII. As Bird has pointed out, in Chapter 3, my EDSIII symptoms including increased joint pain, tissue laxity, and bladder and bowel problems might all have been exacerbated by my endometriosis and my endometriosis might have had a return effect on my EDSIII symptoms owing to hormonal changes. However, until research shows otherwise, neither condition is in any way linked.

What is endometriosis?

Endometriosis is a condition in which the endometrium (the lining of the uterus) escapes into the surrounding pelvis and elsewhere (Henderson and Wood 2000). It is a condition that is so far poorly understood. The shed endometrium causes pain and inflammation as the cells attach themselves to other parts of the pelvis and grow in response to the women's menstrual cycle. One of the likeliest reasons for endometriosis occurring was discovered by Dr Sampson in the 1920s, who developed the theory of 'retrograde menstruation' (Mills and Vernon 1999). More recent arguments to explain the causes of endometriosis include immune factors, blood and lymph transportation theories, and genetic and pollutant factors (Henderson and Wood 2000).

Endometriosis can be found in any area of the pelvis including the bladder and bowels. It can also be found (rarely) in the lungs, kidney and diaphragm (Hamilton-Fairley 2004).

Symptoms of endometriosis (Mears 1996)

- Period pain (dysmenorrhoea).
- Painful intercourse (dyspareunia).
- Painful ovulation.
- Infertility.
- Painful urination.
- Painful bowel movements.
- Back pain.
- Digestive complaints.
- Fatigue.
- Depression.
- Psychological – poor memory and concentration.

Some women will experience only one or two symptoms, whereas others will experience a whole spectrum of symptoms. Considering this range of symptoms it is not difficult to see why some women might suffer problems, but this might depend upon the severity of symptoms. It has been widely accepted that the 'amount' of endometriosis a women has does not necessarily relate to the amount of pain that she experiences.

Diagnosis

The 'gold standard' (evidence level III) diagnosis for endometriosis is with a laparoscopy (Kennedy and Gazvani 2000). The amount of endometriosis (if any) and its location can be found during a laparoscopy. If appropriate, a surgeon may also remove any cysts or lesions that are found by laser or diathermy.

Management of endometriosis

Endometriosis is often a complicated condition to manage, so I am separating pain management from medical management.

MEDICAL MANAGEMENT

Some women might find that they experience less pain after a laparoscopy, particularly when they have had some treatment (Ballweg 2003). Some women might even find they can finally conceive. Both these are positive outcomes of surgery. For other women the symptoms of endometriosis can reappear again, even quite a short time after surgery. This is because whilst normal menstruation continues, any remaining endometriosis, or new endometriosis, continues to be fed by the woman's hormones during the natural menstrual cycle.

There are a few well-known methods and established drug therapies that can be used to medically manage endometriosis. One is through using the oral contraceptive pill, sometimes tricycling packets (combining three months' medication at a time) so that a woman has fewer episodes of menstruation (Proctor and Farquhar 2006). Another method is through use of Danazol. This method results in some unpleasant side effects. Some women are treated using Depo-Provera, a form of progesterone, but again this also causes side effects and is less commonly used these days. Lastly, a group of drugs known as GnRH analogues are often used in the treatment of endometriosis. These work by reducing the FS (follicle stimulating) and LH (luteinising) hormones and lead to lower levels of oestrogen. Since it is the oestrogen that 'feeds' the endometriosis, this means that its growth is inhibited. HRT is given in the form of 'add-back' therapy to minimise the pseudo-menopausal symptoms incurred by this drug regime and to ensure that bone density is retained, as far as possible.

One of the problems with any of these drug regimes is that they cannot be used for indefinite periods. In particular, the use of GnRH analogues is not usually recommended for longer than 6 to 12 months because of concerns about osteoporosis and lack of bone density.

The long-term usage (continuous usage over many years) of GnRH analogues requires further investigation.

This all means that medical treatments for endometriosis are fairly short-term, so that even if a woman is experiencing good pain relief and improvement in her symptoms, just as she starts to possibly feel well again the drugs are often stopped. This can be very frustrating, especially if the treatment has been successful.

PAIN MANAGEMENT

Pain management for endometriosis is difficult because of the wide range of symptoms that it encompasses. A range of analgesia may be used including paracetamol, aspirin, NSAIDs and codeine-related products. Some women who are in severe pain are occasionally hospitalised and offered morphine-related drugs. The use of a TENS machine has been helpful to some women with chronic pelvic pain and endometriosis. Electrical stimulation on the skin via a TENS machine distracts the pain signals and can give relief.

A nutritious diet is also important. One high in fish oils and vitamins B and E, zinc and magnesium can help with the inflammation of endometriosis (Mills and Vernon 1999). Some women also find complementary medicine can be helpful in their management of endometriosis – for example, herbal medicine, homeopathy and acupuncture.

When pain becomes chronic, as it is estimated by Latthe to be with a prevalence of 38 per 1000 women aged 15 to 73, some women might need to be referred to a pain management team for further support (Latthe, Hills and Khan 2006).

Some women with endometriosis find support groups helpful, such as those run by the National Endometriosis Society, whilst others will find helplines or website forums useful. These support factors are vital in managing what can often be a very lonely and isolating condition, as many women find it hard to talk about gynaecological conditions.

My quality of life was very poor. I came across something I had written prior to my last surgery for endometriosis. It is just as relevant to all the other symptoms I was experiencing – for example, fatigue and depression. It is not a happy piece of writing, but I would say it was a frighteningly accurate statement of how I felt about myself and my body a lot of the time.

Debilitating pain to depression: one woman's continuous struggle with endometriosis

When it first happened, I thought that the blood would be bright red. Nobody told me that it might look an old, rusty brown colour. I was just twelve and a half. It was my first menstrual period.

At first the pain wasn't too bad. In fact, my overriding memory at the start is of having to wear my PE kit one Friday afternoon because my flimsy school summer dress was soiled in blood.

Whilst I had no interest in sports at school, I used to do a lot of classical ballet and could easily do many of the 'recommended' stretches for relieving menstrual cramps.

By the time it came for me to do my GCSE exams, I had already spent several monthly mornings in Sick Bay. I had already tried the first line in basic 'home' pain management, Paracetamol and hot baths.

When it came to my A-levels, my then GP was more than happy to prescribe the Pill. I remember my mother saying that she could not believe that there was nothing better for period pain (having suffered herself). This was in 1993.

I then tried various forms of the Contraceptive Pill whilst at university. I would find them successful if they did not make me want to eat cake all week, or if I could physically stand up without crumpling in pain when my period was due.

My first visit to a gynaecologist was in 1994. I was just nineteen. He was quite an old man. I remember him saying that I just had 'Primary Dysmenorrhoea' (Pre-childbirth period pain) and that it would all improve when I had a baby. It was a horrible and degrading experience.

Not long after I graduated in 1997 I remember having some 'period pain' so bad that I passed out. The pain was so intense that I was completely incapacitated. It didn't take my first employer long to realise that I was taking half and full days off on a rather cyclical basis. It was humiliating to say the least to have to explain to the Chief Executive (a man in his late 50s) why I was absent on a monthly basis. I was urged to 'do something about it'.

My latest GP by this time also thought that having a baby would solve all my problems. I was only twenty three by this time, and had only just started my career.

I saw another gynaecologist who gave me a scan, which showed nothing, and also did a laparoscopy where she casually mentioned that she found 'tiny amounts' of endometriosis, but that there was nothing that could be done, and that it might be worth me following a low-wheat diet, and keep taking the painkillers.

I tried the 'healthy and nutritious' diet approach. I also tried a range of complementary and alternative therapies.

Another gynaecologist suggested a hysterectomy (and laughed), and then said, 'Why not try a progesterone only pill?' I hated it, put on weight and was still in pain.

In 2000, another gynaecologist said after doing a laparoscopy that she couldn't find anything other than old and dead endometriosis. I was told that my problem was psychological, and was sent to a Pain Management Consultant.

In 2002 I saw a gynaecologist who diagnosed that I had Moderate–Severe Endometriosis. It was also found to be in my bladder and later in my bowel. In 2003 I was diagnosed with 'Moderate Clinical Depression', and who can blame me?

Endometriosis is as yet a little-known and poorly understood condition where the menstrual flow escapes the uterus and is often found in other areas of the pelvis, and rarely elsewhere in the body. It can affect a woman's fertility and cause a great deal of pain.

Isobel Knight, February 2007

Post-operative report

In March 2007, I saw another gynaecologist who let me remain on Zoladex until I had surgery in September 2007.

So yet another laparoscopy was performed and more endometriosis found and completely lasered away, meaning that nothing was left by the end of this operation. At the same time, a Mirena coil was inserted as this is believed to reduce periods significantly and because it is progesterone based, and also inhibits any new endometriosis.

Just over two months after this surgery, I started to bleed a tiny amount and suffer terrible pain. I was seen as an out patient where it was determined the Mirena was a possible cause, and indeed was no longer in my uterus when it was moved, hence the level of pain I suffered.

At this point in time, the consultant expressed concern that I still had pain, since the endometriosis had been removed. I begged to be allowed to return to Zoladex, a regime which had truly worked for me, but strong doubts were cast upon this in the light of concerns about my bone density.

July 2012

I have now been on Zoladex injections with add-back tibolone (HRT) for four years. This is significantly longer than the drug is usually licensed for (six months) and, although lowered bone density and osteoporosis are risk factors, we don't yet know the implications there might be for my prolonged usage of this drug. Although my bone density has dipped into osteoporotic status, the most recent test in February 2012 showed that I am still in the 'normal' range – I might be managing to retain this with weight-bearing exercise and a diet that has adequate calcium and vitamin D. However, for me the quality of life afforded by this treatment so far outweighs any such risks of being on long-term Zoladex and HRT. My bone density is monitored annually and I am reviewed annually by gynaecologists. I am now in my late thirties. However, I am still potentially 15 years or so away from the menopause, so a decision will need to be made about whether I re-try having periods again or consider a more final treatment such as a total (including ovaries) hysterectomy. My own feeling remains that quality of life is the most important, overriding factor.

In terms of my EDS symptoms and based on discussions with Howard Bird and his writing about hormones, it is now clear to me that progesterone medications seemed to have a worse effect on my EDS symptoms, resulting in more tissue laxity and therefore an increase in pain. Although the medication I am now on may not be ideal in the long term, it is more oestrogen based and is providing me with a much higher quality of life, and a seemingly more stabilising effect on my EDS symptoms.

CHAPTER 11

Sleep and fatigue

I went to sleep at half seven last night and awoke at three this morning, been up ever since, my sleep pattern is appalling!!!!!! I just go on auto pilot!!!!

EDSIII patient, Facebook

It takes me hours to get to sleep and I seem to get my best sleep during daylight hours! I've had a really bad couple of nights then last night I went to bed early, still took a couple of hrs to get to sleep then woke up about 2pm!! I hate it, seems like the days fly by but if I force myself to get up early then I'm in more pain and too tired to do anything useful.

EDSIII patient, Facebook

Sleep deprivation is a known problem in patients with EDSIII and fibromyalgia FM (Berne 2002; Rahman and Holman 2010). Chronic pain has a resultant negative effect on sleep (Shaikh, Hakim and Shenker 2010) and in children and adolescents; growing pains can also impede sleep (Middleditch 2010; Shaikh *et al.* 2010). Sleep is crucial to repair and maintenance and, if inadequate, will lead to sleep deprivation which might also contribute to daytime sleepiness and impaired cognitive function (Berne 2002; Wolfson and Carskadon 1998). A study by Wolfson and Carskadon (1998) looking at (healthy) adolescent students, 13 to 19 years old, showed that sleep loss was due to increasingly late bedtimes and that those struggling academically also showed greater weekend delays of sleep. Self-report in the study showed that sleep problems contributed to daytime sleepiness, depressive mood and sleep/wake behavioural problems. Research by Fredriksen *et al.* (2004) also showed that (healthy) adolescents who obtained less sleep over time reported higher levels of depressive symptoms and decreased self-esteem.

Research has shown that patients with fibromyalgia (FM) indicate that poorer sleep contributes to higher levels of psychological distress (Shaver *et al.* 1997). In particular, Shaver and colleagues report that less stable sleep in the early night suggests that night-time hormone (growth hormone) is a contributing factor. Jones *et al.* (2007) suggest that replacement of growth hormone using insulin-like growth factor led to an improvement of symptoms in patients with fibromyalgia (Jones *et al.*, as cited in Shaikh *et al.* 2010). Berne writes that:

> Deep sleep is restorative, associated with respiration, blood pressure, growth hormone secretion, and other regulatory functions. Lack of deep sleep has been associated with altered immune function... Sleep deprivation causes significant deregulation of bodily functioning and is associated with pain, daytime drowsiness, cognitive dysfunction, decreased alertness and irritability.

Berne 2002, p.151

Berne describes some critical factors which apply not only in the treatment of FM, but also to EDSIII, particularly in adolescence, and, if the patient is rehabilitated promptly, might prevent full-scale FM or symptomatic EDSIII, and prevent the implications for the adult patient, such as low back pain and chronic pain syndromes (Murray 2006). The challenge lies in interpreting the symptoms correctly, and assessing all the physiological and psychosocial factors, of which sleep is crucial (Murray 2006). Of particular relevance to EDSIII is the fact that blood pressure is regulated during deep sleep and those symptoms of disruption to blood pressure – POTS (postural orthostatic tachycardia syndrome) – might be implicated in patients who report having difficulties with sleep. In an adolescent who is not growing sufficiently, the physician should also look at sleeping patterns and sufficient sleep, since the lack of deep sleep is likely to impede the release of human growth hormone. Research suggests that the lack of adequate growth hormone in FM patients is treatable (Bennett 2002; Jones *et al.* 2007). It is, however, abundantly clear that lack of sleep contributes to chaos and huge effects to the ANS and therefore a lack of physiological homeostasis – so we are back to our Maslow Hierarchy of Needs (Chapter 5).

These are accounts of my own insomnia:

I am not sleeping again and it is very miserable. I had seen such an improvement in sleep and not needing the bathroom so much at night that it is very tedious to return to being restless, not sleeping, feeling manic and busy head and a real depression. This has been going on for several weeks and I have had to get myself up this morning even though it is a) Saturday, b) I am feeling jet-lagged and exhausted.

Diary, 17.3.2012

Another night of no sleep so far, despite medications. Thank God for the Internet then and the TV!

Diary, 22.3.2012

There is a real difference between being tired and having fatigue, as can be seen in more detail in Chapter 12. However, here Dr Alan Hakim describes fatigue.

FATIGUE
Dr Alan Hakim

Fatigue is a common and disabling finding in many musculoskeletal conditions. It may be associated with anaemia, endocrine disorders such as underactive thyroid, prolonged infections, low vitamin levels, cancer, and organ disorders such as kidney or liver disease.

Fatigue is often a feature of chronic pain syndromes such as fibromyalgia (FM) and EDS. The cause for such profound symptoms is unclear and may be related to complex neurochemical imbalances in the brain that are as yet ill understood in EDS, autonomic dysfunction and poor sleep patterns and sleep quality (Bravo *et al.* 2010). In these circumstances the tiredness experienced is not that typical after exercise or a busy day at work, but is often an overwhelming lack of energy that may appear after even the most minimal period of activity.

As part of the management of fatigue, diseases associated with it need to be excluded.

There is little published evidence in support of treatments for fatigue. Antidepressants, anti-anxiety drugs, sleep aids and analgesics have been tried with variable success in chronic fatigue syndrome,

FM and EDS. Lifestyle changes including pacing, changing sleep pattern, exercise, and even change of job or hours of work may help.

There is also limited scientific evidence supporting the use of nutritional supplements other than replacing deficiencies of B vitamins and trace minerals (e.g. zinc, selenium and manganese). Carnitine, coenzyme Q10 and 5-HTP are considered to be effective in boosting the immune system, raising energy levels and improving cognitive functioning.

CHAPTER 12

Fatigue and unexpected responses to treatment and incidents

Fatigue is different to not sleeping or being tired. In Chapter 11, Hakim explained fatigue as 'a feature of chronic pain syndromes... autonomic dysfunction and poor sleep patterns and sleep quality'. Sometimes I am too tired to sleep. This is not uncommon.

Fibromyalgia – The beast with a thousand spikes[1]
Tortuous!
A thousand sharps evilly spike my body
Each a shrieking shrill pitched scream

I am a wounded porcupine grounded by agonies,
My muscles just won't stop.
I am fighting sirens of emergency,
My body is on red alert.

Just as a flattened hedgehog,
Casualty to an injury,
I am crushed to death;
The beast with a thousand spikes.

Constraints to progress
Owing to the sheer complexity of EDSIII and a challenging medical history, there have been times when progress has been impeded. Much of this has stemmed from a lack of homeostasis (POTS and autonomic dysfunction), restorative sleep and continuing problems with bowel and excretion, as well as other traumas and overuse situations. The relationship between sleep and fatigue is not conclusive from my subjective graphs (see Figure 12.1; for more information see

---

1   Copyright © Isobel Knight, 2011

Chapter 33) and there is not a direct relationship between them. I would have expected that if sleep is good (low score) that fatigue would also be low, but this is not always the case.

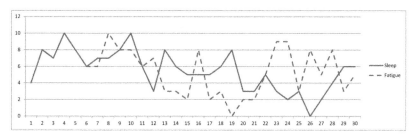

FIGURE 12.1: RELATIONSHIP BETWEEN SLEEP AND FATIGUE

Maslow

It is abundantly clear that the management of sleep is crucial to keeping flare-ups to a minimum and for optimum function. This would be the case for everybody but far more so in this type of patient. Maslow writes that 'If all the (physiological) needs are unsatisfied, and the organism is then dominated by the physiological needs, all other needs may become simply non-existent or be pushed into the background.' (1970, p.37).

Clearly, the type of sleep is also a critical factor, and it is known that patients with fibromyalgia don't always go into the correct sleep cycles (Berne 2002; Shaver *et al.* 1997)– I think this is the critical factor causative of all the huge pain, fatigue and disruption. I blogged the following:

> I often wondered if I knew the difference between being tired and fatigued because of my general lack of sleep – but there is a difference. Being tired is quite gentle and at the end of the day it can feel nice and relaxing and is about being weary. Mentally one perhaps starts to feel 'slower' and not able to retain new things. Fatigue is, by contrast, a much more extreme, sudden and violent form of being tired. It as is if someone has pulled the plug on you. My muscles all ache, my postural control sharply diminishes – particularly in thoracic spine and shoulders. My body craves sleep and being in bed [is] like a state emergency. Last night became one of those.

Yesterday, during ballet, I started to feel 'tired'. This could have been because I went for a long walk in the afternoon and then had relaxed in the warm sunshine, and had just started on annual leave from work. Additionally, I had just been given some new exercises from my physio, particularly focusing on spinal extension work, and all these factors combined could have contributed to feeling tired. The studio was warm, and my lumbar spine was really hurting. I did a 'good' class and a great deal of allegro, pushing into a real training zone and getting a good cardiovascular workout – something I haven't been able to achieve for a long time.

Straight after class, I usually feel quite 'high' and buzzy, but I started to feel fatigued almost immediately and wanted to get straight home. I ate supper and watched the TV, struggling to keep awake until 9pm, then had a hot bath as I had done a lot of exercise, including spending a good 5–10 minutes in spinal extension (seated, cross-legged). My back hurt a lot, but because I was so fatigued, I thought the fatigue would drown out the pain.

I woke 3 times in the night and was in bed for over 12 hours, but still feel wiped out today. That is fatigue.

Blog, 10.4.2011

The signs of the fatigue (the prelude)

I came up with my own personal preludes to fatigue which included:

- feeling 'tired' and unable to wake up in the mornings – even if sleep has been relatively good

- brain getting foggy, things harder to remember and learn

- body aching – in a mild capacity

- alignment potentially less stable – my physio had asked me to observe myself daily to see at a snapshot what might not look so acceptable to her. This time it was neck and shoulders.

Blog, 23.3.2011

Chaos and crisis

As time went on in my treatment I started to get wiser about preludes to crisis and what going into crisis and chaos actually meant. There are a number of potential reasons for going into crisis and, in a broader sense, these included:

- reaction to treatment
- unexpected trauma (e.g. bicycle landing on foot)
- introduction of new movement pattern/overuse (see Part III).

Reaction to treatment

From my experience as a Bowen therapist and in treating other patients, I always hope that patients will respond to treatment, preferably positively for the condition they have attended for. Sometimes there will be a reaction to treatment, and this might be mild muscular pain, but if the reaction is severe it might encompass more severe pain and/or feeling wiped out. In Bowen terms this would count as an overreaction to treatment and quite possibly an indication that the therapist has unfortunately overdone treatment. Fortunately, this does not happen often (to my patients), but when it occasionally does it reminds me that it is sometimes prudent to do less the next time around and in some groups, especially those with chronic fatigue, fibromyalgia or EDSIII.

There have been times when I have had very big reactions to treatment. This was particularly in my earlier days, in treatment with my physio when she was getting to know me and my body better, and the reactions were very often vascular, relating to POTS and problems with the ANS. I tried to explain this in an email to my physio:

> I am sorry I am causing you such a lot of trouble as a patient. It is difficult because I don't want to be unproductive at the end of my session and have it affect my working day. Clearly something is going on. The change in heart rate and pulse variation yesterday was unpleasant. I was suffering from pins and needles and extreme weakness in the left arm especially. I felt 'detached', very, very emotional. I was close to tears at several points in the day, and then felt absolutely exhausted. The (propriospinal) muscle spasm continued intermittently for the rest of the day and at night. I got home, ate some soup and went to bed c8.30pm. I was then too tired to sleep (this happens too),

but then did go into a deep sleep. I ached everywhere from the pelvis and above, with some tender points, particularly bad in the arms.

This morning was exhausted. Have headache, very sore arms, pain across all upper body and feel foggy headed and glands all up again (pelvis and below = fine). I do (as discussed) seem to manage to override the fatigue, but it is getting harder and harder to do this, and because I am in pain or rather sore.

Email to physiotherapist, 22.1.2010

Unexpected trauma

One of the best documented examples I have of an unexpected trauma causing absolute chaos relates to an episode when a Brompton fold-up bicycle dropped on my left foot. I was just sitting having a drink with a friend in a bar and someone's bicycle fell and landed on my left foot. It hurt a lot at the time, even though I had consumed several glasses of wine at this point, but the pain I was in was disproportionate to the level of trauma that was incurred. I recall a huge sense of vibration in my body for hours after the event and there was bruising, but then there was a huge amount of spasming and twitching and an overwhelming fatigue.

I explain, via my blog:

When the bicycle landed on my left foot (previously sprained and injured), my body went into attack the next day and I could not manage Pilates because I was having spasms, pain in my pelvis, back, hips – and then my upper body muscles were 'shaking' because they were too fatigued to work properly. It was a nightmare and I had to resort to curtailing my session. I felt 'out of my body' and was having vascular changes including feeling extremely cold. As I type now, one of my hands is as warm as toast, whilst the other is like a block of ice. Why? What is going on that is causing such things to occur? My physio gave me a triage session at lunchtime. She confirmed my foot was just bruised. Why I felt it could be fractured is interesting, but the pain was 'out of proportion' to the level of trauma that I suffered.

Blog, 24.9.2010

CHAPTER 13

Crisis, flare-ups and management

Oh dear! For some reason I am in a big flare-up. Potential cause – Pilates – new stuff + overreaching + Physio (going into Thoracic spine). I am in 'nodal' pain just about everywhere from tip to toe. I am aching like mad and at the moment – 'hypomobile' factor in a severe attack of IBS (actually resorted to medication), feeling incredibly depressed with a very low energy and you might just get an idea of how I am feeling. I tried to do a bit of shopping but felt dizzy and 'unreal' and felt like I was dragging a lead chain and ball around.

Blog, 21.8.2010

I started to get more interested in what I classified as 'crisis' or 'flare-up' and came up with some signs and symptoms that would suggest preludes. A flare-up might be distinguished by the longevity of the 'attack' and could range from a few days to, in some cases, weeks and months. This was my personal list:

- lapses in concentration and reduced attention span
- inability to follow instructions with accuracy
- memory problems
- brain fog
- unable to explain things with usual clarity
- making unusual mistakes/inaccuracies – e.g. typing errors
- poor coordination/balance
- being more clumsy – dropping things
- feeling very restless and agitated – manic
- feeling anxious

- feeling overloaded/over stimulated
- feeling as if the battery is about to run out
- feeling wired/running on overdrive
- sudden 'emergency' needs – e.g. hunger/needing the bathroom
- behaving like a child – 'demanding' – behaviour similar to overtired child
- showing impatience and irritation – tutting, puffing!
- poor decision making – or inability to make sensible/rational decisions
- being injured already and/or compensating for an injured body part (distraction).

All these symptoms point towards a *fatigue* or, at best, yield point of endurance.

I then put a posting on the Hypermobility Syndrome Association (HMSA) Forum requesting responses from other patients and came up with a diverse list of body systemic signs and symptoms, and the results are below. Most of my responses could easily be dovetailed into this list, making me autoethnographically and socially a cultural representative of the EDS community.

Crisis/flare-up: themes from HMSA members
Digestive
- Upset stomach – I assume I'm reacting to the extra nausea.
- I'll usually start to drop a little weight.
- Stomach problems get worse.

Energy/fatigue
- Total exhaustion kicks in.
- Need loads more sleep than I would usually for some days and then 'crash' for a few weeks – pain very bad, need lots more sleep.
- I am so exhausted I can barely get the energy to lift my feet enough to take a step.

- My only warning that all this is about to happen is the extreme exhaustion and sometimes mini-tremors.
- It's all I can do to drink a little tea and lie there. I don't eat because it takes too much energy.
- I am horribly depressed from the exhaustion of having to try even harder than normal to hold my body together.
- My energy levels go through the floor, my sleeping patterns go haywire. I get very tired.
- I am a poor sleeper but get so tired. Even holding my head up is tiring.

Pain

- Pain levels go through the roof.
- I have pain on a subconscious level.
- I get bad head and neck pain, dizzy and the knee pain becomes leg pain.

Balance and coordination

- Balance is completely off.
- I get very wobbly before the onset of each bendy week.
- I start dropping things.
- My balance goes completely so I stagger like a drunk.
- I start dropping things.
- I always go extra clumsy before and during a flare-up.

POTS

- My POTS symptoms are worse too with more tachy episodes and ectopic heartbeats.
- Even worse temperature control.
- I started to feel colder all the time. I always had cold hands and feet.
- I start to feel cold (even when everyone else was warm).

- I tend to get all the autonomic problems flare up, one at a time: circulation, sweating, gut problems, reflux, palpitations, faintness/dizziness, and confusion, etc. but in no particular order.
- I get neck pain and dizziness.

Restless/fidgeting/shaking and tremors

- I become decidedly fidgety.
- I seem first to be so 'flushed with adrenaline' that I can't stop and can barely function.
- On really bad days my legs start to shake; sometimes the arms shake too.
- The shaking is not visible but it is a deep level in the arms and legs. Now I often take the cyclobenzaprine and go to lie down when I get the mini-tremors.
- I have other neurological symptoms for a few days (non-specified).

Mood

- I often get very depressed just before it starts.
- I become more withdrawn and anxious as I try to hold it all together as well, though I can't see that myself from the inside. I'll become tearful as well. I don't often cry so that's a pretty good indicator for me that I'm more 'under it' than I realise.
- All this makes me angry and I feel like crying.
- I tend to generally be more irritable.
- I am horribly depressed from the exhaustion of having to try even harder than normal to hold my body together.
- First thing I'll notice is the crushing mood and slowness to achieve even getting up, and tearfulness/snappiness with others.
- My body has told me I am done and I can't win this fight.

Feeling unwell

- I also feel bizarrely fluey.

Memory/concentration

- My brain is too tired to find words.
- I also get forgetful, mix up or forget words when speaking.

Overuse/overdoing things

- I am overdoing it.
- I am overusing the muscles.

Skin

- My skin starts cutting and splitting more easily.
- Stress on my body shows in my skin and nails.
- If it is related to bendy week my skin and gums tear and bleed more easily.

This diverse list of symptoms shows just how truly multisystemic EDSIII is and also the complete 'chaos' in the body – so where is this chaos stemming from and what precisely is triggering it? What goes 'wrong' first or becomes the anticipant to the chaos? (see Figure 13.1.)

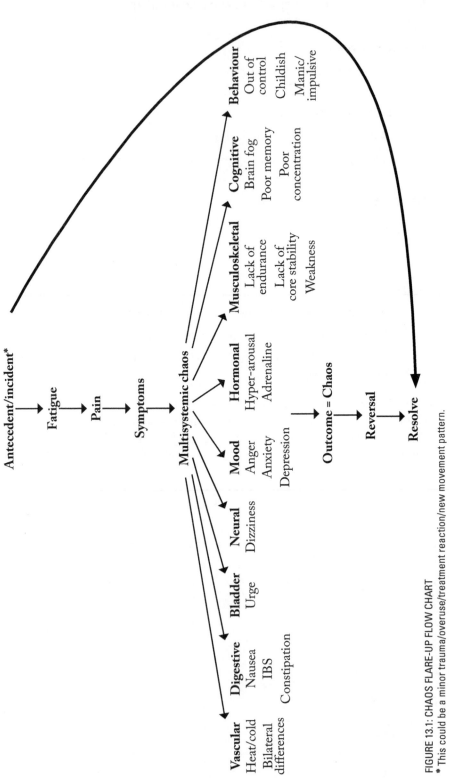

FIGURE 13.1: CHAOS FLARE-UP FLOW CHART

* This could be a minor trauma/overuse/treatment reaction/new movement pattern.

Managing flare-ups

For me the time aspect of flare-ups and the psychological effects of them are harder to cope with and endure than the actual physical symptoms because it is all so uncertain and unpredictable, and I am afraid it will become a permanent thing, even though it often doesn't. Sometimes it is difficult to know when 'rock bottom' has been reached during a flare-up or chaotic crisis before it is possible to start contemplating when reversal takes place.

Sleep is a crucial factor in chaos theory and in reversing resultant flare-up symptoms. The madness reaches its peak when pain is at a crescendo, by which time most body systems might also appear to be affected. The following steps need to be taken following flare-ups before the chaos can be stabilised and subsequently reversed. Psychologically there has to be some kind of acceptance on behalf of the patient before any attempt can be made to stabilise and manage the flare-up. This is what I call 'squaring the circle' (see Figure 13.2).

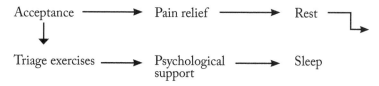

FIGURE 13.2: SQUARING THE CIRCLE – RECOVERY

Ultimately it seems that the key to recovery is sleep, and that until restorative sleep begins there is no real possibility of resetting the autonomic nervous system (ANS) and reversing autonomic dysfunction. I explain the following via a blog entry:

> I have now had three nights in a row of continuous, uninterrupted (by bladder) sleep. In very recent months I had started to have a few odd nights of sleeping through the night, but this is the best it has got so far. I have not slept through since I was a very young child. It feels amazing! I am so much calmer and relaxed – but yet I am still tired, so I suspect that I am still in a sleep deficit after three nights. My life will be transformed if I can sleep right the way through the night most of the time. I am not totally unrealistic. Most normal people have the odd bad night of sleep and are woken by worry, busy head (perhaps bladder after heavy drinking session). It seems that physiotherapy has really made the difference in stopping the nocturia – but quite why I am now sleeping through is still a mystery. I have been on

some diazepam, but last night I didn't take it at all and still slept through. When I have been like this for more than a week I think the pattern might have been corrected and I am sleeping. It will make such a difference to my quality of life, my energy, brain function and pain.

Blog, 9.4.2011

Conclusions about flare-ups

As time has passed and as I have learnt more and more about my condition(s) and how to manage them, I am finding that my time in crisis reduces unless provoked by unusual events or the impact of something more invasive such as surgery. I spend a little less time in periods of fatigue and in fatigue, and the spells are becoming shorter-lived (24–48 hours). I am more skilled at managing them, and this has been helped by a psychological acceptance of what is going on and for me to stop fighting. If I do not battle, I seem to win much more quickly. I rest and relax and wait. Although it is a cliché, time is a healer. It seems that my focus now needs to be drawn to looking at my behaviour and feelings of anger, which might also be perpetuating a cycle of fatigue and adrenalin-driven perfectionist behaviour.

CHAPTER 14

The chronic complex patient and pain management

Chronic complex patient

Chiropractor was seeing me twice a week for almost a year and just kept commenting on how 'this' was back out of place again and to do 'these' exercises. I gave up on him but he had given up on me long before that... just wanted to keep an appointment rolling in. The GP that I was seeing years ago gave up on me and told me I was abusing my Ultram which was 1–2 50mg daily (a joke for a large amount of pain) and handed me Cymbalta and sent me on my way. The Neurologist was stumped. The next GP referred me to my Rheumatologist who then referred me to physical therapy for a strengthening program. They had NO idea I wasn't supposed to turn and twist in such awkward positions and then move heavy weights that way. BAD idea! I had an OBGYN give up on me too. So now it is two physicians, one rheumatologist who is insanely hard to get into, and myself... Once I request my medical records from my journey, I better get the biggest three ring binder available...

EDSIII patient, Facebook

After looking at Maslow's Hierarchy of Needs it seemed that the most basic physiological processes were not functioning optimally. Pain is another factor that might be considered to impede physiological and, indeed, psychological wellbeing.

Pain management

Being in pain is a huge factor involved in the lives of those with EDSIII, fibromyalgia and many other chronic complex conditions. The physiology behind pain management is extremely complex; Dr Alan Hakim explains. Additionally, readers are directed to the references in the footnote below.[1]

PAIN

Dr Alan Hakim

Pain is a mixture of complex experiences. It can be:

- physical, leading to changes such as stiffness and reduced mobility
- emotional, driving anxiety and depression, and may be driven by depression
- behavioural, stopping doing certain things, or responding to the environment in a different way
- 'acute' or 'chronic', often flaring on a background of chronic pain.

Acute pain is typically sharp and sudden. There is often an obvious cause and it gets better fairly quickly. It will usually respond to a pain killer.

Chronic pain is lingering, dull and oppressive. It appears in 'fits and starts', 'comes and goes', and there are 'good days and bad'. The cause is not necessarily obvious and it may not respond well to medication. Chronic pain is associated with fatigue and anxiety.

In an acute pain the nerve mechanisms are relatively straightforward. A local messenger at the site of damage sends a message via 'peripheral' pain fibres to the spinal cord. The spinal cord does three things:

1. It sends a message back telling the local sensors what to do – e.g. 'get that hand out of that fire NOW!' – a quick reflex response.
2. It sends a message to the brain asking for 'help'. The response is often a combination of something physical, something verbal and often something emotional.

---

1   Beighton *et al.* (2012); Hakim *et al.* (2010); Keer and Grahame (2003); Knight (2011).

3. The 'gateways' in the spinal cord respond to signals coming down from the brain in such a way that signals from the periphery become blocked, reducing the messages back to the brain. This is how many analgesics work, and how a person can influence their 'pain threshold'.

Chronic pain is much more complicated:

1. The triggers from the periphery are not well understood and there is often evidence of a hypersensitivity to the simplest of stimuli. A pat on the back can be painful! The triggers in EDS are not understood but may, for example, include nerve irritation from being overstretched, or confused signals from joints that have lost their proprioception (awareness of position) where 'pain' may be the only message the joint can send, or even recurrent microscopic injuries in the soft tissues sending multiple signals – these are conjecture.

2. It appears that the gateway controls are no longer as effective as they should be so that not only do the simplest of stimuli induce pain but also the signals get through the spinal cord, flood the brain, and the brain is not able to stop the upward flow of data.

3. The brain can respond with a number of potentially abnormal messages that can lead to over-perception of pain, changes in mood, changes in the autonomic system and changes in behaviour. Some of these changes are beginning to be understood and related to imbalances in neurochemicals in the brain.

It is for all these reasons that a number of techniques are used to help combat chronic pain, including pain psychology, physical therapies, pacing, behavioural therapies, and analgesic classes such as anti-depressants and neuropathics such as amitriptyline and pregabalin respectively.

I blogged the following 'dark' entries about my experiences of being in pain:

I am in one of the most severe flare-ups I have possibly ever had in relation to pain and FM+HMS. I am so fatigued I had to sleep between the people I was working with today. I had to take a taxi home. I have had two long hot baths in less than four hours and taken diazepam, codeine, oramorph and anti-sickness medication. I have tried stretches, doing my physio exercises, relaxation, watching TV, but the pain is searing, sharp, and in nodules in my neck, shoulders, hips, calves, hands, arms, feet, virtually everywhere. I feel so isolated. I just want someone to hold me. I have cried, I have held my cat. I have eaten chocolate. I feel under huge pressure to be at work tomorrow because I am the only person on duty in my department.

Blog, 17.11.2011

I sometimes wonder if I was very bad in my previous life. Anything that might just explain why I am continuing to suffer so much in my present life. No matter how much I try, what exercises I do, how hard I work (at work); it so often feels as though I get punched back in the face. Today is one of those days. I wonder how much more I can take of this. When I am well (as for anybody) it feels fantastic. No one should take good health for granted. It is a real gift, and just lately, I have had a taste of it. So it now feels so bitter to be in so much pain I want to vomit, so much pain I want to curl up and die, and in so much pain I wish for someone to plunge a needle in me to end the suffering, just as I was able to do for my dear cat only a few weeks ago. This time, there could be a simple solution. I could 'just' be suffering from a kidney infection. Since my urine was tested positively for a UTI, as it always seems to every single time it is tested (last week in urology was no exception), I could be 'measurably' ill with a medically explainable problem. However I more than suspect it is not. That although there is severe pain in my spine, loins, central abdomen and iliac fossa (right and left) no one will help me – the doctors might give me some morphine, but no one will really 'do' anything, until the next time, and the next time and the next time. Maybe I have just become cynical. I have so much I could give and do. I have achieved so much but could do infinitely more, but I am tired. Exhausted. Fighting at times with a force that is bigger than I can cope with and hospital upon hospital appointment and being sent for more and more tests because there are more and more things that are wrong. I want to get off this merry-go-round of hell and just float off into the sunset. Not in this body, but a long way from it. Humans can't be 'put down' – but I wish I could. That would be humane. This is not humane. I will wake up again and want to fight, but at what continued cost to me and the NHS? I can contribute to the lives of others and actively want to help and support others, but I have reached my lowest ebb because I can't see things ever really changing. Ever so once in a while they do – to tease me, and then I get this. Again. I don't want to wallow in self-pity which is why I keep trying to work around this condition writing about it and offering help to others. I rarely get so incensed on here – but pain is highly emotive. Tomorrow might be a different and better day. Like many others with chronic painful conditions, I will keep plodding on. I just hope there isn't a next life.

Blog, 16.1.2012

A few months ago I went to see my GP because I was experiencing such an acute and sudden flare-up of pain. She asked me, 'What do you want me to do about it?' For a moment I was thrown by her bluntness – but actually she was right. What did I really think she could do about it? She was never going to be able to wave a magic wand and make my pain go away forever. Only I had the tools to know how to manage it after all this time. We talked about what I could do whilst in this flare-up. There were of course the different levels of drugs I could take and different types of medications for different things. She agreed I could temporarily increase my diazepam and could take dihydrocodeine as well as naproxen and paracetamol. Then there was oramorph if I was so up against it that all the other drugs failed. I also considered my other non-medicinal strategies such as writing, having lots of hot baths, hot water bottles and seeing a friend or just hanging out and watching a film. The next day my pain score had reduced from 8/10 to almost zero. I will not know where that flare-up came from and all the countless others I have endured over the years. I let others know on Facebook I had been suffering during this time. No one can ever do anything and the drugs merely provide temporary respite but never solve the problem.

Chronic pain can be infuriating and make you very angry – if you continue to let it. However, my experience is that the angrier one becomes and the more one fights it, the more it increases. It is, however, a very hard concept to accept. It is changes in the brain which subsequently cause sensations of pain to continue in varying intensities and for the sufferer to become increasingly sensitised to pain (Shaikh *et al.* 2010). It is no wonder then that if I feel down my muscles are more likely to mimic this and are accordingly achy and sore. The psychology of the situation is so intertwined with the physical and this is what makes it all so complex. Many patients in the same situation get very angry about it all because (rightly) no one can ever 'see' their suffering or understand that they are in pain. This is the difficulty of a rare and invisible condition – of which fibromyalgia and chronic fatigue are obviously close relatives to EDSIII. There are many other excellent books on the topic of pain management and it is beyond the remit of this book to discuss pain in any further detail.

Conclusion to Part II: Physiology

Our bodies try to keep us in a state of physiological equilibrium or homeostasis. According to Maslow's Hierarchy of Needs, if these basic fundamental physiological needs are not met then there is little hope of satisfactorily achieving higher levels of human need (see Chapter 5). It seems to me that many of the difficulties for EDSIII (and other chronic complex patients) relate to autonomic dysfunction, as Hakim explains in Chapter 6. It is this imbalance in ANS function or autonomic dysfunction that seems to create so many difficulties with sleep and other bodily functions including pulse rate, temperature, breathing, digestion and bladder function. If only this were to be adequately addressed and at least managed then the person experiencing these symptoms might have an improved quality of life. In my own case, although I am experiencing improvements, I would not consider my resultant autonomic dysfunction entirely managed, but any progress could be deemed as a positive step in the right direction to achieving baseline physiological health, balance and, ultimately, homeostasis.

PART III
PSYCHOLOGY

Preface to Part III: Psychology

I had endured a week of 'chaos and flare-up' and had emailed my physio a few times. With respect to this physiotherapist, it was the first time he had experienced a succession of emails from me within the six months he had been treating me. In one email I wrote:

> Really don't know what has happened, but am in a real state. So fatigued had to take a taxi home. Sharp, fibro pain everywhere. Arms/hands bad. Still splitting headache, and cannot nod my head or put head in forward flexion. It has got stuck. Hard tilting head to right. Something is jammed in left. Neck feels in solid spasm. Weepy. Emotional. Cannot process information. Whole fibro-fog. Earache. Cold. I think this will be the worst you have seen me...
>
> *Email to physiotherapist, 23.8.2012*

I saw my physio on 27 August 2012 and we discussed what had happened to cause all of this. I had drawn a diagram flow chart, much like the one in Chapter 13, and we discussed my diagram. What was written in my diary was the word 'angry', which appeared twice, which I hadn't realised. My physio thought that the antecedent was actually before my last treatment and might have correlated with me being in a really good state, in a period of relaxation, and that I had let my guard down. This was a theory.

My physio then shocked me by telling me how he had felt about receiving my email. He said he felt rather helpless, overwhelmed and had no idea how to start or respond. He said he had to sit down in quiet for 20 minutes before he could discuss the situation with a colleague. He recognised that if he felt slightly bad about what he was reading it was a drop in the ocean compared to what I would be going through. It was a real eye-opener and a massive surprise to me that my physio could be just as overwhelmed by my experiences. It made me reflect upon my previous physio who had endured months of these types of emails. Therapists have limits, and it was helpful for me to hear my physio's response. He then probed further and asked me if I was angry at him. I hesitated, but then admitted that part of my anger was directed at him when things had been so perfect. Upon reflection now, another aspect of my anger involves my body behaving badly when I should be past this point (in treatment). I was also angry because I needed my body to be perfect whilst in a new job, and this whole lack of control and devastating fatigue threatened that. I was also angry because I had (partly) missed out on some social events.

My physio looked at me and realised how bilaterally split I was. My right side was nice and relaxed – the direction I want to go in – whilst the left side was held, taut, angry, aggressive. We did some side-to-side pelvic movements. When the movements were taken to the left things felt 'secure', whereas movements to the right made me twitch all over the place and felt very insecure and vulnerable. A further suggestion was made for me to clench and release my muscles – anywhere in the body, imagining a dimmer switch to increase or decrease tension as I felt able to. We also talked about breathing, because it was not something I was doing with a great deal of ease whilst hanging on to all these unpleasant feelings.

We talked more about anger and how I felt unable to release mine and that I had taken this out on myself using self-harm (see Chapter 23), but my head controlled everything and my body didn't have a chance. I also admitted that I could not forgive myself for not exercising even when I felt so exhausted. This is another thing to contemplate this week in 'not doing'. I recognise how driven I am and admitted that when I didn't have things to fuel my adrenalin (book, new job, big challenges) I felt bored and dull, yet I am perpetually overdriven and in an energy-depleting cycle. My physio has now suggested we look at some affirmations for when I get into states like this week and goals for changing my behaviours and responses to things. It is no good having me physically in a better state if I keep on winding things up behaviourally. I realise this now, but it is going to be a new part of my story, and one that goes even beyond the end of this book.

My physio and I will keep checking in about my goals and behaviour. We are hoping that dance movement therapy and psychotherapy might benefit me more than counselling has alone, that movement itself might help me to find a voice to safely channel my anger kinetically, rather than at myself. I now realise why I have been such a huge psychological challenge to work with because my behaviour is fuelled by a stubborn and perfectionist streak. Not every chronic patient will present in quite this way, but some patients might have complex psychological issues. It is up to the skill of the therapist to manage their patient and to seek their own advice and support when and where necessary so that they themselves are not unduly overloaded or overwhelmed. This part of the book will tap into some of the psychology involved in working with chronic complex patients.

Introduction

Part III explores working with the chronic complex patient in a psychological context. The fact that it is so large indicates how crucial it is in working with this patient cohort. It discusses many aspects of the relationship between the patient and physiotherapist as well as doctors and patients. Goal-setting is discussed and the difficulties of working with this type of patient and types of 'challenging' behaviour. It explores more worrying behaviours such as self-harm as well as anxiety and depression. The use of cognitive analytical therapy is discussed as a means of supporting those who self-harm and for different mood-states. Dr Andrew Lucas, a consultant lead health psychologist at the Royal National Orthopaedic Hospital (RNOH), describes in Chapter 27 what happens to patients who attend the programme at the RNOH. Part III begins with my own insight as a Bowen therapist in terms of working with EDSIII and other chronic complex conditions.

CHAPTER 15

Isobel's experience of working with EDSIII patients as a Bowen therapist

What is the Bowen technique?

The Bowen technique is a form of complementary medicine. The therapy was founded by the late Tom Bowen in the 1960s in Australia, and is a 'gentle' form of soft tissue therapy. Bowen is a holistic therapy working at all tissue levels of the body, and primarily 'fascia'. It involves a series of gentle 'rolling-type' moves across muscle and tendon fibres, which generates an integrating healing response, and working on the muscle feedback mechanism. It might address a wide range of conditions including postural changes. John Wilks, Bowen instructor and author, goes into far more technical detail about the therapy and how it works in Chapter 38. In Part III I describe my own experiences of working with EDS/FM patients as they now form the majority of my patient cohort.

Working with chronic complex patients as a Bowen therapist

In my ten years' experience as a Bowen therapist, it has become clear that there are a particular cohort of patients who present very differently from all other patients. There are acute patients who I perhaps see between one and three visits and their notes are very simple, usually presenting with minimal previous medical history. Another group might have a longer medical history, but again they still may not require many sessions and their psychology is generally uncomplicated. They may have a few ailments, and there may be some presenting anxiety, but they usually respond in an 'expected' manner. Then there is the 'chronic complex' patient cohort. These patients just present differently. For a start they will frequently send a very long email or require an excessively long telephone consultation before actually attending for treatment. I understand the reasons for this very clearly. These patients have often been abandoned by other therapists or many people have given up on them in the past. They need to know whether it is worth their while investing in a new therapeutic relationship.

Upon arrival for their first consultation session, the chronic, complex patient (and I will use EDSIII and fibromyalgia [FM] as examples) frequently presents in quite a flustered and anxious manner. They will arrive bang on time and usually early, but appear as if they have just rushed in from a late bus or train. They will sit down and, when I ask whether they have completed my client information sheet, will provide a dossier of notes for me to wade through, often with offers of MRI documentation. The latter I usually politely refuse as I am not a medical doctor. They frequently sit in a very restless manner and fidget, their hips swinging all over the place and hands twisted and gesturing. They often start by talking about how they are right now and most often there is pain in numerous random places in the body. Then we look at the medical history. In a Bowen consultation I am also interested in other aspects such as pure water intake (to assess overall hydration, as Bowen works better if the tissues – particularly fascia – are well hydrated). I ask questions pertaining to a patient's energy levels as this is crucial to the amount of Bowen work a patient will be able to take. Often the energy levels in this patient group are very low and so one approaches them in a very cautious manner. The Bowen adage of 'less is more' is critical to this group since they will certainly not trust a therapist who causes them pain or gives them an overreaction.

Medical history

The medical history is usually long and painstaking. Numerous investigations have often taken place, usually with no confirmed diagnosis or abnormality found. There are often frequent injuries going back to childhood. There is pain and poor sleep. Many body systems are involved. All the while there is an undercurrent of fear and anxiety, and depression is never far away. Some may even be weepy upon presentation. These people are often intelligent and have high-performing work histories or are high achievers. They want to understand why they are in such a bad state of health and whether I am going to be able to help them. At this point, if I have any inkling that there is a possibility of EDSIII, I might surreptitiously conduct a Beighton/Brighton score and make notes. We discuss previous hobbies and interests, and it frequently transpires that in those I suspect of hypermobility syndrome or EDSIII there is a history of interest in dance or performing arts, where there is a high prevalence of hypermobility (Bird 2004; McCormack *et al.* 2004). I sometimes press them to find out if they know whether they are mobile or not – this is easily done by just asking them whether they could do the splits or achieve any interesting body postures, either now or in the past (see Appendix 1). I have usually observed that they are by this point; I just need to hear this from them. Depending upon their knowledge I might mention the word 'hypermobility' to them if they weren't already aware of it. At this stage I don't take things any further for the obvious reasons that I am not a medical doctor and I want to see what else emerges from the first session or two before I take things any further (which would involve talking to them a little bit about EDSIII and that their GP would need to see them and refer them to a consultant rheumatologist). However, I would *only* do this if I thought the patient might be ready to hear it and was already quite aware of their hypermobility. However, even if they did present with a diagnosis of EDSIII or FM, the way in which I treated them (with that information) would be the same as if there were no confirmed diagnosis. It is worth noting I have referred a few patients on for diagnosis, not just for EDSIII, but for more sinister conditions where I suspected cancer and sent them for immediate medical referral. It would be professionally responsible and therefore essential for me to do this – and has been life-saving on more than one occasion.

Many of the EDS, chronic pain patients present as frightened and anxious. They have been rejected and ridiculed by many other medical professionals and therapists and some have been told their problems are psychosomatic. They have not been believed. They have to invest so much trust in a new therapist and then they very often become exhausted in having to tell their very long and complicated stories again – and why are you (as a medical professional/therapist) going to be any different to all the others? Thus it is easy to see why the psychology in treating this patient cohort is so important. They need to be listened to very carefully and spoken to in a very gentle and reassuring way. They need to tell their story and are often anxious that you believe it and believe in them. Having had some counsellor skills training I often find that reflecting back to them what they have said is a helpful strategy – 'So when Dr X said you had Y, what happened next?' or 'How did you feel about that?'

We discuss previous treatments and what has helped/what hasn't. There is often anger at the way the medical profession have treated and dismissed them. They are frequently on many different types of medication and the crux of the matter seems to be that many are not very effective. As discussed in Part II, the physiology and homeostasis of these patients is often lacking. They don't sleep, they can't excrete properly. Their quality of life is very poor. Yet despite all of this there is an underlying streak of hope that makes them press on in their quest either for a cure or indeed for something that will help them. When we reach this point I have to be honest and say that they are presenting with many things and that Bowen therapy might help with sleep, energy levels and perhaps pain. As with any treatment there is no guarantee of success, but if they sleep better, or have less pain in any particular area or better energy, for example, then this would be an indication and an objective measure that the Bowen therapy is effective.

Preparing for treatment

When I further explain Bowen, and that the work is very gentle, they are often quite happy as many of them have been badly hurt by other therapists – especially osteopaths and chiropractors who have handled them roughly and caused them more pain – particularly if they have had manipulation. I am able to reassure them that Bowen is very gentle, with breaks in between each series of moves so the body can rest and respond to the work. When my patients are lying on the couch (they start lying prone) we ensure they are comfortable – so use of pillows or anything else that ensures their comfort is paramount. For those unable to lie on a couch, it is possible to treat patients seated. The ambiance of the room is important. The lighting is very low so as not to arouse the sympathetic nervous system – this is absolutely essential in this group as they sometimes present in a 'startled' way. There is no music in the background. I wrap my patients with towels/rugs and make sure they are warm and, most importantly, feel safe. Compared to other patients who usually fall asleep (or are at best very relaxed after a few Bowen moves) this group very rarely settle. They are usually looking around the room (even lying prone).

When I come back into the room having left them for a few minutes (to allow the body time to rest and for the muscle spindle feedback mechanism to respond) they might start to talk to me again, but I discourage any further dialogue since this means they are not relaxing and disengaging. I ask them to keep any questions for the end of the session. I am, however, interested if they suddenly become very cold or hot or appear to be reacting to treatment. If they suddenly report many sensations then this is a time for me to stop and leave them for a much longer time. I explain carefully to them that we are interrupting a physiological response and that it is deterimental to give the body even more information when it is already processing something.

By the time we get to the end of the treatment, which may be quite short in the beginning with such patients, they have usually visibly calmed down and look less startled and anxious and 'more in their bodies'. We then discuss sensations they might have experienced and how this feels. They are usually happy because the Bowen work has not caused them pain and I have been very gentle with them, so their fear of touch is reduced. We discuss after-care, which involves drinking more water, avoiding sitting for too long (so the body has time to adjust to any alignment changes, since Bowen primarily addresses the fascia), and trying to walk a little over the coming days. This sometimes worries them a little, but I just request they try to do what they are comfortably able to manage.

Contact between sessions

The chronic, complex patients are by far the most likely to make contact within the week between treatments. They might also contact me by phone. Sometimes this is because they are worried about a flare-up of a new symptom or because they are able to tell me they slept better. When they reappear for treatment they are often more difficult to assess for progress than any other patient group. They are quite negative and sometimes can't see their own progress. For example, if in their first appointment they said their lower back pain was the worst thing for them and then in the second appointment they say 'I still have headaches', 'I am still not sleeping well', 'My bowels are bad', 'I am feeling depressed', etc., then I ask them about their back and they will casually say, 'Oh, that hasn't hurt much this week.' I can then say, 'Oh, well that is an improvement then!', and then they can see that too. They nearly always present with a new symptom in the second appointment, or one they forgot to mention in the first session. I often find that their pain 'bounces' about the body from session to session, which makes it hard to track very easily. One symptom might improve against another declining. It is difficult. After a few sessions (three or four) I will ask them how they are finding Bowen. I have no wish to keep treating a patient for whom there is no improvement or response. I have mostly found (though, of course, not always) that they like Bowen and have found the work gentle and that has helped a little bit with some of their symptoms (e.g. sleep, perhaps IBS). Then they are happy to continue or perhaps have treatment once a month owing to financial constraints and the fact thatBowen is only covered by one health cash-back plan.

Patients intuitively seem to like and trust me. I am always honest with them. If I felt it better to refer them on to someone else or a different therapist, I would explain this carefully to them. People cannot afford to pay for treatments that are not helping and I do not wish to waste patients' money. Trust is absolutely essential in this patient group. This patient group is complicated, and I am not afraid of this, but understand why they come with so much psychological baggage. They will need careful listening and time – I often allow more like 75 minutes for these patients – particularly in their first appointment.

Leading EDSIII physiotherapist Rosemary Keer writes the following in terms of both communicating with and listening to patients with EDSIII, which also backs up my own therapeutic comments in working with this patient cohort and my own experience (described in Chapter 16) as a patient.

COMMUNICATING AND LISTENING
Rosemary Keer

Communicating
Patients frequently come with a history of problems covering many years. Additionally they have often seen numerous professionals, often with little tangible success. They are angry, frustrated and have a lot to say or shout. Any therapeutic intervention will get off to a better start if the patient is allowed to tell their story. It is often beneficial to extend the duration of the appointment to allow sufficient time. It may be helpful to encourage the patient to write a list of all the salient points in chronological order and send this to the therapist

ahead of time. This allows the therapist to obtain a good overview before meeting the patient and the consultation can then focus on gaining further insight and detail on the particular points they feel are important.

We also know that there is greater benefit and cost effectiveness when patients, who expressed a preference, received their preferred treatment (Preference Collaborative Review Group 2008). It may be that their preferred treatment is not appropriate or possibly even contra-indicated. In this case the therapist will need to engage the patient in a discussion on the topic to decide on more appropriate treatment. Nevertheless, it should be a joint decision based on the best available evidence.

Communication, while rated very highly in a qualitative study exploring perceptions of physical therapy in chronic low back pain (Cooper, Smith and Hancock 2008), is fraught with misunderstandings, amply illustrated by a cartoon appearing in *Vertebral Manipulation* by G. Maitland (1986): 'I know that you believe you understand what you think I said, but, I am not sure you realise that what you heard is not what I meant!'

It is often a good idea for the therapist to repeat back to the patient a précis of what they think the patient has said, to ensure that what was said was indeed what was meant. It is also very reassuring for the patient to get concrete evidence that the therapist has a good understanding of their problems.

Giving a patient time to ask questions, to talk about their fears and worries, can be very revealing and invaluable in directing treatment.

Listening

Listening involves communication, both verbal and non-verbal. Picking up on key words and knowing how to establish a rapport with our patients are important components of effective communication. But in the busy medical world, it would appear that we are not always very good at it. As Geoff Maitland wrote in 1986: 'it is amazing how often doctors and physiotherapists do not listen, nor listen carefully enough, nor listen sensitively enough, nor listen at sufficient depth to their patients'.

Listening is an art. Listening is active not passive, and we should give it sufficient attention to gain as much insight into the patient's problem as we can.

Hypermobile patients frequently have long and complex histories. Conversely, they may appear to look well and move well (Keer 2003) and so their physical examination can often be at odds with their physical complaints. In many cases this can lead to reports of patients feeling that they are not believed, having their complaints dismissed, ignored or worse labelled with a psychological disorder with comments such as 'it is all in the mind' (Child 1986). A survey of UK-based consultant rheumatologists carried out in 2000 (Grahame and Bird 2001) would seem to concur with these reports, finding that 72 per cent of respondents did not consider joint hypermobility syndrome to be a major contribution to the overall burden of rheumatic disease. This current text and others over the years (Gurley-Green 2001; Hakim *et al.* 2010; Keer and Grahame 2003; Knight 2011; Tinkle 2008, 2010) are slowly changing these perceptions, but ultimately we must believe our patients' subtle comments and remarks. 'We must listen, we must search and we must believe' (Maitland 1986) is a catchphrase we should all adhere to.

'Physiotherapists allow me to play an active part in my treatment and have taught me to use my muscles to protect my joints' (Gawthrop *et al.* 2007). Every person is an individual, and although many individuals will have the same diagnosis, it is how it is affecting them, their life, essentially their story, that is the important feature. Working *with* the patient will ensure greater compliance, self-esteem and satisfaction and ultimately better results.

CHAPTER 16

The physiotherapist and patient relationship

Dear Physiotherapist

I have often wondered why this book wasn't called *Dear Physiotherapist* because, from my point of view, I had written my physio so many letters and emails over the past three years, not to mention blog entries. Of course, when I very first met my physio in April 2008, I had no idea just how important and significant she would become in my life as my time in physiotherapy unfolded.

I very clearly remember my first appointment with my physio, when I produced an A4 piece of paper outlining my previous injuries and traumas. I recall my physio assessing me, as one might expect, but then giving me a series of exercises to do. I don't remember her doing any 'hands on' physical work on me, but unbeknown to me at the time I had put out a very strong message that my physio was not to work on me 'hands on'. However, during my first appointment I instantly remember liking my physio straight away. She had a very warm and welcoming manner and she listened carefully to what I had to say – even as a body worker myself, I was oblivious to the complexity of my case and how my presentation with a (by then) healing grade 2 medial gastrocnemious tear of the right calf was the least of my physio's worries. I was prescribed exercises to do and, after that first appointment, there was an interval of approximately four to six weeks before my next appointment. This was in part owing to my financial situation at that time, and I had no health insurance. So let us reflect upon what makes the beginning of a patient/therapist relationship so important.

Rapport and communication

As Keer wrote in Chapter 15, communication is very important. The way that the physiotherapist greets the patient sets the whole tone for the way in which the therapeutic relationship begins. Smiling, being friendly, making eye contact and using open body language are crucial starting points before any therapeutic work even starts. The ambiance and environment of the clinic room are all important, including the hygiene of the physiotherapist (Potter, Gordon and Hamer 2003b). The physiotherapist showing an interest and listening, as Keer also suggests in Chapter 15, are vital skills which are essential in gaining the trust and confidence of the patient. A qualitative study conducted by Hemmings and Povey (2002) highlights the importance of a positive attitude and good listening skills as highly important skills in physiotherapists in their research surveying the perceptions of chartered physiotherapists in England with respect to the psychological content of their practice. Qualitative research conducted by Potter, Gordon and Hamer (2003a), involving group interviews with a cohort of 26 patients, indentified some common themes in what patients viewed as 'good' physiotherapy, in terms of their experience of private physiotherapy. Common themes included:

> listening, body language, building trust and demonstrating empathy…that the physiotherapist was caring, friendly and inspired confidence…that the physiotherapist put the patient first…that the physiotherapist was punctual and created a pleasant and welcoming environment within the practice… [and that] the physiotherapist was clean and hygienic.
>
> *Potter et al. 2003a, p.197*

This was all before diagnosis and treatment. With respect to what constituted 'good' physiotherapy, responses were defined in three main categories. 'These were the physiotherapist's communication ability, other attributes of the physiotherapist, and the characteristics of the service provided by the physiotherapist' (Potter *et al.* 2003a, p.197). If this paper provided a benchmark for what patients defined as 'good' physiotherapy, then my physio modelled being a 'good' physiotherapist.

I have encountered some 'bad' physiotherapy in the past. Indeed, Potter *et al.* write that 'the main commonality of bad experiences related to the service provided and then ineffective communication skills on the part of the physiotherapist' (2003a, p.200). However, the research is based on private practice, and my prior experience of physiotherapy had been within the NHS, and it might have been time constraints that were the primary problem in dealing with a patient as complex as myself. Six sessions of physiotherapy, whenever I managed to obtain six sessions, were a drop in the ocean compared with what I needed. I was also frequently treated by different physiotherapists within multidisciplinary teams. The physiotherapists were not 'bad' people by any stretch of the imagination, and some were doing the very best they could, reflectively, but frequently they had no positive effect on my pain, or at times made detrimental comments that I have never forgotten, such as 'your back is horrendous'. When progress was made, I was simply discharged from the service and then just put 'back into the system'. Nobody (at the time) ever asked what I hoped to get out of treatment or what my treatment goals were.

Patient-centred physiotherapy

I believe that aside from having good interpersonal skills, my physio was a successful physiotherapist because she worked with a very patient-centred approach, and wanted to know my treatment goals. Potter *et al.* explain, with respect to patient-centred physiotherapy, the importance of gaining an understanding of the social and psychological context of the patient's world rather than just focusing on diagnostics. They write that 'a key issue in the success of a patient-centred approach involves the practitioner and patient reaching a mutual understanding of the problem as well as goals and priorities for management.' (2003a, p.195). This is where my physio was originally successful. My physiotherapist wanted to know what I wanted from treatment, and goal-setting was an important component, as discussed in Chapter 17.

Goal-setting and patient review

My physio knew from the very first time that she met me that my goal was to get back to doing allegro in classical ballet classes, following my calf tear. These are some reviewed goals almost two years into treatment.

Isobel's goals in physiotherapy

New goals

Short-term (acute)

1. Manage neck pain and headaches.

2. Fatigue (resulting from the above) and resultant upper body/'hand' pain.

3. Improve upper abdominals and neck stability.

4. Knee tracking – constant clicking of both knees, particularly left.

Medium-term

1. Further improve lumbar spine stability at hinging level (go even deeper than I am now – will need time).

2. Develop mobility in thoracic spine whilst continuing to strengthen cervical spine.

3. Continue to develop strength in gluteals, hamstrings and adductors so calf release can begin.

4. Shoulder stability/arm strengthening work

Long-term/future

1. Improved overall functioning with less fatigue.

2. Greater control and stability in my most hypermobile areas.

3.   More flexibility in the tighter areas.

4.   Able to manage 'full' allegro again in ballet (this goal is still not yet attained).

Blog, 26.3.2010

It was not until almost three years later that I realised that my physio needed to keep up a certain level of pretence with me with respect to my goals (which I was achieving to a certain degree) because it was a way in which she could continue to motivate me whilst we were generally rehabilitating me for basic postural functions such as sitting and standing. My physio was not being devious. I was simply incredibly unrealistic in my expectations, which made me very complicated to deal with, so we were dealing with a complete dichotomy. On the one hand my physio was getting me to sit up properly and I wanted to be able to do something on completely the other end of the movement and motor spectrum. Classical ballet is one of the most sophisticated and complicated forms of dancing. It was a huge gap to bridge. However, we were still working towards this end goal, and despite everything, I was already successfully managing to jump (at some level) by the second year of treatment.

Patient review

All medical professionals will have their own way of recording patient progress, usually bound by NHS regulations or the regulations outlined by their own body of practice (e.g. the Chartered Society of Physiotherapists). Goal-setting could be a useful strategy, keeping the treatment plan very patient-centred. (See Appendix 2.)

In addition, I also decided to create a SWOT analysis (strengths, weaknesses, opportunities and threats) as another way to monitor my progress and identify continuing difficulties/threats as they emerged (see Table 17.1).

TABLE 17.1: Isobel Knight's 'SWOT' analysis	
Strengths	**Weaknesses**
• How far I have come. • Inner strength and resilience despite what I sometimes think. • Expertise of my physio. • Local medical expertise – e.g. Prof G/B. • Personal expertise and research. • Team support from Pilates and ballet teacher. • I am ambitious and stubborn(!)	• Time. • Change in body is hard to cope with and feels chaotic and disorganised. • Lack of understanding from others – lack of support. • Feeling frightened and lonely during difficult metamorphosis periods. • Wonder how far I am going? • I work too hard and don't like rests. • Pacing!
Opportunities	**Threats**
• How the 'end' result will improve overall life quality and functioning.	• Time taken and personal cost (and financial). • Ever feeling or being completely normal. • What happens next?

Dr Andrew Lucas, consultant lead health psychologist, explains below his approach to goal-setting in his work with patients at the Royal National Orthopaedic Hospital.

GOAL ATTAINMENT SCALING: THERAPEUTIC USE OF GOAL-SETTING IN ENCOURAGING AND MEASURING IMPROVEMENT
Dr Andrew Lucas

It is essential that patients are discharged with a clear plan to achieve further progress, and at the Royal National Orthopaedic Hospital we utilise a method called *Goal Attainment Scaling* (GAS) (Kiresuk, Smith and Cardillo 1994). This is a technique for goal-setting, and typically patients will set goals around physical exercise, stretch, pursuing activities of daily living, hobbies and interests, but also goals to improve communication and assertion skills. GAS allows for multiple individualised goals and the conversion to standardised scores, which allows for direct comparisons between individuals or groups of patients. GAS also allows for calibration of degrees of success, recognising partial attainment of a goal, as opposed to the 'all or nothing' approach of other goal-setting approaches.

Goals can reflect different disciplines and can be functional, physical or psychological; for example, goals can be set to increase activities around the house, improve walking tolerance and showing less anger towards a partner by shouting less often. An example of a completed goal sheet is shown in Figure 17.1 and is taken from my clinical practice.

Goal Sheet

Name A. Jones	Therapist A. Lucas	Discharge date 15 June 2012	Follow-up date	
	Goal 1 Increase walking	Goal 2 Improve function	Goal 3 Socialising	Goal 4 College course
-2 Much less than expected	Can walk less than 20m unaided	Never wash and dress independently	Sees friend less than 1 × monthly	Give up any hope of going to college
-1 Somewhat less than expected	Can walk 20–39m unaided	Wash and dress 1–2 times a week independently	Sees friend 1 × monthly	Wants to investigate college course
0 Expected level of outcome	Can walk 40–59m unaided	As above 3–4 times weekly	Sees friend 2 × monthly	Visit college and collect prospectus
+1 Somewhat more than expected	Can walk 60–79m unaided	As above 5–6 times weekly	Sees friend 3 × monthly	View prospectus and decide on course
+2 Much more than expected	Can walk 80m unaided	Wash and dress every day independently	Sees friend 4 × monthly	Arrange to start course and do it!

FIGURE 17.1: EXAMPLE OF COMPLETED GOAL SHEET

The multidimensional nature of EDS/HMS needs a flexible individualised measurement tool that focuses on patient priorities. It could be argued that GAS meets the criteria for such an instrument. GAS provides meaningful information, is relatively easy to use and does not require expensive technology. GAS has been shown to be useful in both programme evaluation and clinical and therapeutic settings (Fisher and Hardie 2002).

As well as making treatment as patient-centred as possible (see Chapter 16) and focusing on patient goals, the therapist also needs to build trust in working with the patient, as can be seen in Chapter 18.

CHAPTER 18

Trust

I tested my physio to the limit, but I believe I had a reason to do this. In the past, almost all medical professionals have either given up on me, or failed to address or manage my resultant symptoms. Some had run a mile ('your back is horrendous'). To her great credit, my physio worked with me for a considerable length of time. I had perhaps tested her as a leap of faith, without having this level of devious thought – it is just that I expected her to consider abandoning me just as everyone else had in the past. Potter *et al.* write that patients with behavioural problems tend to be more problematic and 'deliberately deviant' (2003a, p.58). These (behavioural) patients, they argue, are difficult related to the extra time required to treat patients with multiple physical problems and the pain associated with multiple injuries. Over time, I let down my guard and allowed my physio into my complex life history and multisystemic symptoms.

I believe that my physio was so successful with me because she listened to me and gained my trust. She was extremely positive, which spread into other areas of my life, gradually improving my self-confidence – certainly in a physical sense, if not yet in a mental capacity. I became more confident about my body and started to show some control over my body rather than constantly being at the mercy of it. My physio listened to me, which had been crucial in my case, far more than she might have realised. As a result I eventually shared with her things that I had not discussed with other medical professionals before because I didn't think they could help (e.g. night-time micturition). I believe that she took a very patient-centred approach in her work with me and she tried very hard to gain a social and psychological context of my world rather than continuing to focus on the diagnostic process (Potter *et al.* 2003a, p.195).

EDSIII physiotherapist Rosemary Keer comments on the importance of trust in the context of working with EDSIII patients.

TRUST

Rosemary Keer

Trust is an essential component of the patient–doctor/therapist relationship. The patient wants to feel confident that they will be listened to, that they will be believed and that the doctor or therapist will have some understanding of their condition. They need to feel safe – in the knowledge that their fears won't be dismissed and their joints won't be pushed harder or further than they are comfortable with.

The therapeutic intervention should be a partnership between the patient and the therapist. No one person has all the answers and no one knows their own body better than the patient. A therapist who shows patience, interest, compassion and an openness to learn will encourage patients to engage fully in the rehabilitative process and not be fearful of saying how they feel. There is no magic bullet here; finding what form of treatment or exercise works for someone can be a case of trial and error. Many hypermobiles have lost confidence in their body's capabilities. But in a sense they have the answers. They need to listen to what their body is telling them and try to convey this to the therapist. The therapist, through an active process, listens and interprets what is being said and in the light of their experience and knowledge works with the patient to solve their problems. The solutions or suggestions have to make sense to the patient in order that they can confidently work with them.

Amanda Sperritt, describing what it is like to live with EDSIII, amply illustrates this when she writes: '…the most helpful professionals treat me as a partner in the management of the condition…listen… support…help…make life that bit easier' (Gawthrop *et al.* 2007).

CHAPTER 19

The challenging patient

By my own admission I could certainly be classed as a challenging, perhaps 'difficult' patient. Below are some examples of my behaviour:

I was jumping before my ballet teacher got there and doing split runs before I had even warmed up. I was being outrageous. I can be quite (ahem) rebellious! If someone asks me to go right, I will go left and I can be incredibly stubborn and difficult to move. I suppose my behaviour is quite defensive at times, but sometimes I am bloody minded and just determined to do things, at whatever cost!

Physiotherapy, 5.1.2011

My body is very naughty – it is like a naughty child. As soon as you want to go in and do something else with it, it turns round and says, 'no', I am not having any of it!

Physiotherapy, 1.3.2011

In a qualitative study about difficult patients in private practice, Potter *et al.* (2003b) describe key characteristics of difficult patients including those with complex medical problems, social and environmental factors and patient behaviours (e.g. demanding, manipulative). Thirty-seven physiotherapists took part in the study and a number of difficult patient behaviours were identified, including:

patients who had an inability to rest and overdid things... patients who arrived late...dependent patients who expect us to do everything for them...patients with bad experience of other physiotherapists...[and] patients who think they know more than you do.

Potter et al. 2003b, p.57

One key theme to emerge from this research was that difficult patients required more time and that those with behavioural problems were more difficult to deal with than those with complex medical problems. Furthermore, more time was required with those with multiple physical problems and injuries (Potter *et al.* 2003b, p.58).

Physiotherapy contract

I came up with and created this sample contract that a physiotherapist could possibly use and adapt. Unfortunately I never shared this document with my physio at the time, but it could have been useful had I done so with mutual agreement to a respected contract.

Physiotherapy contract, March 2011

I, Isobel Knight, will try to:

- self-manage standard symptoms and pain using the appropriate resources (including medication) in between physiotherapy sessions

- avoid unnecessarily texting and emailing my physio unless there is an out-of-context emergency or acute incident resulting in a new or a different trauma (e.g. ending up in hospital)

- respect my physio's right to privacy and time out from my case, including vacation/weekends when she is otherwise unavailable to me

- in an emergency seek advice from other medical professionals/present to A&E, as appropriate within the context of the situation

- negotiate with my physio the type of psychological/ emotional support that she is comfortably and clinically able to offer me at an appropriate time

- look at my other resource banks/alternative support bases to avoid unnecessarily fatiguing my physio but not seek other physiotherapy, unless my physio is away and I am in crisis.

I, Physio, will try to:

- avoid introducing IK to particularly new/risky movement patterns that are likely to cause flare-ups or acute symptoms when either she or I are going to be unavailable for support (e.g. vacation times)

- support IK as I continue to challenge psychological and physical patterns that are likely to be either raw for her or new movement patterns that are likely to cause temporary chaos

- support IK towards greater independence of self-management (in line with what IK is going to try and do), to avoid feeling guilty if IK ends up in pain or crisis when I am unavailable to her and IK feeling guilty for needing support and help from me

- continue to support IK with behaviour modification in physiotherapy (e.g. not jumping off couches) and, as appropriate, in the wider context (e.g. work/life)

- tell IK when it is not appropriate for her to contact me (e.g. vacation) and to remind her about email overload, if required again, and reset boundaries.

A sample contract can be found in Appendix 2.

Timing

Keer wrote in Chapters 15 and 18 that EDSIII patients often require a lot of time. I have often needed a great deal of time from my physio, which must have been at times hugely overwhelming for her. Eventually we crossed the time barrier and during my third year in treatment I started to have 'double' physiotherapy sessions. However, this hardly made up for the huge demands I otherwise placed upon my physio in terms of emailing or by requesting her to keep up with my online blog. The other reasons I have needed so much more 'time' are that my condition is very complex, and even reporting back my weekly subjective (see Table 19.1) update took a good 5 to 10 minutes before treatment for that session could commence.

TABLE 19.1: Extract from subjective update		
Acute summary	**Musculoskeletal**	**Sleep**
Mild fatigue on Saturday, this is a pattern. I also link feeling overwhelmed with fatigue. • Calves!! • Temporomandibular joint (TMJ). • Left knee. • Upper traps. I am calmer than I was, so much so I feel I am out of adrenalin. Weird.	All is quiet on the Western front. Left knee clicky. You will have to go back whence you came on that! TMJ!! Lumbar spine etc. all much better. Neck OK. Tsp OK! ☺	Better, and had Friday night with no drugs, slept 7 hours, went back again for another 2 and still woke feeling tired and un-refreshed. Had to sleep again after being up 2 hours!! (Fatigue.) Slept on the way to ballet! (Should I have gone??) ☺ Bladder – better.
POTS/asthma	**Skin/harm**	**Chronic**
Throat sore again (really low down) and dry cough again. This keeps coming back.	Self-harm is ongoing, but not significantly worse. Back is a mess.	Left eye spasm.
Exercise	**Ballet**	**Digestive**
Doing well with new exercises. I can also do head-nodding, thoracic roll-down and adductors – so fighting all my demons. Neck ex with breathing is v difficult as can't keep the neck muscles active.	Leg in extension issues and jamming my first position. Grand battements devant much better – improved height owing to improved hip flexion. Doing significantly more demi-pointe and 2–2 feet allegro – probably explains calf pain.	Weight gradually going down. Digestion – was better but IBS bit worse again.
Gynaecology	**Psychology**	**Support**
Nil to report.	I think I am feeling strange because I actually have some control of my body. Highly significant!!! I spasmed whilst watching a film! Triggering images.	Calves, TMJ, ITB Sleep, IBS, etc.

Resultant rehabilitation has been very holistic and body-systemic, and all this needs to be accounted for in the session and for the physiotherapist to assess and produce an ongoing treatment plan. As a patient I am hugely aware that I demand a lot of attention and time, but that is because it is very difficult to discuss my hidden condition with anybody else who is either uninterested (when is it interesting listening to someone's ailments?) or because they really don't understand. My physio has had to endure me patiently and help me to piece together my very difficult body. Additionally, I had frequently been ignored and dismissed in the past by other medical professionals who had left me alone to try to assimilate any information, or cope with rejection and lack of understanding or empathy with very little support. My physio has had to manage years of my hidden and bottled-up feelings about my body. None of this is entirely realistic or actually possible within the constraints of the conventional 30-minute physiotherapy slot. It is therefore understandable in Potter *et al.*'s (2003b) paper that the time the 'difficult patient' demands requires thought by the physiotherapist who manages that patient and that putting them at the end of the clinic might be a reasonable solution.

Crisis support management plan

I came up with my own 'crisis support management plan' that can be found in Appendix 2. This is obviously personal to me – but it is a strategy other medical practitioners could develop with their own patients.

Complex medical problems

Unfortunately for my physio I had complex medical problems, multiple physical problems, injuries and psychological difficulties. As we built up more trust in each other, my physio was gradually able to begin to tackle some of my psychological and behavioural difficulties, which were also supported by my having Cognitive Analytical Therapy. However, she was doing most of this herself in listening to me and making appropriate and reasonable suggestions for ways forward. As her confidence increased, my physio was more able to tackle some of the odd behaviour I exhibited during physiotherapy sessions – for example I had a very bad habit of jumping off the couch without warning (more below), which was dangerous from her point of view as well as being very disconcerting. I gradually got better and asked her if I needed to move or to fidget, since I was constantly fidgeting, which must have made treating me very difficult indeed. There is no doubt that I fit into the category of 'difficult patient' by my own admission, and therefore my physio is to be congratulated for having stuck with me long after anyone else would have given up. I continue to be challenging for my present physio and we continue to work on reviewing my goals and fatigue-driven behaviours.

Working hands on

One of the greatest difficulties my physiotherapist had originally faced was in working 'hands on' with me, since unbeknown to me I put out a very strong message that this was not going to be a possibility. This was partly fear-driven because I had been hurt by previous manual therapists, and also because I didn't want my physio to work on my lower back, which I now considered to be 'stable' and relatively pain-free. This meant that she had to approach me in a different way, and started instead by giving me exercises, with physiotherapy sessions several weeks apart. This went on for some months before sufficient trust was gained and it became apparent that progress would be hampered without manual intervention.

I was also a challenge to treat because of other ways in which I behaved during physiotherapy (which all improved significantly over time). For example, as already mentioned, if I felt threatened or anxious about something or fearful in general, I sometimes jumped off the couch at inappropriate times. I also had some issues with bright lights. In the rest of this chapter I discuss some of my behaviour.

Jumping off the couch

At times I have physically jumped off the couch, which has potentially been dangerous, because if I was not wearing my glasses and I did not realise how high up the couch was, I have jumped off at my peril. My physio eventually started to assert some control in my escape from the couch and requested that I 'hold on'. The extracts below are summaries of incidents during physiotherapy treatments:

(Working on a trigger point) Don't jump off the bed…I won't…
Well done, well done!

Physiotherapy, 5.1.2012

As my physio was working into my left thoracic spine, T8, observing that Left T1 was 'horrible' I said ouch and looked liked I was about to jump off the couch. My physio said that we need some control and that I now had to do as she requested – it being a New Year's resolution!

Physiotherapy, 5.1.2011

I asked my physio if I could get off the couch because things hurt, I felt out of control and needed to earth myself. I said it all felt horrible and that my calf felt as though it was going to go into cramp. The interesting thing about this was that my physio had been releasing subscapularis and latissimus dorsi, which had certainly had a curious effect!

Physiotherapy, 2.6.2011

Darkness/light

I find bright lighting in a treatment session very stressful. Bright lighting didn't bother me during my early physiotherapy sessions when I wasn't having 'hands on' treatment, but it certainly began to stress me out, especially when my physio worked on my neck, TMJ or face. I felt very exposed in those areas and overwhelmed and wanted to hide away. I frequently felt a need to hide or escape during treatment – when sensations become too intense for me or perhaps too difficult to cope with, I found myself wishing I could either hide under the couch or simply run away.

I asked if we could have the lights switched off. We discussed the reasons people don't like bright lights – or can be hypersensitive to it. My physiotherapist said it was fine to lower the lights!

Physiotherapy, 13.1.2011

My physio asked me if I wanted the lights off. I decided I did. We discussed how I was now funny about that and that it had now become 'one of my things' when it hadn't been in the past.

Physiotherapy, 8.2.2011

Heightened sensitivity and pain response and fear

Quite often, whenever I felt 'threatened' or my physio did anything that related to my calves, including any intention of palpation of them, I would simply cross my legs just like a barrier. It was a strong piece of body language from my point of view, but as I now understand it, the pain overflow signals will constantly fire back into my calves because of their years of repeated micro-trauma. This was hypersensitivity as a result of changes to my pain system and sensitised sensation. It was another thing my physio had to work around.

> My physio asked me if I was alright because she noticed I was lying prone with my legs crossed. She wanted to understand why I did this. I explained that I did it to protect calf and so I could get more control over it. In the same session I asked her if I could get up and she said I could do whatever I liked. She sensed I didn't like what was going on. I admitted it was like running away, but I needed to earth myself. My physio commented I was now better about not running off!
>
> *Physiotherapy, 17.2.2011*

> My physio asked me if she was going to be allowed to palpate my calf, and I found it really awful so I crossed my legs. My physio asked if I could manage not to do that since this was going to make it difficult for her to palpate them. It turned out this was one of the first times I had allowed her to palpate them (three years into treatment). She acknowledged I was doing incredibly well.
>
> *Physiotherapy, 1.3.2011*

Now, almost 18 months after my physio's original attempts to work on my calves, things are radically different, but this has taken a huge amount of time and trust.

> I had an interesting physio session today. My physio decided to work down my right lower limb and then up the left lower limb. He is working on various spiralling patterning in me. All this lower limb work involved a lot of calf work and I coped really well and in fact it was the first time for me that it was finally hardly an issue. I got through any difficulties with use of breath for relaxation. The fact that my physio had explained to me some weeks ago that my sensitisation of (an overly) sensitised

central nervous system aka chronic pain would bottleneck in my calves (due to previous traumas) has really helped me to understand when and why they become 'wired'. However it is a huge breakthrough that I am now allowing my physio to work on them properly without throwing the kind of fit I would have done not so long ago. For me understanding things is the key to breaking through these kinds of issues. A lot of work has been done on the whole calf issue over the past few years. Latest measurement of calves now leave only 2cm between right (38cm) and left (40cm) legs. Our hope is to reduce this gap by a further 1cm, which would be normal.

Blog, 30.7.2012

In the next chapter, the difficulties of communicating to doctors are explored in relation to a series of real examples.

CHAPTER 20

The doctor/patient relationship and treatment of chronic complex patients

In a condition like EDS, and having 'chronic pain', there is often a strong psychological element at play which the medical profession seem to pounce on. This means that I have often been ignored in the past by many doctors and my plight has not been taken seriously, even when I have really been suffering. I am very definitely not the only patient who will have experienced this problem, but as soon as doctors get wind of previous medical problems and chronic pain, they stop looking for ways of treating the presenting symptoms, which is incredibly damaging and fatiguing for the patient. None of us wants to be a burden, but I have just as much right to request help from a doctor when I am in pain as the next patient, even with a complicated medical history. Locker (1997) suggests that individuals are encouraged into dependency to manage their condition, and supports living as normal a life as possible, and I agree with this, but the medical profession must also respect the individual who is the expert on their own body (Richards 2008). Part of the problem is that dramatic symptoms are more likely to receive prompt medical treatment and be interpreted as 'real' illness than less obscure symptoms (Scambler 1997). The difficulty for the 'chronic' patient is that sometimes the presenting symptoms are 'obscure' and difficult to verify scientifically, which leads the medical profession at times to be dismissive and at worst completely disregard the patient.

Examples of the doctor/patient relationship

The following are autoethnographical representations. The first forms the basis of a letter of complaint to a hospital, but the other two examples illustrate the complexity of dealing with a patient who suffers from chronic medical conditions and the apparent subsequent symptomatic mismatch.

Example 1

On the afternoon of Thursday 9 December 2010 I was sent to Hospital 'X' A&E by my physio owing to neurological symptoms and severe head and neck pain. I have a medical condition called Ehlers-Danlos (EDS) type III – hypermobility syndrome (EDSIII) which is a genetically inherited connective tissue disorder causing systemic collagenous tissue laxity and excessive joint range of movement. EDSIII is a multisystemic condition which causes chronic pain and frequent soft-tissue trauma owing to both fragile tissues and ligamentous laxity. The condition has a holistic effect, hence it is called a multisystemic condition, and asthma, irritable bowel syndrome (IBS), fluctuations in temperature, blood pressure and pulse rate, headaches, joint dislocations, bursitis and tendonitis are examples of some of the physical complaints related to this medical condition.

My physio suspected that I might have cervical instability, which is a clinical condition which might have been related to my EDSIII, since blood vessels can be compromised in EDS and even burst owing to tissue laxity in some forms of EDSIII (there are many different 'types'). I was sent to A&E as I had had a sudden onset of neurological symptoms which the physiotherapist was concerned about, notably severe nausea, blurred vision, extreme headache, dizziness, changes in temperature and pulse rate (which can also be related to EDS). Unbeknown to me at the time, my physiotherapist was concerned about the possibility that I might have a blood clot or some serious vascular incident. She sent a colleague to attend with me with instructions as to what the A&E doctors might check in her absence.

When I arrived at A&E I was struggling to walk, let alone sit upright owing to my tissue laxity and extreme neck and head pain. I arrived in a temporary cervical collar which I borrowed from work. The A&E doctor was not particularly pleasant or helpful and did not seem to treat my plight very seriously. In particular he was reluctant to talk to my physiotherapist who would have proved invaluable as she had treated me for over

2.5 years and knew me very well and would have been able to advise him on her informed medical concerns as to the nature of my condition and its sudden neurological change. It seemed to take some convincing to even request an X-ray and the doctor was very rough in examination with me. One of the problems is that many patients with EDS are very weak owing to poor muscle tone at the helm of the extreme tissue laxity. I struggled to do a 'push and pull' test on this day and it set me off having a series of other muscular spasms and twitches. I was also asked to do a urine test which seemed unrelated to the matter at hand, but I complied with this request.

I was strapped in a neck brace for the X-ray and when sent for X-ray the same doctor also roughly pulled my arms, which was too much for me. I was then sent back to the ward area whilst the results were processed. My colleague (who had accompanied me) had noticed a group of the doctors poking fun at EDS and saying 'they are the people who can do this' and showing the joint positions that some patients can manage to achieve. When the doctor came back he said that there were no subluxations in my cervical spine, although my cervical spine appeared to be 'very straight'. We did not need to know about subluxations since my physiotherapist already knew there were none. The doctor then said very publicly, in front of my colleague who had kindly attended with me, that I had a urinary tract infection (UTI) and that was why I was feeling sick and nauseous. One of the problems with EDSIII is that it can provoke the autonomic nervous system so that things such as bladder function might change – for example, one might pass urine more frequently, or pulse or blood pressure might change. I know that this is what had happened to me, not that I had a UTI (as was proved the next day when I attended Y Hospital, and no infection was found!). The doctor had no desire to find out any more about either myself or about my medical condition, or to speak to an expert (my physiotherapist) so that the correct tests could be carried out. He maintained that (correctly) he was the doctor (and I entirely agree), but he was not prepared to listen or to hear any more or to help with any of my symptoms or pain. I left the hospital feeling rather angry about his attitude, his lack of support or ability to listen, empathise or learn.

I was no better at all the next day and was sent to Y Hospital where I was treated with far better respect and taken far more seriously, the outcome being that I am now waiting for an MRI scan. A CT scan was conducted at Y Hospital and admission offered. The doctors there listened to me, sought advice from my physiotherapist and I was treated with compassion and dignity.

I thoroughly realise that EDSIII is a complex and chronic and rather specialist rheumatological condition, but surely it would have been all the more reason for the doctor to take my concerns seriously and to listen and investigate the complaint rather than insisting he was the expert. There are times when a patient becomes quite informed about their condition and what sort of advice and help they need. If I had already known I was well, there would certainly have been no need to bother your doctor or his team at A&E.

In order that EDSIII patients are better treated in the future, I would certainly be most happy to talk to your staff, or would suggest that they update their policy and treatment approach with hypermobile patients. I would therefore recommend that they might contact the Hypermobility Syndrome Association, or review the latest research on EDSIII hypermobility type. There was a recent publication called *Hypermobility, Fibromyalgia and Chronic Pain* (2010) by A. Hakim, R. Keer and Prof. R. Grahame. I would certainly like your team to review the way in which they treat EDSIII/EDS patients and hope that you will share my letter with them. I would be interested to receive feedback about this incident and an ongoing forward resolve.

Example 2

At the beginning of the year I managed to completely baffle my GP and local Accident and Emergency Dept. I had a very audibly wheezy chest and was given steroid tablets and increasingly stronger inhalers, but my 'peak flow', which measures lung capacity on exhalation, was not showing particularly low – my average reading seemed to be 350 (my usual reading is 500). After a few days of increasing steroid intakes and no major changes to my peak flow, but no changes to my wheezy chest, my GP put me on a nebuliser, measured my peak flow again, which had decreased, and then gave me a second nebuliser treatment. There was no change or improvement. She then decided to put me on a course of antibiotics and suggested I attended A&E if there were no further improvements. She was contemplating sending me there directly, but we decided to see if the antibiotics worked. My GP said she was quite puzzled by my lack of response to the nebulisers and even started to wonder if I was allergic to one of the drugs administered. The next morning I felt slightly worse again and so went to A&E, as advised. The A&E doctors were equally baffled. They could hear my very audibly wheezy chest and yet as before my peak flow wasn't disastrous. I mentioned that I had EDSIII, but they failed to make any connections between that and asthma. They questioned whether I was indeed experiencing asthma and discharged me without taking any further action. Two days later I returned to my GP and she sent me for a chest X-ray which was normal. I mentioned to my GP about EDSIII and an article I had found on asthma and airway collapse in heritable disorders of connective tissue (Bird 2007; Morgan *et al.* 2007) but my GP didn't seem to be particularly interested or could not make the connection. An informal discussion with my rheumatologist confirmed that the unusual peak flow and my slightly strange response to medication did seem related to the EDSIII and an increased lung capacity owing to systemic collagen laxity.

From Knight 2011

Example 3

A visit to my local Accident and Emergency Department ended inconclusively (again) at the helm of another EDS-related symptom. One day I was in a meeting at work and I was not feeling well. I was not caffeinated, stressed or anxious. During the middle of the meeting I felt a sudden surge of heat up to my brain followed by a change in pulse rate and temperature accompanied by immediate brain-fogging and feeling as though I had been put on 'pause'. I tried to continue the rest of the meeting as calmly as possible, but developed a sudden headache and feeling of 'pressure' in my head. I didn't know what was happening to me, but it was extremely unpleasant. I managed to complete my meeting and then had to go into another one almost straight away. I managed to conduct the second meeting in a matter of minutes and alluded to feeling unwell. I then managed to get back to the clinic rooms at work – working in the health department has its advantages. Several other things happened simultaneously. I began to have very large and systemic muscle spasms that again stemmed from my spine, and was twitching away. I felt extremely cold and was shivering (it was a very muggy July day) and became very clammy. Not feeling very comfortable about things, I asked one of my colleagues to sit with me and requested them to ask for two of the Pilates staff who knew about my muscle spasms and my condition in general. Very unfortunately, my physiotherapist was away.

The Pilates staff arrived and couldn't believe what they were seeing. I was arching all over the place right the way through my whole spine. It looked like I was having a major seizure. Sitting up seemed to improve things a bit, but the spasms and muscular 'twitches' continued. After a further hour with nothing stopping them and a very nasty headache, my colleagues felt that I should be checked out in hospital. I was generally very resistant to the idea because I didn't think that they would be able to 'do' anything. However, later, my colleagues disclosed they had anxieties about me because of the severe headaches and wanted to ensure that nothing more sinister was going on (stroke).

When we arrived at Accident and Emergency it was apparent that there was going to be a long wait – even early on a Thursday afternoon when nothing remarkable was surely going on! I was eventually given a thorough MOT and had an ECG done and full blood and infection counts done which were all normal. I was given a drip of fluids and salts and my urine was tested and revealed the beginnings of a possible infection, but nothing remarkable. Blood pressure was apparently normal including pressure taken on lying down and standing. There was nothing in my chemistry that could apparently account for this strange course of events, which were behaving in the manner of POTS. The doctors could not believe the spasms and had no idea what was causing them and why they were continuing so relentlessly. I had to convince them this was not a panic attack! They discharged me because this was Accident and Emergency and they had achieved their role in eliminating anything life-threatening or sinister. They suggested plenty of rest, painkillers and fluids and no work next day. They also suggested that my GP refer me to be reviewed by my rheumatologist sooner rather than later to investigate the cause of the muscle spasms. Yet again, this was another example of peculiar EDSIII-related symptoms, but a total lack of knowledge from medical doctors who were unable to allude to the cause and solution of muscle spasms and waves of twitches. I had known that it would be a waste of time in attending Accident and Emergency, but needed to appease my work of nothing more serious going on.

From Knight 2011

Clinical justification

In each situation it is not reasonable to criticise the medical profession for negligence – the doctors used the appropriate and conventional clinical methodology and testing which did not show anything 'wrong' as such, and yet there appears to be a complete mismatch. The patient attends the A&E department and has an array of symptoms. The testing outcome is normal and yet symptomatically something is very wrong, or at best 'abnormal'.

In the first example, a CT and later an MRI scan were clear and normal. However, symptomatically something is very wrong. The cervical spine is not functioning normally (see Chapter 36). There is profound ligamentous laxity and muscle weakness, yet these are not assessed in a medical examination. The reasons underlying the neurological abnormalities are not examined and a cause not found – other than conjecture that ligamentous laxity and muscle weakness are wholly responsible.

In the second example, it appears that the conventional medical measures for asthma are potentially inappropriate in these patients, or that different testing and measuring guidelines are required. The patient attends with severe wheezing symptoms which are not responding to conventional treatment; the patient is clearly symptomatic, but is not receiving the appropriate treatment to resolve the symptoms. The patient is discharged because the situation is not considered life-threatening, and yet symptoms persist.

In the final example, the doctors are clearly baffled by the situation and by what is happening in the case of the muscle spasms and twitches. Conventional medical testing rules out the possibility of anything life-threatening or sinister, but the patient's symptoms persist and she remains in distress. In sum, no one can really help her.

In the neck example there are functional abnormalities which are not uncovered by conventional testing. In the asthma example, the peak flow suggests a 'reasonable' reading, but the testing is inadequate in matching the level of wheeze and symptoms experienced by the patient, and in the third example, no testing can explain the patient's symptoms, but vital signs and testing – for example ECG – are all deemed clinically normal. (See Figure 20.1.)

EDS patient + conventional testing + 'normal' results = symptom mismatch

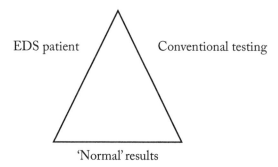

FIGURE 20.1: CONVENTIONAL TESTING AND SYMPTOM MISMATCH

The patient is clearly symptomatic but it appears that the medical testing for 'normomobiles' might not be appropriate and/or sensitive enough to measure in a patient with genetically inherited connective tissue disorders, where the collagens are abnormally lax systemically (Ferrell and Ferrell 2010). Does this therefore mean that the testing objective and criteria for the EDS patient need to be amended, for example in the case of peak flow measurements? Would EDS patients require different peak flow measures to reflect the tissue laxity which will be found in the lungs (Bird 2007; Morgan *et al.* 2007)? The way in which the medical profession addresses the management of EDSIII patients might require some revisions and further specificity given the continuance of the patient's symptoms. Further accounts of other patients' experiences of A&E suggest these are not isolated examples, but equally the medical profession cannot be entirely to blame; certainly not in their duty of care – it is rather more the case that conventional testing cannot always find the answers for all symptoms, or explain the occurrence.

The A&E system in particular needs to be aware of this type of patient and consider other ways of managing symptoms that might not be excluded by conventional medical testing. In the first case, the patient had severe neurological symptoms which were excluded by both CT and MRI, yet how can this be classified as normal when the symptoms were anything but 'normal'? On the part of the patient this leads to a feeling of failure, of being a burden to the system and being completely mismanaged. At worst she is considered as either a woman with anxiety, who is having 'panic attacks' (in the asthma example), or, in the third example, as a woman they can't really understand or help with what is going on. The patient is not in a life-threatening situation, so 'do nothing'. This patient group is frequently labelled as hypochondriacs, or their symptoms are 'psychosomatic', and yet clearly the doctors were aware something was going on: 'they could hear the audible wheeze in my chest' and 'observe the muscular spasm/twitches going on'. When such patients present at A&E, it might be that doctors need to consider additional and alternative approaches to management and look at actively managing the symptoms that have appeared, particularly where conventional measures appear to fail. Symptoms appear alarming and the patient needs help, but they are often discharged feeling psychologically worse than when they arrived at A&E. 'I knew it would be a waste of time', and with no resolution of the medical symptoms, it feels like medical mismanagement.

This is a really true and accurate representation of what is going on, and care is very poorly coordinated – particularly following on from A&E presentations (see Chapter 1).

Psychological consideration

Consultant lead health psychologist Dr Andrew Lucas writes the following about the psychological profile of EDSIII patients and working with them, including communicating with other medical professionals and, crucially, support for medical professionals working with the chronic complex patient. Patients most often only think of their own problems without factoring in the way they might come across to the medical professional they are facing and that medical professionals need support too. I now unhappily realise that I did not fully appreciate this in terms of both the physiotherapists who have worked so hard to support me. A little more thought from me (even in times of distress) might have been appreciated.

A PSYCHOLOGICAL PROFILE OF PATIENTS WITH EDS/HMS

Dr Andrew Lucas

Regarding the psychological profile, it has been reported that elevated anxiety and panic disorder has been found in EDS type III. A study by Bulbena *et al.* (2011) reported that joint hypermobility syndrome is a risk factor for developing anxiety disorders and was also found to be a risk factor for social phobia and simple phobia. They further reported that anxiolitic drug use was nearly fourfold higher amongst HMS sufferers compared to non-HMS participants. More precisely the increased risk of suffering from anxiety disorders in patients with HMS is 22 times higher than in non-HMS individuals. It has been hypothesised that the relationship between anxiety disorders and HMS may have a disautonomic basis when symptoms such as palpitations, light-headedness, hyperventilation and fatigue are commonly reported for individuals with HMS. Similarly, postural orthostatic tachycardia syndrome or POTS was reported in 78 per cent of the HMS participants compared to 10 per cent of controlled participants. The authors in the Bulbena *et al.* (2011) study strongly recommend screening for joint hypermobility in routine health assessment for teenagers and those in early adulthood.

I have compared the EDS/HMS group to my other patients with chronic pain, for example chronic low back pain. I collect data on the following domains: pain, pain-related disability, anxiety, depression, emotional distress, pain-related self-efficacy (self-confidence), fear avoidance and quality of life. The profiles are very similar apart from higher pain-related disability, lower pain-related self-efficacy (self-confidence) and poorer quality of life. This preliminary analysis suggests that patients with EDSIII report higher disability, lower confidence and poorer quality of life compared to other patients with musculoskeletal chronic pain.

There needs to be a description of the psychological sequelae of not being believed or being taken seriously, and these difficulties can begin at an early age. A common finding has been seen when the young patient complains of pain and dislocation or subluxation. The parents undertake a number of visits to health professionals when no major pathology was found. There was a danger of the patients being labelled as attention-seekers or suffering with a psychiatric illness. In my clinical work I have found, and not uncommonly, that many parents suffer guilt in following the advice of health professionals who simply told their child to get on with it. An extreme clinical example illustrates this well when a patient told me how she would be struggling to get out of bed to go to school, and her father, believing she was faking or exaggerating her symptoms, would pull her out of bed and order her to get dressed and go to school. This behaviour (although with the best intentions) actually increased subluxing and shoulder dislocation. Of course, in this situation the patient's father was simply doing what he thought to be the right thing in encouraging his daughter to go to school, and indeed was following the advice of the health professionals who described his daughter as 'an attention-seeker'.

One surprising feature of working with this patient group has been the increased occurrence of experiencing guilt compared to other patient groups. This guilt can often be felt by parents, who in hindsight now recognise that they could have done more to support their child, particularly during the teenage years. One can imagine that after taking your child to a number of medical consultations and who is then labelled as an attention-seeker, the advice to parents might be to ignore the symptoms and carry on as normal. In my opinion both patients and family usually cope in the best way they know how and do their best to make sense of a very difficult set of circumstances.

Patients with EDS/HMS can have their school years significantly disrupted, which in turn can have long-lasting consequences for their quality of life. It has been a surprise that in working with patients with EDS and their families time may need to be devoted to exploring and changing feelings of guilt and shame.

With regard to the psychological consequences of not being believed I have found that many patients with EDS/HMS are defensive and hypersensitive to being challenged. In particular, finding out that I am a health psychologist often fits into their previous experience of being dismissed or labelled as simply a psychiatric or psychological concern. During my first session I often have to spend time reassuring the patient that they have not been asked to see me because anyone thinks the pain is in their head or imagined. In order to move forward both patient and therapist will need to collaborate while being wary of making value judgements and erroneous assumptions. Unfortunately, some patients are too guarded and resistant to change, perhaps as a result of fighting for credibility, and so may sabotage the therapeutic rapport. I believe that ability to change is influenced by many factors, including the patient's own characteristics and behaviour. Conversely, no doubt at times I have shown a lack of compassion and understanding when becoming frustrated with what I perceive as 'difficult behaviour' that has also led to attenuating the therapeutic relationship. Clearly, greater understanding and improved communication on both sides of my desk would improve our outcomes.

Communication with health professionals

It is clear to me that many patients with EDS/HMS struggle for recognition and acceptance of their condition, particularly when, over the years, they have encountered health professionals who, at best, are sympathetic but unhelpful and, at worst, patronising and insulting. I firmly believe that in order to help patients move forward with their condition there is a clear need to communicate effectively and assertively with health care providers.

It can be imagined that if a patient has typically been dismissed from previous health care interactions they might bring a certain prejudice or attitude into any future consultations. This might be seen when the patient displays passive aggressive behaviour, for example being flippant or sarcastic in their replies to my questions. No doubt this type of behaviour can be seen in both health care provider and patient.

I often experience a new patient making erroneous assumptions about my role and involvement in their care, for example believing that I am there to confirm a mental health diagnosis or a label of attention-seeking behaviour. I find it helpful to describe my role as trying to support a patient in improving their coping style with a complex long-term condition. Patients are far better informed and may well come to the initial appointment with a file of printouts from various websites. I also adopt the position that it is patients who are most familiar with their condition, and in order to improve coping there needs to be a collaborative and shared approach. It is important for both sides in this collaboration to be open and respectful of each other's knowledge and experience.

Unfortunately, I have observed some patients who enter the consultation with an attitude that is both provocative and a barrier to effective communication, although I reject the notion of 'difficult patients' as it is pejorative, judgemental and labelling, and I prefer the term 'difficult problems'. For example, the patient tries to 'test me out', checking on my knowledge, experience and approach to treating patients with EDS/HMS. Some of my colleagues on the rehabilitation team have also observed such behaviour. It is almost as if the patient is deliberately trying to sabotage the consultation by trying to trick the therapist into showing weakness or lack of experience. The health care professional will be well advised to consider their communication style and be wary of making similarly erroneous assumptions and appearing judgemental, which might be considered provocative and put the patient in a defensive frame of mind. Effective communication must be a two-way process, with both sides playing their part in trying to maximise a successful outcome.

Supporting other health professionals working with EDS/HMS patients

The rehabilitation therapy team at the Royal National Orthopaedic Hospital changes every six months due to staff rotation. Some colleagues embrace the model and others struggle with the 'hands off' approach. Rather than relying on input from health professionals, the patients are encouraged to become self-managing with support from the health professions. Problems can occur when more experienced members may be resistant to new ideas introduced by less experienced or newer members of the team. Although staff rotation can be difficult, it can also be an opportunity to review the team dynamic and be an impetus for positive development. Orientating new members of staff is essential. Taking time to explain their specific role and those of the rest of the team, and how the team delivers the service, can help to integrate new team members.

Working in chronic pain management is very demanding, and it could be argued that 'burnout' is a risk factor for cohesive team working. Burnout in chronic pain settings can lead to high levels of absenteeism and high staff turnover (Spanswick and Parker 2000). Peer support helps to prevent burnout. Trying to help patients who can often be highly distressed, demanding and fearful can drain the therapist's own coping and leave them vulnerable to stress-related concerns. Many changes have occurred in the structure of the rehabilitation team, and clearly some colleagues find the work very rewarding while others struggle, are frustrated and may move on to other posts. New members may struggle adapting to working in a multidisciplinary team. There is clearly pressure to 'do something' when medical treatment options are limited. Some EDS/HMS patients consider the rehabilitation programme as their last chance for help, and this burden of responsibility can weigh heavily on members of the therapy team. Support systems should be available to help team members working with such challenging conditions and, in the words of Spanswick and Parker (2000, p.354) when describing patients with musculoskeletal chronic pain, 'cope with the emotional pressures that can occur when working with such a demanding group of patients'.

Effective communication skills are essential for cohesive team working, although colleagues have described how their unidisciplinary training has poorly equipped them and thus failed to enable them to develop such skills. The rehabilitation team have seen how patients can exploit a weakness in the team, such as poor communication. To offer support to my colleagues, I deliver in-service workshops to develop skills and reflect on practice, including 'Effective communication' and 'Dealing with challenging situations'. Conflict within the team is always possible and needs confronting and managing rather than retreating and ignoring the problem which can lead to fracturing, protectionism and suspicion, and ultimately compromise patient care. Interpersonal problems can occur when areas of professional overlap lead to conflict between different disciplines. Professional and interdiscipline rivalry can lead to a lack of respect for other disciplines' training and qualifications, or some members of the team perceiving themselves as more important than others. Fragmenting of the team can be avoided by ensuring good communication, controlling the size of the team and encouraging group cohesiveness by collaborating on service development (Spanswick and Parker 2000).

Robust structures and procedures can help the team deal with conflict. It has been found useful to devise clearly defined protocols and procedures and to agree the operating model of care delivery (Adams 1997; Parker, Dumat and Booker 2000). When difficult situations occur, I have encouraged debriefing and reflective learning as useful strategies for improving future practice. Encouraging all members of the team to be responsible for outcomes helps to ensure collaborative working. Time needs to be set aside for team development and team building, which can be achieved through staff training and ensuring effective communication channels. Effective communication can prevent many interpersonal problems, and early intervention can help resolve and improve communication problems. The dynamic within the team is constantly changing and needs monitoring to ensure good practice. Regular meetings can help avoid feelings of isolation, but equally can be frustrating when not productive. These meetings can enable individual team members to express concerns and develop improved practice by identifying the source of any concern and devising written strategies for resolution.

CHAPTER 21

Learning styles and learning 'difficulties'

So far, we have explored the therapeutic relationship in great detail – including communication, listening, trust, rapport, goal-setting, difficult and challenging patients and medical miscommunication, as well as looking at the psychological profile of EDSIII (and other chronic complex patients) and support for medical professionals. In this chapter we look at patient learning styles and learning difficulties, some of which are anecdotal difficulties whilst others (e.g. development coordination disorder or dyspraxia) are shown to be linked to EDSIII (Kirby and Davies 2007; Kirby, Davies and Bryant 2005). We start by exploring patient learning styles and how this has helped me personally in physiotherapy sessions.

Patient learning styles – using MP3

From September 2010, and in agreement with my physio, I decided that I wanted to audio-record some of my physiotherapy sessions. Partly this was because at that particular point in time there was so much going on in a POTS capacity during treatment and also because I thought it might be interesting just to see what was going on during treatment and if there was anything that we could use, perhaps in a research capacity or to share with other physiotherapists. In fact, the use of an MP3 audio recorder has proved incredibly valuable in many ways because my predominant learning sense is auditory. This meant that I could later play the recordings and extrapolate what I needed to do for the different exercises that my physio gave me. Hearing the instructions again reminded me exactly about what I needed to do. The recordings have also given me insight into my own behaviour at times and a permanent auditory record for my physio in the work that she has done on my body, particularly when extraordinary things have occurred.

Pritchard writes that:

> Auditory learners prefer to learn by listening. They have good auditory memory and benefit from discussion, lectures, interviewing, hearing stories and audio tapes, for example. They like sequence, repetition and summary, and when recalling memories tend to tilt their head and use level eye movements.
>
> *Pritchard 2009, p.45*

The use of MP3 has been so significant for me that it felt very important to alert other medical professionals to ensure that other learners' support needs are met during physiotherapy sessions as there are several learning styles encompassing visual learners who learn by seeing. This group might benefit from diagrams – for example of exercises issued during physiotherapy sessions (Pritchard 2009). Another group of learners, known as kinaesthetic learners, learn by doing. Pritchard writes that 'this group are good at recalling events and associate feelings or physical experiences with memory. They enjoy physical activity...and other practical first-hand experience' (Pritchard 2009, p.46). In a physiotherapy setting it is imperative that this group actually 'move' to learn movement or exercises that might be set as homework.

Learning difficulties

I was a late walker, and had been a bottom shuffler in terms of movement development. This is not uncommon in hypermobile patients (Maillard and Murray 2003). In terms of our family history, this was insignificant – but perhaps other things should have been picked up on. For example, apparently I had very poor hand-to-eye coordination and difficulties in writing and drawing. I also had many problems with using scissors, which appears is a common finding. Research by Kirby *et al.* (2005) showed that 66 per cent of 114 children experienced problems with using scissors and 69 per cent had difficulties with writing.

I love the report my art teacher wrote when I was 13 years old (see Figure 21.1). It was one reason why I gave up art classes at the time.

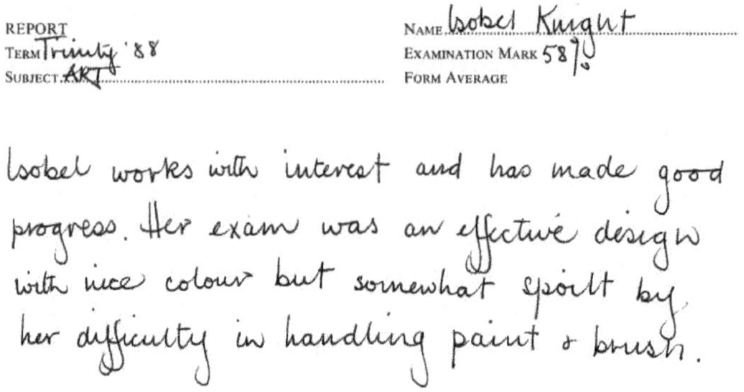

REPORT
TERM Trinity '88
SUBJECT: ART

NAME Isobel Knight
EXAMINATION MARK 58/0
FORM AVERAGE

Isobel works with interest and has made good progress. Her exam was an effective design with nice colour but somewhat spoilt by her difficulty in handling paint + brush.

FIGURE 21.1 ISOBEL'S ART REPORT FROM SCHOOL (AGED 13)

However, as well as art, my handwriting was, and still is, appalling. I have difficulty holding pens and cannot write for long at all without enduring fatigue. The coordination problems certainly link to development coordination disorder (DCD), and although it is not something I ever had, early research shows some prevalence of DCD amongst some EDSIII patients (Kirby and Davies 2007; Kirby *et al.* 2005). Indeed, and anecdotally, many patients seem to have movement difficulties, as other EDSIII patients have written on Facebook:

> I had dyspraxia. The only sport I could do was swimming. If I tried to run I would fall over, my ankles were so unstable. I could not catch a ball because my hand–eye coordination was so bad. I struggled with shoelaces and ties. Thankfully, I grew out of it but my hand–eye coordination still isn't the best.

> Dyslexic, and very clumsy! I was always falling over, but in other ways was always climbing and running everywhere! The world was my play ground! Lol!

> I was very clumsy in terms of gross motor skills but oddly my fine motor skills were/are excellent. My youngest is exactly the same: rubbish at PE, good at Art. My eldest has poor gross and fine motor skills and a diagnosis of dyspraxia. The one thing that is odd about her dyspraxia diagnosis (according to the OT) is that her visual skills were on the 75th percentile leading me to think this is fundamentally a bendy issue.

It has always amazed me that for someone who has such ineptitude in the sportsfield I can manage to do something as motor-controlled and as sophisticated as classical ballet. In my earlier book (Knight

2011) I wrote at length about classical ballet, and have less room to do so here, but I surmise that because of my hypermobility and therefore hip range of movement, lateral turnout is of little effort for me, and that my limbs achieve the lines and extensions required of classical ballet more easily than those without hypermobility. In this sense it is a great asset – but as to why I can coordinate myself in a ballet class and not on a sports field remained a mystery until I realised that music was possibly part of the key to managing this type of movement. I have been reading several of the renowned neurologist Dr Oliver Sacks' books with great interest, particularly *Musicophilia* (2011). There are a number of descriptions of people with movement disorders who suddenly become more 'organised' in a movement capacity when music is played. It is as if their tics or poorly executed movement patterns disappear or improve. In many ways this makes great sense. I am now managing to run, but I know I run 'even better' if I am listening to music at the same time, or something with rhythm – for example the sound of the waves on a beach.

I listen to music all the time – rhythm is organised, and I recall doing 'rhythmical handwriting' when I was at primary school. I managed to do this quite well and can only think it was the music that helped me. I type along to music in a similar way – if the music is appropriate. I know I have quite an amazing ear for music and can replicate tunes (usually on a recorder) or play along with them from memory. I can often tell what key a piece of music is played in and have a very strong sense of harmony. Although I have been taught to read music, I really struggle with it, so it was once a great surprise when I was presented with a piece of music and I looked at it as if it were a foreign language, and was then told, 'You just played that piece of music along to a CD five minutes ago!' I was stunned.

They say that music and mathematics go along together and that many people who are good at maths are also good at music. Here, I struggle. I don't think that dyscalculia existed or was very much known about when I was at school – people were beginning to become more aware of dyslexia, but dyscalculia and attention deficit disorder (ADD) were not really known about. Had they been, I would have certainly qualified for dyscalculia, and quite possibly dyspraxia or development coordination disorder (Kirby and Davies 2007; Kirby *et al.* 2005). I may have even qualified for ADD – but only because of the constant fidgeting. This may be the case for some EDSIII patients.

Coordination can be a problem for some EDSIII patients. I described doing a 'cat movement' exercise during physiotherapy:

> I was doing a cat-movement in physiotherapy. My physio had asked me to go back down in the movement and I moved away from her. She knew I hadn't liked it because I had disobeyed her – as often happened if I didn't 'like' doing something. However my physio knew I hadn't been deliberately defiant. She understood that at that moment I was pleasingly in the flow of movement and it was hard for me to stop, the realisation being that stopping mid-flow was more of a coordination problem for me.
>
> *Physiotherapy, 8.12.2010*

It is very fair to say that I found mathematics a great challenge and still struggle with my times table now – things that should be automatic are just not. Algebra held no logic at all for me – although I was better at geometry. I struggle with 'reasoning' and still can't cope with numerical work or other spatial concepts (e.g. map reading). I am, much to my own amazement, good with organising my own personal finances and can even manage financial computer packages, but statistics were a great challenge during my MSc and sometimes graphs I have selected to use at work have apparently been 'meaningless' in a data capacity – although I thought I did a great job with colourful graphs on Excel.

I find words so much more appealing and powerful – and I am a good communicator, so work with numbers as little as possible. I do not find them meaningful, and had a huge struggle to gain a GCSE grade C, which I needed in order to train as a primary school teacher (and rightly so). I had similarly to repeat my MSc statistics exam about three times in order to pass it. Whether this links at all into anything significant in terms of my brain-processing capacity and EDSIII I will not know. The following extract describes some of my thoughts about 'maths'. However, some other EDSIII patients also have similar specific problems with maths as well as with writing or dyslexia. Considerably more research is required into learning disorders or abilities and connective tissue disorders that do have links with movement difficulties – more understandably, DCD, but why not dyslexia or dyscalculia? I describe my anxieties in mathematics on the next page:

I found myself in Class Five with half of a class that I didn't know and felt lost, vulnerable and confused. To add to the stress of the situation we had the Headmaster, Mr Brown on Friday mornings before lunch for maths. I quickly learned to dread Friday mornings and for me this was the start of nervous stomach feelings and other behavioural difficulties. I used to get so stressed out that I used to nod and shake my head, as if straining to understand and pay attention, especially if I was asked a question. Then I would always get it wrong. Mr Brown would shout and get angry. His face would go red like an over-ripe tomato and he appeared to be about twice as large as any of the female teachers. The more that I panicked about maths, the more mistakes and difficulties I experienced. It wasn't long before I was taking maths home as a punishment and would spend lunch hours crying over my maths with my mum, who also couldn't understand why I was quite so stupid either. The maths issue remained forever in my life, later on.

Knight 2006

Other EDSIII patients comment on Facebook:

My maths was appalling. Could never grasp the concepts as they were explained and only just scraped through my exam by the skin of my teeth.

My maths was and is terrible. I didn't really understand it, or science. I understand a bit better now, but would say I am still much below average with the maths!

Yes same as some others my maths was and still is shocking and I always messed about doing silly stuff acting the clown etc, even now when I see a word I can mistake it for another, my head still goes 100 miles an hour though the body can't!

The last comment picks up on dyslexia which is something that a number of EDSIII patients seem to have; but again, there is not research to formally explain links between dyslexia, dyscalculia and connective tissue disorders, although there is some research linking EDSIII and DCD (Kirby and Davies 2007; Kirby *et al.* 2005). One possible (but personal) theory, which links into difficulties with short-term memory processing (common to all three learning difficulties), is that perhaps it just takes people with EDSIII a little longer to process and organise information, just as it does in their bodies. Perhaps there is a time delay (owing to tissue laxity) that takes longer for the information to be processed in the brain in this particular patient cohort. Until more research is conducted, we will simply not know whether or not there is a higher than normal prevalence of such learning difficulties within the EDSIII population (including attention deficit disorder). So, until such time, these theories can only be conjecture and speculation from the author, rather than considered proven research! Other EDSIII patients on Facebook further comment:

> I was shy and quiet; day dreamed a lot, found it difficult with maths and English. Afternoons I would be useless cos info won't go in. My memory is rubbish short term, long term can be ok. I get my words back to front and muddled up.

> I am dyslexic: not too much trouble reading but I am a rotten speller and have trouble with tasks that, like spelling, require sequencing. I have trouble with left and right and reading maps too. My maths was erratic: I was really good at equations but terrible at spatial things such as graph work.

CHAPTER 22

Social media, forums and support groups

In recent years the introduction of online support groups and Facebook, which are all forms of social media, have become an increasingly important way for people with chronic complex conditions to communicate with each other from the comfort of their own homes. When I raised this topic on my Facebook page, I received some of the following responses:

> I love the friends I have made through the online HMS groups, and it does help to have people who truly understand. I think it makes the condition a lot less isolating, especially if your mobility is limited.

> It is so much easier to get support and information via online groups/forums, but I find I spend so much time on them that I end up following only one or two and the others get neglected. It is great to know they are there though and if I need something I know I have plenty of places to go to find it. I agree as well that if you have limited mobility or even feel you have to forego more social events due to fatigue or any of the other associated problems, these groups provide a lot of solace and I love knowing that there are people to talk to here and it does make me feel less isolated.

> I've only just fully accepted that my HMS is a long-term thing that I have to come to terms with and make changes for…and the forums have already been brilliant, full of actual experiences and descriptions of the little things as well as the major symptoms: you have to look to find the information but there is loads there. I felt quite lonely in my pain before, very few people without it really understand so in real life I feel I have to explain myself

constantly. On the forum I've only posted a couple of times and the members have been so welcoming and full of suggestions that it has really helped me and given me ideas...

The themes that seem to unite people on social media are a reduction of a feeling of isolation and a sense of community belonging in that other people understand what is going on. It does seem to be invaluable for those who are immobile and cannot physically leave their homes to meet other people face-to-face. The danger is that perhaps it is only the very sickest members who use the online forums or Facebook for this level of support – meaning that there is a less balanced viewpoint and people are only discussing/seeing people not getting any better. There have been elements of competitiveness in symptoms and some people dismissing mine, for example, because of a flattering picture of me dancing and suggesting that my symptoms could not be as bad as theirs. Maybe not – but then it is all relative. It is important that there are balanced and positive threads on forums and Facebook to keep a balance of the good and bad aspects of managing chronic conditions. Nevertheless, they really are a lifeline for the most seriously affected, and even those of us who are 'better' still might need to check in from time to time for advice and support. The Hypermobility Syndrome Association (HMSA) forum is very well moderated and there are positive threads, but of course no forum discussions can possibly substitute official medical advice.

Consultant lead health psychologist Dr Andrew Lucas has the following comments to make about social media.

ONLINE COMMUNITY SUPPORT
Dr Andrew Lucas

In the last few years the role of online chat rooms and looking at the EDS community in general has, in my opinion, increased in profile. Most patients in my experience are likely to research their condition online, although that does not mean that the information is accurate or well researched. Patients will often attend my clinic having printed reams of information from various website addresses, which could prove useful or equally contribute to ill-informed opinion.

Regarding the online forums, the patients I see generally fall into two categories. The first are those who value the online community support and who gain confidence from sharing experiences with other people who have been diagnosed with EDS/HMS. In my experience many patients welcome the opportunity to be part of a larger community, which helps to reduce a sense of isolation. The second group are those who deliberately distance themselves from the online community. A number of patients have told me how they have viewed some online conversations and felt uncomfortable with what they describe as 'the self-pitying statements' and what I have described as 'competing for misery'. It is understandable that common symptomatology is discussed but I have noted how some patients will compete for the greatest number of symptoms, the greatest number of interventions and the widest range of medications. Coping with long-term physical health problems is multifactorial, but I believe that for some patients focusing on their symptoms and the negative consequences of their condition could be viewed as part of their coping style. Equally I have met patients who tried to live their life at the other extreme, not acknowledging their problems and coping by gritting their teeth, being fiercely independent and trying to lead a productive lifestyle. I would argue that both extreme positions are ultimately unhelpful in managing their EDS/HMS. Shared commonalities for both of these extreme positions are the difficulties that patients have had with credibility and appropriate diagnosis.

One can only speculate on the psychological sequelae of repeated medical consultations from various specialists with each offering an opinion and possible diagnosis. I would term this experience as 'fighting for credibility'.

Support groups

Recently I was asked if I would volunteer to run the London Support Group for the HMSA. I agreed to do this having had previous experience of running support groups and facilitation skills from my teaching background. Although the group has only met twice so far I know that it is something that members find highly beneficial and they appear to be so grateful that something is organised in a public space (usually a public house) where they can meet with other patients who have the same condition. So far the meetings have been very informal and HMSA members have had the chance to talk to other members about their condition and share stories. Rather than being negative, people had positive ideas for management of the different problems encountered, and there was a general sense of not going through their symptoms alone – that others understood this too was very powerful. The group situation is invaluable for the newly diagnosed, some of whom are a little overwhelmed by their diagnosis and require support in their future journey in living with EDSIII. As a group facilitator I find running the group a very rewarding thing to do, although I have discovered that I cannot possibly be ill because the members now see me as a beacon of hope, which is a double-edged sword. However, I ensure that I have both support and supervision so that I am not too overloaded.

Members say on Facebook:

I went to my first one a few weeks ago and it was great to finally meet the people I talk to all the time, people who know and understand exactly how I feel and just get it! Never been in a room with so many bendies since I did gymnastics!

I think that there is a huge value to being involved in support groups, whether they are online or physical. The benefit of being with people who actually do understand what you are going through is invaluable.

CHAPTER 23

Self-harm, anxiety and depression

This chapter explores self-harm, anxiety and depression in terms of the chronic complex patient. It is essential to point out that there are no proven links with either self-harm or depression and EDSIII, so some of this is personal to the author. However, self-harm in general might be linked to some aspects of the wider spectrum of the chronic complex patient and maladaptive coping mechanisms. On a very personal note and at the risk of autoethnographical self-exposure (Chang 2008), I also felt that it was important to bring the issue of self-harm into the public domain so that mental health issues can be discussed and people informed, rather than hidden and stigmatised.

Skin-picking

I started to pick my skin at a very young age – I think I was about five years old. I had eczema as a child which I used to get in the joints of my skin, mainly in the joints of my elbows and knees, which, I hadn't reflected on until now, are all my hypermobile joints. However, the relationship between the eczema and hypermobility can only be conjecture. It stands to reason that the areas would have been 'stressed', and research is beginning to suggest that the skin heals less well in hypermobile patients (Russek 1999; Simpson 2006; Tinkle 2010). I hated my skin feeling rough, and gradually when I received other skin assaults – for example, a mosquito bite – I would start to pick at those and any scabs on my body, as my poem so clearly explains. I felt a sense of calm after I had picked my skin.

I think that at one level when I first started skin-picking it was simply about removing a source of irritation (a scab), but that eventually I was using it as a 'soother' or way to reduce both feelings of anger and anxiety. As I got older, the 'hit' needed to reduce both these feelings increased, so I started to pick more and more; firstly on sites on my limbs, but eventually this spread to my face. I will never know what caused the start of incidents on my face, but the damage I inflicted was serious and I looked a mess.

My parents couldn't understand my behaviour, about why I was picking or the underlying cause. GPs did nothing (until much later) and neither did my school help in any way, even though I was being bullied by the age of eight. My parents moved me to another school in Year 5, but I didn't stop picking. It might have been predictable that when my father died very suddenly during that same school year (I was ten years old), my picking got worse, and my mum became more frustrated and angry about it during my pre-adolescent years. I still didn't stop skin-picking. However, the skin-picking had by this time become an ingrained pattern of behaviour and most likely compulsive – but a very wrong way of coping with strong emotions of anxiety and anger.

By the time I was 15 I had stopped picking my face, but picked my scalp and pulled my hair instead. The self-harm continued until my early thirties when I had Cognitive Analytical Therapy (CAT; discussed in Chapter 24), which was an enormous help, and completely stopped me self-harming in the form of skin-picking.

Although I think that I was skin-picking and therefore self-harming to cope with feelings of anger and anxiety which I was unable to express in a normal fashion, I also think I felt quite disconnected and 'out of my body'. With the knowledge that I now have about my body, hypermobility and joint proprioception, I do wonder whether the instability and lack of control I felt in my body certainly contributed to use of inappropriate behaviour to cope with these feelings. I never quite knew where I was. Lucas suggests (in this chapter) that even behaviours such as 'over-exercising' might be considered self-harm, but if I go into these types of states I now have the psychological skills to change my behaviour using CAT skills and I am still having to work on some of my more extreme behavioural states and belief-systems (e.g. I have to exercise every day!).

Self-harm: skin-picking

Skin-picking can be a common behaviour, which shows little increase in those with dermatological conditions compared to a student population (Keuthen *et al.* 2001). Skin-picking can range in intensity to include scarring and disfigurement and even death (Keuthen *et al.*

2001). Those who skin-pick self-injuriously report fewer feelings of social anxiety and embarrassment and avoidance compared to those who are non-injurious skin-pickers (Keuthen *et al.* 2001). Keuthen *et al.* suggest that this is owing to comorbid anxiety and mood symptoms, but this is conjecture. However, both groups (injurious and non-injurious) use clothing and skin-camouflaging cosmetics to cover up their habit, and skin-picking does impact upon quality of life including leisure, clothing and sporting choices (Keuthen *et al.* 2001). Skin-picking might also occur in trichotillomania, body dysmorphic disorder and borderline personality disorder (Keuthen *et al.* 2001; Klonsky, Oltmanns and Turkheimer 2003).

It is difficult to determine why self-harming behaviour commences, but some suggestions and studies include a link between deliberate self-harm and childhood trauma (Klonsky *et al.* 2003; Paris 2005). The strongest association for self-harming behaviour appears to link to coping with feelings of anxiety (Haw *et al.* 2001; Klonsky *et al.* 2003), which superseded depression in Klonsky *et al.*'s (2003) research and, interestingly, there are not always gender differences (Haw *et al.* 2001), with males and females being at equal risk. It appears then that childhood trauma and anxiety all increase risk factors for self-harm, but further research would need to be undertaken to examine any such links with self-harm and chronic complex medical conditions; although anxiety could certainly be related to these. Anecdotally there might well be self-harm in the EDS and complex patient cohort, but this can only be a personal view since there is insufficient research data to draw any firm conclusions. My self-harm is now thankfully in the past.

Jess Glenny, a moving body teacher, facilitator and therapist, has EDSIII and was anorexic for 11 years. She shares her story below. Jess and I shared a similar feeling of disconnection from our bodies. Jess writes:

> I have Ehlers Danlos Hypermobility Syndrome and was anorexic from the age of about 17 to 27. Anorexia has a complex fabric of causation, but for me one of the strands was clearly hypermobility and the need to establish a more reliable body boundary. Anorexia seemed to me to be a solution to an ongoing sense of physical fragmentation, dispersal and disintegration, which started when I was aged five and convinced my big toes were falling off. As a child, I loved cut-out dolls because they

had a black line around their body. Hunger gave me a sense of securely existing. Reducing myself down to the minimum, condensing myself to an essence, similarly enabled me to feel contained. The body boundary issues in hypermobility are little discussed and in my experience very significant. Today, aged 49, I still struggle to know reliably that I exist. However, I now understand that the origins of this feeling are biological, rather than psychological or philosophical.

Dr Andrew Lucas, consultant lead health psychologist, writes the following.

SELF-HARM AND EDSIII PATIENTS
Dr Andrew Lucas

The role of self-harm within this patient group demands mention. I am clinically intrigued by the various forms of self-harm displayed by patients and this can manifest in many overt and more subtle behaviours. For example, self-harm behaviour can vary from cutting or striking oneself to deliberate over activity in the knowledge that an exacerbation of symptoms is the likely outcome. The causes of self-harm in this patient group are beyond my expertise, although I can offer a few thoughts. Many patients struggle with the uncertainty of their physical ability and the varying intensity of their symptoms. It could be argued that the self-harm is a display of control in an unstable health condition. Perhaps the frustration expressed by many patients is eased by self-harm? Perhaps the self-harm is about punishment, shame or guilt associated with their condition? Anecdotal evidence suggests to me that the frequency of self-harm incidents is elevated in this patient group, but further research may provide empirical support which might then justify further attention and targeted interventions.

The poem below describes feelings of anxiety.

The worry organ[1]

It is located in the fleshy part, below the sternum.
The size of my heart, with the flatness of my hand.
Dark, purple and constant,
Fluttering with the eloquence of a toad.

Pressure tightens across my worry organ,
It is as subtle as a blunt vegetable knife.
All consuming, it sucks the calm out of me,
A nest of anxieties keeps me buzzing.

Moods: anxiety

On this subject I draw on my previous book (Knight 2011). There is increasing evidence to suggest links with anxiety and hypermobility (Beighton *et al.* 2012; Eccles *et al.* 2012; Martin-Santos, Bulbena and Crippa 2010; Russek 1999). Research by Martin-Santos and colleagues (1998) suggests that patients with anxiety disorder were over 16 times more likely than control subjects to have joint laxity. However, Martin-Santos and colleagues found little evidence to support the fact that panic leads to hypermobility, so it was presupposed that the hypermobility condition came first. Martin-Santos and colleagues were unclear as to the reasons why patients with hypermobility were likely to suffer from anxiety. However, frequent pain and joint instability might explain why patients do exhibit anxiety (Harding 2003; Russek 1999).

A further study in 2004 by Bulbena and colleagues found evidence to suggest that there is a genetic link between joint hypermobility syndrome and panic (2004, p.435). State anxiety may be defined as 'feelings of tension and apprehension, associated with arousal of the autonomic nervous system' (Spielberger, as cited in Hardy, Jones and Gould 1996, p.141), whilst trait anxiety refers to 'a general disposition that certain individuals possess to respond to a variety of (relatively unthreatening) situations with high levels of state anxiety'. Additionally, Bulbena and colleagues (2004) found that scores for trait anxiety and to a lesser extent state anxiety were significantly higher for subjects with hypermobility, suggesting that hypermobility could

---

1   Copyright © Isobel Knight 2009.

be linked to an innate form of excessive response to fear. It could perhaps be hypothesised that there is something in the hypermobility that leads to anxiety, possibly related to the need to exhibit some control over chaotic tissue laxity. A constant feeling of vulnerability over unstable joints could indeed explain why some hypermobile patients develop anxiety. However, a study by Ercolani and colleagues questions even that point.

Looking into the psychological features of hypermobility in patients who were pain-free at evaluation, Ercolani *et al.* (2008) found that hypermobile subjects were obtaining statistically higher mean scores than the healthy group on all of the nine scales of the SCL-90R Illness Behaviour Questionnaire. The SCL-90R scales measure psychological symptoms. Ercolani and colleagues theorise that the reasons behind those results are linked to the group 'giving more attention to bodily symptoms, perhaps as related to self-perceived weakness and fragility' (2008, p.253). There is, it seems, a link between the instability associated with hypermobility and the range of bodily symptoms, anxiety and general psychological distress. Indeed, Ercolani and colleagues (2008) recommend that physicians should not ignore these symptoms, which might have been dismissed in some hypermobile patients as hypochondria, and lead to a resentment (from patients) towards the medical profession (Grahame 2009; Harding 2003; Keer 2003).

What is particularly interesting and significant about the Ercolani study was that the hypermobile group were all asymptomatic and not aware of their diagnosis, and still scored highly on anxiety and other aspects of health psychology behaviour. The fact that the hypermobile group was not injured thus suggests that anxiety and hypermobility are perhaps very much related and that anxiety might be genetically related to hypermobility (Bulbena *et al.* 2004). Therefore it might imply that anxiety is less relevant in relation to patients who are already injured if, as the literature suggests, the anxiety is already there, perhaps by default (Bulbena *et al.* 2004; Ercolani *et al.* 2008).

It is no wonder that patients with EDSIII end up feeling more anxious when they frequently injure, are regularly in pain and suffer from psychosomatic disorders such as IBS and POTS (Eccles *et al.* 2012). Patients with EDSIII often experience poor proprioception, or an awareness of the body in space, owing to their hypermobility (Ferrell and Ferrell 2010; Ferrell *et al.* 2004), which can be frightening and disorientating. If one then factors in the increased likelihood that one is not going to be believed by medical professionals (or others) it is not hard to understand why anxiety is so prevalent within this patient group. Depression is not shown to be linked to hypermobility, but is shown to be linked to chronic pain, another manifestation of both EDSIII and conditions such as fibromyalgia.

Shades of black[2]

I can't stand this terrible flatness, of feeling sunken, empty and colourless.
I detest feeling indecisive.
I loathe not wanting to do anything, my concentration like a butterfly.
I can't bear this feeling of horrific boredom, of only wanting to sleep.
I wish someone could let me die.

I remember once wanting to do things, but not any more.
For a long time now I just want to sleep – there is nothing to do.
To do anything is a superhuman effort.

Moods: depression

Depression is not linked to EDSIII, but is nevertheless one of the worst feelings to endure for those who experience it. Depression can vary on a scale from perhaps feeling a bit low because it never stops raining (summer 2012), but become so serious that one might contemplate death. It can certainly be a very draining emotion which is very difficult to disengage from. There has been considerable research in linking chronic pain with depression (Banks and Kerns 1996; Fishbain *et al.* 1997; Hendler 1984; Katon and Sullivan 1990; Romano and Turner 1985). It is therefore no wonder that many EDSIII, FM and chronic complex patients find themselves in a state of depression owing to their pain, but also because their quality of life is poor – both physiologically (see Chapter 5) and also psychologically.

For some patients medication will be essential (Martin-Santos *et al.* 2010), but other therapeutic therapy may also be invaluable in the form of counselling and psychotherapy, or behavioural therapies such as cognitive behavioural therapy (CBT) and/or cognitive analytical therapy (CAT) (Daniel 2010). Psychologists on pain management courses such as the one that Lucas describes in Chapter 27 are essential in helping patients to cope with, and manage depression.

---

2   Copyright © Isobel Knight 2009.

If the depression is dealt with, it might also help with symptoms of pain given the overlap (Banks and Kerns 1996; Fishbain *et al.* 1997; Hendler 1984; Katon and Sullivan 1990; Romano and Turner 1985).

Conclusion
It is essential that any medical professional working with a patient showing signs of self-harm, anxiety or depression intervenes early and arranges appropriate ongoing therapeutic advice.

CHAPTER 24

Cognitive analytical therapy (CAT)

In 2006 I was referred for CAT for treatment of both self-harming behaviour and mood swings. Denman defines CAT as 'a brief focal therapy informed by cognitive therapy, psychodynamic psychotherapy and certain developments in cognitive psychology...it has turned its attention to the treatment of personality disorders, specifically borderline personality disorder' (Denman 2001, p.256). In CAT, one goes about addressing repeated behavioural patterns which have undesirable results and outcomes. Anthony Ryle, who was the founder of CAT, describes these 'faulty procedures'. He describes 'traps' as:

> repetitive cycles of behaviour in which the consequences of the behaviour feed back into its perpetuation... The second kind of faulty procedure is the 'dilemma' which involves the representation of false choices or unduly narrowed options... The final maladaptive procedural sequence is the 'snag': the subtle negative aspect of goals. Snags are anticipations of the future consequences of actions that are so negative that they are capable of halting a procedure before it ever runs.
>
> *Denman 2001, p.257*

The number of CAT sessions that a patient is going to have is set in advance – usually between 16 and 24 sessions (Denman 2001). The way that CAT therapy starts out is perhaps similar to other therapies in that the therapist needs to establish trust and build a therapeutic relationship. The patient's story is gathered. At some point, usually between the third and fifth sessions, the therapist writes a letter to the patient. This is unique to CAT. Denman writes that 'the reformulation letter most often begins with a narrative account of the patient's life story, because this account makes clear the developmental origins of repetitive patterns' (2001, p.247). The rest of the sessions concentrate on changing this maladaptive behaviour. CAT then concludes with a goodbye letter written from patient to therapist (about what has been learned and changed) and from therapist to patient about what they too have changed and will hopefully continue to modify in the future (Denman 2001).

My CAT treatment

I had two episodes of CAT – the first in 2006 when I had the full 24 sessions, and then in early 2011 I had a further eight sessions with a completely different therapist to remind myself how to avoid harming behaviour and to revise how to use the therapies and remind myself about the previous patterns and mood-states identified in 2006 (see Figures 24.1 and 24.2).

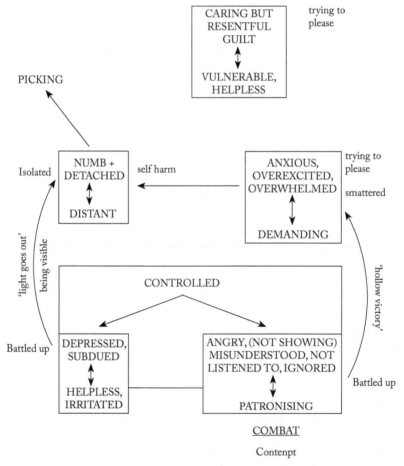

FIGURE 24.1 EXAMPLE ONE OF ISOBEL'S THERAPEUTIC DIAGRAMMATIC DIALOGUE WITH HER CAT THERAPIST LOOKING AT DIFFERENT MOOD-STATES AND STATES WHERE SHE MIGHT SELF-HARM

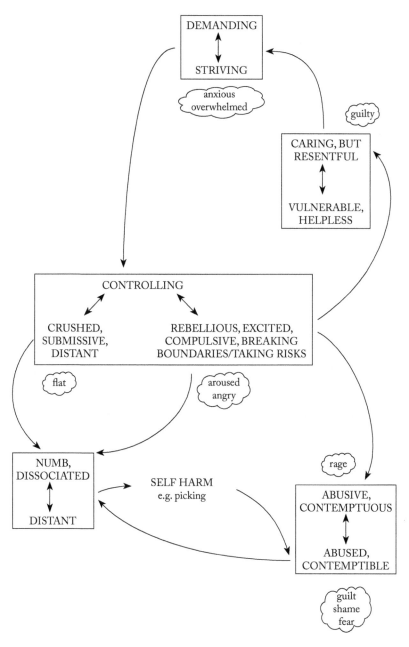

FIGURE 24.2 EXAMPLE TWO OF ISOBEL'S THERAPEUTIC DIAGRAMMATIC DIALOGUE WITH HER CAT THERAPIST LOOKING AT DIFFERENT MOOD-STATES AND STATES WHERE SHE MIGHT SELF-HARM.

Table 24.1 is a table I created based on some of the very opposing mood-states I could find myself 'swinging' between.

TABLE 24.1: Intellectual vs emotional functioning			
Intellectual positive	**Intellectual negative**	**Emotional positive**	**Emotional negative**
Astute	Dull	Clear	Confused
Alive	Dead	Orderly	Chaotic
Clued-up	Disengaged	Logical	Illogical
Switched-on	Turned off	Sensible	Nonsensical
Enthusiastic	Bored	Straightforward	Devious
Clear-thinking	Muddied thinking	No 'game-plan'	Manipulative
		Rational	Irrational
Quick to understand	Slow to understand	Mature	Childish
		Comfortable	Hurt
Happy to be challenged	Unhappy to be challenged	Calm	Distressed
Engrossed	Disinterested	Guilt-free	Guilty
Analytical	Unanalytical	Tempered	Angry
Thriving	Under-performing	Orientated	Disorientated
		Associative	Disassociative
Energised	De-energised	Sociable	Antisocial
Creative	Uncreative	Functioning well	Unable to function
Productive	Unproductive		
Happy	Unhappy	Communicative	Poor communicator
Forward-thinking	Stuck	Elevated	Depressed
Strategic	Poor planning	Non-compulsive	Compulsive
Sharp	Flat		
Focused	Lacks concentration	In my body	Out-of-body
		In control	Out of control
Professional	Unprofessional	Comfortable	Uncomfortable
Motivated	Demotivated		
In the moment	Nowhere		

In CAT, as treatment comes to an end it is common practice for the client and therapist to write a goodbye letter. Here is my 2011 goodbye letter:

CAT goodbye letter

Dear T

When I returned for more CAT earlier in the year it was clear as you so aptly put it (in my 7th session) that things had become covered in dust and that I was not able to see the colours and patterns in my life as clearly as before. This was not a surprise as it has been five years since I last had CAT therapy and I was able to recognise that I was beginning to fall into some familiar traps and unhelpful patterns again. I have been surprised at the fact I have needed so few sessions in order to see the colours again and to be able to nourish my life. 'Spring has sprung' in my life again and I feel much more balanced all round. I found the pen and third-eye analogies particularly helpful and if I can keep all the colours in my one pen running evenly then I should be much more successful and balanced in all aspects of life. That nasty red ink in the form of anger had taken over once again and had more recently started to fuel a small element of self-harming behaviour. Your suggestions in how to manage this have been helpful, and so I will be using dance or perhaps even clay as ways forward to release pent up feelings of unresolved anger. I will try and acknowledge the feelings without allowing them to take up vast amounts of energy or dwell on particular moods for days at a time.

I have enjoyed your stories and drawings on the whiteboard and I particularly remember the biscuit story and it made me reflect that I was no longer having 'biscuit' in my life and in the last two weeks I have made some positive changes to my social life and have suddenly become very popular as a result of whatever message I am putting out and have had a lot of people suddenly want to go for drinks/out with me. This has led to a very positive feeling of self-confidence, value and self-esteem for me as being someone that people want to be with. Having a rest and going out with people has also put an essential balance back into my life where work was having far too great a dominance. It is possible to work and play hard too.

The fact I have been in a very positive, happy and calm state of mind for the last two weeks is something I am going to take, develop, nourish and allow to grow [and] is a lovely way to end our brief time in CAT. You reminded me that the mood didn't need to change because I could keep feeding this positive state of mind. Of course it will rain again, but I can change the seasons, and I don't need to keep getting stuck in the same weather pattern, or colour – e.g. that red anger. I am encouraged that I can have more CAT again if I need to and would like it if you could reflect this in my notes. As you suggested – I might not need any again for another five years and then I might only need just one or two sessions.

Thank you for reminding me what is really possible and that I have the resources to do this myself, which I probably knew all along – I just needed a revision course. I am a little afraid as our work draws to a close because there will be nobody to check back in with. The acid test started yesterday with a 'blue mood' as I fell into serious pain and fatigue. I gave myself permission to cry as I went to bed, but had a very difficult night and did not sleep until 5am. It was hard to pull out of a meeting I very much wanted to attend, but I had to realise that there were others there who could find out what it was about and that I do not have to be superwoman. I allowed myself to follow my care plan, take pain medication and fall asleep until I felt ready to properly get up (not until 11am). The sunshine helped me to feel more relaxed and to indulge in some much needed rest without feeling guilty about work. Although I did some work, I did small amounts [and] only doing what I felt able to manage knowing it would be better to wait until I had fully recovered from the fatigue and pain I was in before I could manage my usual 'tour de force'. Recognising that this state of pain and fatigue will only be temporary (which is usually the case) helped me to reconcile my feelings and to keep calmer about everything. Once I could relax and accept the situation I was able to cope with my day again. There are going to be many more days like this, but I will only get better with practice. I recognise these are traps I fall into, but the better I get at intercepting this, the less I will fall into the same behavioural negative loops that I have been in before. I was also able to acknowledge to both my colleagues that I was very tired and had reacted badly to something that had happened in my absence. I was initially frustrated, but realised it was very trivial to be cross about it, that I had to deal with it, get on with it and manage my frustration. This was better than I had been able to manage only a short time ago.

As I look into the garden, the spring is blooming and so it can in my life too, if I continue to nourish and develop myself and an acceptance of certain states of mind and attending to my behaviour just as I would look after the flowers in the garden.

With very best wishes and many thanks.

Isobel Knight, April 2011

In the next chapter I reflect on the management of chronic, complex patients.

CHAPTER 25

Managing complex patients with psychological issues

Isobel's reflection

When I think back on my life history, I am not surprised that I end up with a label of 'complex' patient. There is layer upon layer of physical, emotional and psychological issues that each weave into and work on the other. Nothing got there by accident, but the fact that so many layers have accumulated over time makes it difficult to unpick and extrapolate, as both Keer and Lucas document in earlier chapters. This is a whole example of 'chicken and egg'. In my case, I wonder what did come first – an 'odd' personality overlaid by a need to 'self-harm' because I was unable to adequately express anger and anxiety by the age of five. Factor in at this point poor physical and hand-to-eye coordination, most likely some element of DCD, and then finding it hard to fit in with others or be picked for the team in PE – so socially excluded quite early on. In addition, factor in a child who adores classical music but is seen as very odd by her class teacher, let alone her peers. It is already really stacked against me before I am six years old, by which time I also stop sleeping properly at night. Then factor in all the knowledge outlined in Part II about Maslow and the body's physiological needs and we have a malfunctioning physiological body, psychologically there are already difficulties, and then we have our first 'serious' physical injury at the age of seven and the domino effect of all the catalogue of other physical problems (Grahame 2010). There is then trauma with my father's death when I was aged ten, and then adolescence brings with it growing pains, very painful dysmenorrhoea and frequent calf tears. By late adolescence we have the beginnings of chronic back pain at a hinge in my spine, also owing to a disc prolapse. Psychologically, self-harming behaviour has continued. We have problems with a highly perfectionist personality and eventually depression and anxiety on top of a host of other physical and somatic conditions such as IBS and endometriosis. The body has taken over and become a very big feature in my life because it is so malfunctioning, but the behaviour and psychological overlay are so important because all these factors feed into the physical body and the way in which the body perceives pain and 'behaves', and is painful or not. I can say this because it is my body and I know it overtook my life. Indeed at times in treatment my physio and I talked about me being very self-centred about this, but it was a necessary self-centredness because most people do not have to think about the implications their actions will have on their bodies later on, but people with EDSIII and other complex pain conditions such as FM do.

As my physiological bodily systems have improved and homeostasis is beginning to be achieved, as my body strengthens, and functions normally with corrected movement patterns, my body becomes less of an importance and a focal point to me. I am a little less distracted by it. My mind is freed up for other things. I am less self-centred and bodily preoccupied. It has taken over four years of treatment to reach this state and a whole range of treatment including physiotherapy, both manual and exercise-related rehabilitation, Bowen therapy, trauma release, CAT therapy, surgical repair, bowel re-training, pain management training, psychiatric treatment for mood swings and gynaecological management of endometriosis. I have additionally required treatment for my temporomandibular joint (TMJ) and even speech therapy work. However, according to Maslow's Hierarchy of Needs I am probably now working at relationship and love needs, but also cognitive and aesthetic needs. None of those would be possible without having some underpinning physiological homeostasis.

The medical professional working with the EDSIII patient needs to be aware that they are very certainly going to encounter much emotional life baggage in dealing with all the myriad of health-related and symptomatic features of a chronic complex medical condition, which both Keer and Lucas are aware of (see Chapters 15 and 20). Some stories will be more complex than others, but the medical professional will invariably face many barriers, of which trust is a major underpinning factor, because the patient will have been disbelieved so many times. It does indeed feel implausible when so many parts of the body do not work well. The most difficult to explain or define are definitely ones where there are multiple pain points (FM) or where POTS symptoms are involved. Medicine has become so specialised that the other difficulty encountered by such patients is that one is sent to so many different specialists that no one is then working with the body holistically or communicating back. The fact that one medical professional tried to rehabilitate the whole of me was an enormous undertaking – in fact, it turned out to be unrealistic and downright impossible for the person to manage because so many bodily systems required additional highly specialist rehabilitation, including surgery. However, having one person try to do this was helpful from my point of view as a patient because I had one point of reference and did not have to keep telling my story hundreds and hundreds of times again.

For the medical professional involved, boundaries are going to be absolutely crucial in working with this type of patient – particularly the person who is their key worker or for someone like a lone therapist or physiotherapist (not attached to a hospital team). It would therefore be prudent for the (physical) therapist to agree on an initial number of sessions, as would be the case for a counsellor or psychotherapist, and then how long each session might be (e.g. one hour, if including exercise rehabilitation, or half an hour for manual therapy). The therapist might want to say how it is acceptable for the patient to reach them in between sessions, and how – for example by phone or email. Such a therapist might well require supervision themselves, particularly if they are not attached to a hospital team. A consideration needs to be made of where your responsibilities start and end – for example if psychological issues come up, do you try and address these, or refer the patient to an appropriate other therapist? The GP or rheumatologist might be the appropriate 'coordinators' of such patients, but there is no doubt that the chronic complex patient attracts many experts and each requires their own support, as Lucas explained in Chapter 20. Holistic packages of care are expensive, but they are what this type of patient requires, though the lone therapist needs to be very clear about where their responsibilities begin and end, according to their own professional code and in terms of their own proficiencies, and when they are going to say, 'No, I can't help you with this – please seek advice from someone else.' As Lucas so clearly describes, medical professionals also need help and support (see Chapter 20).

Invariably most patient programmes involving, for example, pain management have a multidisciplinary team of experts who can support each other. For instance, the pain management programme I attended had a consultant anaesthetist, physiotherapists, clinical psychologists and occupational health therapists. They would meet each other frequently to review each patient so that each member of the team would be alerted if there were issues or difficulties with a particular patient. For example, when I failed to turn up for my circuit training exercises, the physiotherapist and the psychologist went to talk to me to find out what was going on and why. For the rest of that day and week I was asked to 'check in' with the psychologist about why I wasn't going to do my exercises during the week I had my period (it was too painful). A lone therapist doesn't have this luxury or backup. They have to make decisions themselves about what they can do. It is an arduous and a potentially risky journey. They have to be confident of their own ability, but also know their patient very well and build a very strong foundation of trust. The therapist has to be very skilled indeed, but part of this skill involves knowing when they can no longer help or that it might be risky both to them professionally as well as the patient to continue doing so. They must therefore not consider it a weakness if they say, 'For your difficulties with (e.g. self-harm), you need to see a different therapist.'

My physio tried to address my behaviour (very gradually and carefully) over a number of years of working with me in physiotherapy. There were a number of things I did which were unacceptable, for example jumping off the couch at any moment, and it was appropriate for her to address this type of behaviour because it was related to safety in a treatment capacity, but it was also a way she could get me to 'ask first' if I needed to get off the couch or tell her if I felt afraid. Then she knew that things were getting difficult for me and we could either stop and talk about it for a moment, or I could get off the couch to fidget (which was often the main reason) and then we could continue. However, whether it was appropriate for my physio to address other behavioural issues might be considered more contentious, but she had gained trust in me, and I was actually listening to her and her approach was working for me. There were many times when she pointed out things to me I might not have wanted to hear. The dialogue described below illustrates this and concludes this chapter:

My physio said to me that she admired me a huge amount and felt at times she might have overstepped the mark by challenging my behaviour, but I felt it was necessary for her to do this. My physio said that I was very accepting about everything and could have easily felt comments about the way I behave could have been interpreted as unfair. She was impressed that I was positive about any such criticisms, bounced back and worked them out. She said it was impressive and brave. I acknowledged it was hard, but necessary.

Physiotherapy, 26.9.2011

CHAPTER 26

Terminating client relationships

Sometimes patient/therapist relationships go wrong. There can be many reasons for this. In my capacity as a Bowen therapist I decided to reflect upon some of the patients (and colleagues) that I had felt were 'difficult' for me and why this was, as per suggestions Wilks (2007) makes in a chapter about client/therapist relationships. A pattern did emerge. I had difficulties with people who were very negative, grumpy, 'boring' or difficult to 'read' and those who exhibited anger, superiority or who made me feel anxious or nervous, and therefore I then felt relieved when they had gone. I am working out what this says about me – that I am usually a very positive/bright person, so find the opposite very difficult to cope with. I am also a very open person, and probably give away more than I should, so when I cannot 'read' another person or gain any insight about them I find this a challenge. Lastly, I know I find anger difficult, and a combination of anger and people who make me uncomfortable also makes me anxious and nervous. I then just want to get away from them.

I have referred clients on to other therapists before. I have done this when I felt they weren't making sufficient progress in my care, or if I felt they were 'chemically' too difficult to work with. Sometimes nature just takes its course and the patient also feels they have had sufficient sessions and then it is quite a relief when they no longer want to see you for treatment. Fortunately, I have only suggested twice in almost ten years that a patient of mine should see a colleague. This was for personality reasons. It felt the right thing to do and the patient was happy with my suggestion. I told the patient that X knows a lot more about temporomandibular joint (TMJ) problems (as it was) than I do. They were happy. I was happy. It was a good outcome.

In Bowen we do not usually work with clients for very many sessions at a time so it is rarely necessary to refer them on. There are clients with chronic complaints who visit me in clinic regularly and so I have built a rapport with them, and then I have just one patient who I have worked with (on and off) for a whole year. If I had to terminate a client relationship I would handle it with the utmost care – particularly with those I had been working with for some time. Patients do become attached to us. There is sometimes what psychotherapists describe as countertransference (Wilks 2007) between therapists and patients. Patients do need careful preparation if the relationship is going to be terminated. I usually warn them when it is time to reduce their sessions. If they are not ready we talk about how we will do this, so that any dependence is reduced very gradually. It is always sad for both therapist and patient if one moves into another geographical area, but if this is communicated in advance then both patient and therapist understand this. However annoyed I might be by a client, I would never abruptly terminate their treatment without explaining a rationale for so doing. I would speak to them and explain my concerns and provide suggestions for ongoing treatments or a referral to another therapist. To behave in any other way could be considered both unprofessional and quite detrimental in a longer-term patient/client relationship, particularly where the client is vulnerable or has a complex psychological history (Bembry and Ericson 1999; Hunsley *et al.* 1999). This is why counsellors spend such a long time towards the end of the therapeutic relationship on 'endings' and saying 'goodbye' safely (McLeod 1998).

As Lucas describes in Chapter 20, medical professionals also need support, and so the types of supervision that are compulsory for counsellors should also extend to all disciplines of medicine and complementary and alternative medicine.

CHAPTER 27

I'm not mad

I have EDS so why would I need to see a psychologist?

Although I have not personally attended the Royal National Orthopaedic Hospital (RNOH) course, I did attend a pain management course at another leading London hospital in 2006, and described the experience in detail in my previous book (Knight 2011). The experience was invaluable and helped me to move forwards in all aspects of my life, physically and psychologically. This chapter concludes the vast but crucial part of the book on psychology, with consultant lead health psychologist Dr Andrew Lucas explaining what happens at an expert centre in the treatment of chronic complex patients at the RNOH.

I'M NOT MAD: I HAVE EDS SO WHY WOULD I NEED TO SEE A PSYCHOLOGIST?

Dr Andrew Lucas

Introduction

This section will describe my clinical experience of working with patients diagnosed with Ehlers-Danlos type III and hypermobility syndrome as part of my role as lead clinical health psychologist at the Royal National Orthopaedic Hospital. Over the past three years, the Royal National Orthopaedic Hospital rehabilitation team has been at the forefront of delivering improved services for patients with EDS/HMS. I will describe the structure and content of the rehabilitation programme while emphasising the role of family and friends. I will also describe some of the research considering the psychological profile of this patient group.

For the purpose of this section, I will refer to EDSIII and joint hypermobility syndrome interchangeably as 'EDS/HMS' after a paper by Tinkle *et al.* published in 2009, which argued that benign joint hypermobility syndrome and Ehlers-Danlos syndrome hypermobility type represent the same phenotypic group of patients and are not distinguished from each other. They further argue that clinically this group of patients are better served by uniting the two diagnostic labels.

Patient pathway to the rehabilitation programme at the Royal National Orthopaedic Hospital (RNOH)

For over three years most of the hypermobility EDSIII patients have been referred by the rheumatology service at University College London headed by Professor Rodney Grahame and supported by Dr Hana Kazkaz. The collaboration between the two services developed as Professor Grahame visited the RNOH and was confident that the RNOH could take the lead in offering inpatient rehabilitation. Typically, a patient will be seen in Professor Grahame's unit for assessment which will then make a referral to one of the consultant rheumatologists at the RNOH who will undertake further assessment.

In describing the patient pathway the admitting consultant will undertake a medical assessment which may include requesting further investigations and tests, and exploring treatment options which may include changes to the medication, referral to another service and referral to the preadmission clinic.

This pathway may include outpatient work in preparation for a possible admission, and this might include a referral to physiotherapy, occupational therapy or clinical health psychology. If the patient is invited to the preadmission clinic this involves attending with up to eight other patients who first attend for a group presentation that describes the rehabilitation programme, including the structure and content, and a presentation by each of the four disciplines involved in the rehabilitation programme – notably physiotherapy, occupational therapy, clinical health psychology and nursing colleagues. You will note that, at this stage, there is no medical input as, typically, if the patient is admitted onto the rehabilitation programme they will generally not be seen by a medical consultant.

After the group presentation the patient then attends for an individual assessment with members of staff. This is to further assess suitability for the programme, in particular to discuss whether expectations are realistic, whether the patient is ready to engage in exploring self-management strategies and to initially discuss meaningful goals for a possible admission. Often, at the preadmission clinic, goals are also set in preparation for a possible admission – for example, a patient with a very poor structure to their day will struggle to engage in the day-to-day programme, and so the importance of improving their sleep and activity patterns might be discussed. It is worth noting that the most common goal amongst EDS/HMS patients is to gain greater understanding about their condition. If the patient is considered suitable for an admission they are then added to the waiting list for an admission, either to the hotel or the ward-based rehabilitation programme. If the patient needs support with activities of daily living then the admission is planned for the ward. There now follows a description of the rehabilitation programme.

The Royal National Orthopaedic Hospital EDS/HMS rehabilitation programme

The RNOH rehabilitation programme adheres to current best practice and published research for helping patients with chronic musculoskeletal conditions. Chronic pain has been described as a key feature of EDSIII and described as 'a serious complication of the condition with both disabling effects for physical and psychological consequences' (Levy 2012).

It is worth mentioning that often patients are looking for pain relief and amelioration of their symptoms, and it is made clear that this is an unrealistic option and it is more helpful to explore self-management strategies. EDS/HMS is a lifelong condition that needs lifelong management and health investment. This means the patient making changes to their routine and activities and also to their thinking in order to manage their condition more effectively and to reduce the impact that the condition has on their quality of life.

The patients are usually admitted for a period of three weeks, with admissions lasting from Monday to Friday. The patients are encouraged to go home at the weekend to start transferring the skills and knowledge which they have learnt on the programme to their home situation. Typically, a 15-day programme will involve multidisciplinary input that combines group and individual sessions.

Every programme is bespoke and unique to the individual; although all patients attend group sessions, it is the individual therapy sessions that characterise the individualised approach. In my clinical experience HMS can be considered an umbrella term with no two patients the same and each presenting with varying degrees of symptoms and complaints. For example, some will be more troubled with postural orthostatic tachycardia syndrome than others.

It is clear to me that there is a need for physical restoration for patients with EDS/HMS, but it also seems apparent that traditional models of exercise and stretch need redefining with this patient group. For example, a low back pain sufferer whose muscles have weakened through disuse and guarded behaviour would probably benefit from regular and systematic graded stretch. This approach is not as applicable to patients with EDS. Further consideration needs to be made when trying to improve physical conditioning through testing of physical limits, and patients might be caught in a dilemma, as was explained to me by a female patient who described the need to improve physical conditioning by pushing the boundaries, but then risking a one- or two-day flare-up of her pain and fatigue. Simultaneously she recognised that improvement would not occur without pushing the boundaries. This patient also described how a boundary as a limit would vary day to day; exercise tolerance would not be static and the same set of exercises or stretches would have different consequences. In trying to support these patients with such challenges, I would argue for the need for psychological flexibility and the need for acceptance to help cope with this variability in their physical state.

The therapy team comprises physiotherapists, occupational therapists, occupational therapy assistants and clinical health psychologists. There is only medical cover if the patients are admitted to the rehabilitation ward. Individual sessions are mostly delivered in physiotherapy, in addition to occupational therapy and clinical health psychology as appropriate. Group therapy sessions combine educative, guided mastery and discussion. The interdisciplinary input is delivered Monday to Friday from 9am to 4.30pm. Weekend goals are set for the two weekends during the programme. Discharge goals are set and reviewed at the follow-up sessions. Patient progress is reviewed at the standard three- and twelve-month follow-up but *ad hoc* sessions are also arranged. Clinical experience suggests that more than one admission can be useful for many patients. The opportunity for further admissions will be discussed amongst the rehabilitation team.

Group-based cognitive behavioural therapy

Group therapy is an essential component of the rehabilitation programme and includes sessions on assertiveness, family and friends, and managing relapse. I hope it is useful to the reader if I describe these sessions to illuminate group-based cognitive behavioural therapy.

Assertiveness

The session on assertiveness provides a particular challenge as some patients readily admit to lacking assertiveness, while others take the opposite view, believing they are very assertive. It is a challenge when a patient expresses the view, 'This does not apply to me.' Patients are encouraged to consider that improvements or alternatives are always a possibility. Patients will often recognise they can be their 'own worst enemy' with examples such as overdoing activity, allowing oneself to be manipulated or exploited and not speaking up for oneself. A lack of assertiveness is a common theme underpinning being one's own worst enemy. Patients are asked to offer definitions or examples of being assertive.

For some patients, speaking up for themselves is extremely difficult, not only with strangers but close family members also. The session will also provide an exploration of communication styles and suggestions for improving effective communication. Patient examples will be used, and members of the group will make suggestions about how, for example, requests for help can be politely declined. As discussed above, a patient's sense of guilt can underpin a lack of assertiveness. Some patients will not speak openly with family and friends in order to avoid conflict and talk of 'keeping the peace'. Realising that being assertive is not the same as being rude or aggressive can be empowering for many patients. Lack of assertiveness may be explained by the desire to avoid causing conflict. There is usually opportunity to practise being assertive on the programme, and role play can be employed within the session. As with all behavioural experiments, it is essential to try out the behaviour and reflect, review and modify the strategy if needed. Trying out new strategies for improving assertiveness will be easier in the safer environment of the programme.

Family and friends

Closely linked to the assertiveness session is an exploration of the role of family and friends. Long-term health conditions cannot be simply viewed from the patient's perspective, and trying to cope with a long-term chronic health condition will clearly have an influence on the quality of their relationships. Suffering is usually in the public arena and will impact on those closest to the patient. During this session the patients are encouraged to view their condition within a *systems* approach (Bennum 1988), with a collection of reciprocal interactions. Patients are asked to consider how they behave towards family and friends and reflect on how family and friends feel about their condition. The group is asked to think about the rules and characteristics of their family and how they impact on their condition and coping with pain (Williamson, Robinson and Melamed 1997).

The effects of chronic pain on relationships are discussed. Peck and Love (1986) describe how incapacity can lead to a shift in duties to the partner, and fewer joint activities can lead to a less rewarding relationship. A person in pain may withdraw from social interactions or obligations, and the subsequent sense of isolation will augment the suffering. Patients are asked to consider how the pain has affected family life. While some patients withdraw, others try to cope by trying to overcompensate and not 'letting the pain beat me'. Some patients describe how family members will display solicitous behaviour which can absolve the patient of family responsibilities (Flor, Kerns and Turk 1987). By attempting to care for their relative in pain, family members may augment and reinforce disability. Patients are encouraged to review the quality of the relationship and highlight how it might be helping or possibly undermining their ability to cope.

The role of the emotional climate within the family home is also explored. Consolidating an earlier session on stress, patients are asked to identify possible stressors within the family. A review of communication patterns and styles may encourage patients to reflect on their role in difficult familial situations. Many patients come to realise that a particular relationship is causing stress and are determined to improve such a relationship. Some patients realise that a particular friendship is exploitative and attenuating their coping, and leave the programme with the intention of distancing themselves from that friend.

A discussion of familial roles and how those roles may have changed due to pain can also help to improve communication. Patients are encouraged to discuss the programme with family and friends. As previously discussed, the patients return home at the end of weeks one and two and are encouraged to introduce and practise the new coping strategies within their home. One constant concern expressed by patients is questioning the real-life applicability of the programme. Patients acknowledge it is far easier to practise new coping strategies on the programme where they are not distracted by the routine and demands of their home life. Involving close family in achieving discharge goals may help to maintain progress. Family members are invited to attend a group-based session delivered by a consultant nurse to help inform them about the structure and aims of the programme, and provide an open forum for discussion. The rehabilitation team also asks patients to invite family members to visit the programme on an individual basis. Patients are reminded that the programme focuses on achieving change which will have consequences for those closest to the patient. It is hoped these changes will be embraced, but experience suggests that some family members may inadvertently undermine the programme by resisting change.

Maintenance strategies

Marlatt and Gordon (1980) identified four steps in relapse prevention: being aware that relapse is occurring; remaining calm and employing relaxation techniques to prevent exaggerated emotional response; reflecting on the antecedents leading up to the setback; and utilising a setback plan. Keefe and Van Horn (1993) suggest relapse is more likely if symptoms increase in intensity, there is a weakened sense of symptom control, and psychological distress is magnified. They have described four key skills to help patients cope with relapse: practice in identifying high-risk situations that are likely to compromise coping ability; practice in identifying early warnings of relapse; rehearsal of coping skills to these early relapse signs; and training in self-reinforcement for effective coping with early relapse.

The final session is devoted to preparing patients for discharge and maintaining their progress. Patients will usually be optimistic and positive about returning home, and eager to implement newly acquired coping strategies. This final session can be an opportunity to explore any concerns and explore strategies for minimising 'slip-ups' or occasions when progress is not maintained and the patient is in danger of falling back into old maladaptive patterns of behaviour. Common topics for discussion will include such issues as being distracted by family commitments, overactivity or lacking motivation. There will be discussion around strategies to prevent losing focus. Patients will leave with good intentions but are warned to be vigilant of slipping back into old habits, and the group is warned about risk factors that contribute to this. The role of stress, habitual behaviour and lack of support are all common risk factors. Group members are asked to reflect on what risk factors could be relevant to their situation.

Realistic goal-setting is an important strategy for ensuring progress is maintained after discharge. Patients are taught how to set long-term goals such as return to work and that these are more likely to be achieved and to be more sustainable if they set smaller short-term goals. A key question put to the group at this session is, 'What needs to change in order to achieve your goal?' Throughout the programme, patients are encouraged to think about their goals, which are set at discharge and reviewed at the follow-up sessions. Examples of goals from previous programmes are offered to prompt discussion. Long-term goals are suggested, and the group is asked to design the necessary short-term goals. It is interesting to note at this session how easily members in the group will problem-solve the goal-setting exercise.

The final part of the session explores what happens when slip-ups occur or when a patient loses focus. Patients are warned about complacency, and although many patients make significant progress after discharge, others struggle and fall back into old maladaptive behaviours. Setback plans are discussed as strategies for coping with pain flare-ups or loss of focus (Parker *et al.* 2000).

Losing focus should not be greeted with apathy or anger; instead it should be used as an opportunity to reflect, consider why the focus was lost and make plans to recover progress. Being too harsh or judgemental will not encourage refocusing on goals. It is useful to accept the disappointment but not to dwell, and make plans to get back on track. Patients are encouraged to read their programme file, which by discharge should have developed into a health condition management resource. Contact details of the staff are included in the file, and patients are encouraged to use these details if further support is needed.

Characteristics of the group in therapy

It is interesting to note the different roles that some patients assume in group therapy. The *group initiator* is a member taking on responsibility for answering questions and breaking awkward silences. The *group joker* will often diffuse tension or add humour to the discussion. The *group parent* is the patient who takes on a parenting role, offering comfort and support to other members. The *group challenger* may question the model of the programme, expressing doubt about the validity of group therapy. The author considers a key function within the group is to facilitate, challenge, confront and provoke at times. A key focus of the psychology sessions is to encourage introspection and require the patient to ask of themselves, 'How is this material relevant to me?' Although there may be a need to confront, for example, an inflammatory remark from one member to another, the group cohesion needs to be maintained. Proposing an alternative view can often help to diffuse difficult situations. There is also a need to be aware that many core pain beliefs may have been held for many years and alternative explanations need to be presented with sensitivity and discretion.

Problems within group therapy

It is clear from my own evaluation that patients generally find the psychology sessions most challenging. This finding might be explained because patients are encouraged to introspect and consider their role in trying to manage their health and may feel uncomfortable with the process. There is a danger of appearing judgemental and there is a need to try to challenge erroneous assumptions with sensitivity. The author believes part of the role is to facilitate and encourage change, rather than criticise or make value judgements.

A problem commonly seen occurs when a patient's expectation of treatment outcome is not met by the programme. At assessment, patients are clearly told and given supporting literature that pain relief or cure is not the focus of attention. Nevertheless, some patients still hope that pain will be reduced, particularly and possibly encouraged by the hospital-based setting. It could be argued that the community-based programme will help to further de-medicalise the pain problem, and I plan to evaluate the data from the hotel-based programme.

It is important to watch for signs that a patient is not engaging – such as passive aggressive behaviour, vociferous complaints or apathy. It can be useful to speak privately to such a patient and try to offer reassurance and reiterate the core aims of the programme. Some patients may expect group therapy to fail because they view their pain as a problem that can only be helped through medical treatment. These patients may fail to engage in treatment or prematurely drop out of group therapy. Some patients will interfere with the group process. For example, some will attempt to dominate discussions if permitted, or use the time to complain about their frustration with poor medical treatment. Anger and frustration are common sequelae of chronic pain and are regularly displayed within the group.

Family systems

The management of EDS/HMS is still a relatively new science, but it is clear to me that models of care must include involvement of friends and family. I can see how this can be a controversial area and it is not my intention to cause offence or insult, but in my opinion the role of the family is crucial because the type of support may contribute to ineffective coping. Just as individual patients will cope in idiosyncratic ways so will family and friends try to adapt and cope accordingly. Again I believe using a scale can usefully illustrate this issue. At one end a family may be trying to help by over-solicitous behaviour, seen when paying close attention to symptoms and encouraging maladaptive coping, such as leading a very sedentary lifestyle and being over-attentive. At the other end of the scale is the family who adopt a somewhat more resigned way of coping, seen when they believe it is helpful to tell the family member with EDS that they need to pull themselves together and ignore their symptoms. This position can particularly be reinforced by previous medical consultations which may have suggested the symptoms are psychosomatic and the patient is engaging in attention-seeking behaviour. Again I would argue that both extremes are equally unhelpful. I believe that further models of therapy need to be explored involving family and friends.

At the RNOH we have developed ways of working with the family from the initial assessment, as discussed earlier. I find it particularly useful to ask close family members how they believe their relative copes with EDS/HMS and tries to make sense of their condition. It is also useful to ask about lifestyle and structure to their day. We have also developed a family and friends session where family and friends are invited to attend, which is part educational but also gives the family and friends further opportunity to discuss concerns. We also offer an open invitation to family and friends to meet with any of the team on an individual basis, and in the past I have worked closely with partners and the parents of patients with EDS. Although in my opinion, for those patients who would benefit most, it is unfortunate when their family and friends do not attend. This is perhaps indicative of a difficult set of familial dynamics. Even when I have worked with family and friends I have often encountered resistance to change. It is certainly not my intention, but regrettably some family members feel judged and criticised for not coping more effectively with their relative's condition. Of course, not all family and friends are overtly resistant and some of the barriers are more subtle. For example, I have encountered passive aggressive behaviour when parents may show an interest in attending and clearly want to be seen to be doing the best for their child, but actually in hindsight they have been unwilling and unable to change the family dynamics. Unfortunately, both patients and family members may make erroneous assumptions about my role, for example resistance in working with me because there is a belief that the involvement of a psychologist is further evidence of an imagined or psychiatric concern. Some direct quotes may help to illustrate this point.

I have been told, for example, that 'I am not mad so I don't need to see you, the pain is not in my head so I don't need to see you'. Some family members have told their relative with EDS that 'I don't need to see the psychologist because I am not the mad one'. I regularly find that I need to explain my role within the team and feel the most helpful explanation is to explain that the whole team is interested in changing the patient's ability to cope with their EDS/HMS. Indeed, some of the most dramatic improvement has been with the support and inclusion of family and friends.

I have found that encouraging patients to review their relationships can be a helpful start in exploring alternative models of coping and communication style. For example, many patients need to become more assertive with family and friends in trying to meet their needs, and for some patients this will mean asking for more help. For others being more assertive might mean explaining to the family members that actually they are more capable of engaging in activity and what is needed is space and opportunity to explore change and become more independent. As we are still developing our expertise working with this patient group, it is clear to me that we also need to develop expertise in working with family and friends in order to encourage and foster improved coping.

Conclusion

I have tried to describe how the rehabilitation team at the RNOH are currently working to improve the lives of those with EDS/HMS. The views expressed are my own and a personal reflection on my work with this patient group.

Although the RNOH can now be considered the residential rehabilitation centre of excellence in the UK for EDS/HMS patients (personal communication with Professor Grahame), we still have much to learn. I believe that every patient contact is an opportunity to learn more about EDS/HMS. It is clear to me that health professionals need to collaborate with our patients to develop better models of care. Prejudice and erroneous assumptions need to be challenged. The rehabilitation team has embraced the challenge to push the boundaries of knowledge in working with this patient group who have not received the level of care seen in other chronic health conditions. It is hoped that the rehabilitation team at the RNOH will make a substantial contribution to improving the quality of life of those with EDS/HMS.

Acknowledgements

Thanks to Margaret Piper for transcribing, and to my patients, who grant me the privilege of trying to support them in securing a better quality of life.

Conclusion to Part III

When I started to write this book I had no idea just how vast the psychology section would become. There were so many aspects to explore, not just personally as a patient, but also for me to reflect upon professionally as a therapist. In conclusion, the psychology in working with and managing the chronic complex patient or a patient with conditions such as EDSIII or FM is highly significant and deserves careful thought, great attention and emphasis in medical practice. Further research is required to look at any relationships between learning difficulties such as dyslexia, dyscalculia and ADD and connective tissue disorders such as EDS, as well as medical practitioners being alerted to the issue of self-harm and other psychiatric or personality disorders in this patient group and early intervention, support and management. Therapists and medical professionals need to take care of themselves too!

Part IV is all about exercise and rehabilitation, but is also strongly linked to both the physiology and psychology sections.

PART IV
EXERCISE AND REHABILITATION

CHAPTER 28

Exercise and rehabilitation

EDS patient experiences of physiotherapy and Isobel's 'stages' of treatment

Introduction to Part IV

In Part IV we look at my rehabilitation in physiotherapy, and also at other treatment approaches including Pilates, the Feldenkrais Method® and the Bowen Technique. Movement patterning and muscle stiffness are all discussed as well as imaging movement and considering the quality of movement. A return to exercise is discussed and in particular cardiovascular and endurance work. Other aspects of specific rehabilitation are discussed in terms of temporomandibular joint (TMJ) and cervical spine. Issues in relation to trauma, birth trauma and movement disorders are also discussed. Part IV (and the book) ends with a conclusion about the outcome in terms of the management of my EDSIII.

An EDSIII patient wrote on Facebook:

I recently became so overcome with the totality of my diagnosis that I fell into utter despair, depression and anxiety about what my life has become. I quit my job due to pain and depression, I stopped eating, stopped leaving my house pretty much, and COMPLETELY STOPPED EXERCISING. More to the point, I stopped physical activity of any kind and was basically bed-ridden except for bathroom breaks and a few short trips around my house. I watched my muscles atrophy. I could no longer stand without my heart racing. I could not do simple tasks due to weakness. Two weeks ago I decided I cannot give up and I must get stronger. I started walking around my development

– one lap per day and was totally exhausted. I am now up to four laps per day! I was able to take my son grocery shopping yesterday! I am able to do tasks again and am stronger. We need to keep active, no matter how slight the movement may seem. Keep the muscles working, girls!

Exercises and rehabilitation

Physiotherapy is known for its usage of exercises to strengthen and rehabilitate the injured body after injury, and it is often an essential aspect of the treatment (Bassett and Petrie 1999; Hemmings and Povey 2002; Medina-Mirapeix *et al.* 2009). In terms of exercise rehabilitation, I would most probably be considered a model patient since I actively requested exercises that I could do at home and my physio never had any problems in terms of my adherence to exercise, which can be a problem with some patients (Medina-Mirapeix *et al.* 2009). There are two reasons why exercises have worked for me. The first reason is that I was internally motivated to do them and, second, my physio gave me minimal exercises in terms of causing an increase in pain or symptoms, often taking a 'less-is-more' approach, meaning that I was often able to see improvements in a short space of time. The programme has got to be realistic to the patient and their compliance tolerance – for example, what they are likely to realistically manage (Bassett and Petrie 1999; Hemmings and Povey 2002). Again, the manner of the physiotherapist can make all the difference in patient adherence to exercise programmes. In order to fulfil my requirements as an autoethnographical writer, I am using other EDSIII patients as social and cultural representatives. The following text comes from the Hypermobility Syndrome Association (HMSA) forum. An HMSA patient writes:

> The third course [of physiotherapy] was really only to add to the exercises that I already had as I felt I wasn't working certain muscles as well as I could be doing, and as the physio knew all about EDS he was far more helpful than I'd expected! Helped my shoulder instability loads when I'm using my arm (although when I'm at rest it still falls out) and given me lots of 'just in case' exercises for various other parts of my body so if I start to have a problem with that joint (although it's fine now) I can just refer to my folder and there it'll be. He also helped my knee

proprioception and my posture load, and he had the same sense of humour that I do so we had a right laugh!

With respect to the types of exercises given to EDSIII patients, the same member makes the following comments, and I agree, that:

'Normal' physio exercises can be damaging to HMS/EDS patients because some physios don't seem to realise this before it is too late and their patient had been injured. We need gentle, Pilates-type exercises to strengthen our core and minor (stabilising) muscles, then eventually thera-band exercises, exercises to work our bigger muscles and gentle cardio once we have developed the necessary core strength, I just wish more physios realised this!!

Another HMSA forum member pays attention to the need to educate physiotherapists who specifically work with the EDSIII patient group. She writes that:

In my opinion there is a huge need to educate the physiotherapists that do not work specifically in hypermobility clinics. They can do so much damage if they are not aware by inappropriate exercises. Also, something to help with the clumsiness, I have heard that there are specific physio tools you can use but not sure what. My good physio did lack [knowledge] in that he was not fully aware, I believe, of the effects of conditions like POTS, fatigue, stomach problems etc and trying to work on your ability to exercise. Sometimes I felt the amount of exercise 4 times a day was just way too unrealistic and really worsened my dizzy spells. There needs to be more practical realistic advice about how we can incorporate physio into our daily life, with the many other difficulties we face. Ultimately, if we are shown correct and appropriate measures the first time it reduces the chance that we will have to keep 'burdening the NHS'. I also believe there needs to be a huge shift in the attitudes of some physio/doctors just to actually listen to their patients. I work as a nurse in oncology, so I know how stressful NHS can be. But I would never dismiss my patients like that.

In working with the EDS patient group, the physiotherapist needs to work very quickly to build a good rapport and trust with the patient, many of whom have been badly let down in the past by previous therapists, as in this case of the following HMSA member:

I have listed and reviewed the 17 physios I've seen over the last 10 years and they include NHS and private (mostly), this country (mostly) and abroad… None moved me forwards.

It is very much the case that EDS patients are likely to be generally quite a challenging group of patients to work with owing to the complexity of the condition. The physiotherapist who inherits an EDS patient will need to be prepared for a challenge, aside from the fact the patient themselves might have had poor prior experiences to physiotherapy. The following describes what I call my 'phases' of physiotherapy treatment.

Phases of my physiotherapy treatment

Phase one: April 2008–October 2008
Generally exercise based, sessions initially 4–8 weeks apart. Largely 'hands-off'. My musculature begins to change and I am given some gross motor support with improvements to gluteals, adductors, obliques, abdominals and hamstrings and calf.

Psychologically the exercises were incredibly important to me because they gave me a sense of empowerment and control and enabled me to take some responsibility for my own recovery. I could sense the physical improvements through doing the exercises – particularly in the way my musculature started to tone up, which led to an improved perception of my body image and an increase in self-esteem. In terms of the translation of improving my gross muscle groups, I think it took some time for me to embody the usage of the gained control into ballet classes, but in the early stages I still had no sense of just how poor my muscular control was and how unstable my body really was. I think that it wasn't until I started to do the exercises that my physio gave me that I began to understand this concept and there was possibly a whole lot more going on than an injured calf.

Phase two: October 2008–September 2010
Pilates studio sessions started in October 2008. Physiotherapy 'hands on' work started from approx November/December 2008, starting with some lumbar spine work which caused an increase in pain and symptoms. Throughout phase two, different areas of the body were worked on, but there was still a strong exercise-based focus. Progress was actually very slow, although musculature was continuing to change. There were

no improvements to other body systems during this time, and active muscle spasming or twitching started in January 2010. Neck rehabilitation started during that time. Thoracic spine rehabilitation started during August 2010. Pilates work continued and I was often suffering from global muscle pain and fatigue. Progress in general was fairly minimal, but I had built up trust with my physio and although there was much overall change, I wanted to continue having treatment. I thought that Pilates was supplementing change.

Phase three: September 2010–July 2011
I had suffered problems with the new T-Spine range of movement (ROM) that my physio had given me in August which led to a radical increase in POTS symptoms for a while. I stopped Pilates in September owing to price increases. At this point physiotherapy became the mainstay for my treatment. Rehabilitation became very holistic and a more systemic review began. It was a challenging time, and change and progress were hugely accelerated amongst periods of turbulence for me, with particular reference to the problems encountered in treating my neck. This was largely owing to deep muscular weakness which was exposed, initially thought to have been previously rehabilitated, which was not the case. I started to get improvements with bladder function, headaches, POTS, asthma and IBS. Being given new ROM caused an increase in pain and symptoms at times, but the benefits were beginning to outweigh these deficits. I also experienced an increase in stiffness owing to further significant and more sophisticated muscular and neuromuscular control. This stiffness was released as required by my physio and as my strength improved – for example, I gained greater ROM in other body parts, including the first metatarsal joint. I continued to experience waves of extreme fatigue (and pain) during this phase, but perhaps that is of no great consequence, or surprise, given the magnitude and rapidity of change.

Phase four: August 2011–December 2011
I finally conquered walking in true parallel although still experiencing some problems with left ITB relating to continuing abdominal weakness owing to underlying gynaecological and bowel pathologies. I started to respond from crisis far more

rapidly and was in a much more stable state. Although I still suffered from fatigues/crisis these were becoming shorter in duration and I was becoming more predictable and less ANS reactive. Spasms were still there, but again were less rife than before. I was becoming more independent in the management of my EDSIII and at this point began to reduce dependence upon a physiotherapist (as a life-support machine).

Phase five: December 2011–ongoing
I changed physiotherapists at this point and this was a difficult time for me. I started to do cardiovascular exercise, including more swimming, and started to go jogging which has built up significantly over time. Physiotherapy appointments have reduced to an average of one to two appointments per month with new remedial exercises as required. Remaining areas have included exercises to stretch ankle and Achilles, exercises for TMJ and exercises to strengthen psoas and thoracic spine. Manual therapy continues in order to release hip flexor tightness, upper thoracic tightness and trigger points and to continue working on TMJ function. Work continues to address psychological/behavioural patterns which continue to fuel some of my fatigue/pain.

Before I even started some physio exercises, I was using the concept of imaging as a way of rehearsing movement that might not have been possible (initially). The other adage that my physio had was of insisting upon the impeccable quality of movement, especially on initial learning. Thus she advocated a less-is-more approach to movement, as can be seen in Chapter 29.

Imaging exercises and 'less is more'

There are two different kinds of imaging: one whereby someone mentally rehearses (for example) movement, as if they were going to do it for real, but don't. It might be a way for a person to visualise or think through a movement pattern before they commence the activity. This gives the brain an opportunity to rehearse the movement mentally before commencing the actual physical movement. For dancers, it is a particularly common way to practise and think through movement patterns and sequences without the physical activity, thus saving them valuable energy whilst the brain is still receiving the information and motor and muscular patterns continue to be forged. Warner and McNeill write that:

> Mental imagery and mental practice require no special equipment and are easily taught and learned. Physical therapists' implementation of mental imaging and mental practice and other proposed procedures enabled their patients to assist in speeding recovery, create a greater ease of performance, enhance their mental clarity, reduce stress and create a sense of serenity.
>
> *Warner and McNeill 1987, p.520*

The second type of imaging involves use of evocative language provided by dance teachers and movement practitioners, for example physiotherapists and Feldenkrais and Alexander Technique teachers. The words and language used are to facilitate improvements in movement – for instance, 'imagine there is water flowing down your shoulders to release tension in the shoulders and neck'. Movement therapist Eric Franklin writes that:

> When doing exercises under instruction we are apt to think that we move or direct the moving of the muscles. What actually

happens is that we get a picture from the teacher's words or his movements, and the appropriate action takes place within our own bodies to reproduce this picture. The result is successful in proportion to our power of interpretation and amount of experience, but most of all perhaps to the desire to do.

Franklin 1996, p.36

Franklin further suggests that using a variety of sensual feedback can further facilitate the quality and improvement of movement. He writes that:

Often the most powerful imagery is composed of a variety of senses. If you imagine yourself standing under a waterfall you may have the sensory experiences of seeing and feeling the water pouring down your body, hearing it thundering all around you, smelling its fresh scent as well as tasting it in your mouth.

Franklin 1996, p.49

Either way, both mental rehearsing imagery and sensual imagery are both ways of improving the outcome of movement and the eventual quality of it. When working with EDSIII patients, the mental rehearsing is invaluable because it saves the body's already (often) depleted energy levels. Sometimes, when I was learning a new exercise in physio, I was encouraged just to 'image' or rehearse what I intended my body to do without the replication of physical movement. The images that were then provided to improve the quality of that exercise – for example, imagining a feeling of sinking (when putting my head on an overball) – would further assist in replicating the best possible movement I could (realistically) achieve.

Quality and 'less is more'

One of the problems for EDSIII patients and patients of other related conditions such as FM or chronic fatigue syndrome (CFS) is that they fatigue very quickly and so, as discussed, imaging and mental rehearsal are effective strategies for practising new movement patterns, but when the actual movement is attempted for real 'less is more'. One really quality repetition of a movement in a series, for example pelvic tilt, is far better than ten badly executed pelvic tilts. The body needs to learn the correct movement pattern, so in fact by doing less the body has a much clearer idea of what is expected with endurance with one repetition which is performed with excellence than with copious repetitions where quality of movement declines significantly unless the patient is being very carefully observed. I am thinking more here about exercises that patients are required to do at home. Obviously, though, as the movement is learned correctly and well, then repetitions can be gradually increased over time. However, quality absolutely must supersede quantity. This was something that was a consideration in my Pilates work, described in Chapter 30.

Pilates, physiolates and core stability

In my previous book *A Guide to Living with Hypermobility Syndrome* (Knight 2011) I recommended Pilates to the reader, because at the time of writing that book I had every reason to believe that doing Pilates was the correct approach for someone with HMS/EDSIII, if the whole premise behind Pilates is to strengthen core stability. I explained that:

> I started to do Pilates which I hoped would give me the abdominal muscles I had always dreamed of and more technically, improve my core stability so that my painful back might have more muscular support. Joseph Pilates created the Pilates Method based on allowing people to optimize their health and physical wellbeing and correcting imbalances and weaknesses (Friedman and Eisen 1980).
>
> *Knight 2011, p.94*

Not long before I completed my first book, the prices rose sharply in the Pilates studio and it made it too costly for me to continue (on top of paying for physiotherapy, etc.). In some ways this might have been useful, because when I reflect back over the time I was doing both physiotherapy and Pilates, I appeared to be making less progress and there are a number of hypothetical reasons as to rationalise why.

Quite often after Pilates I would feel far more fatigued and would end up in more pain. I had previously always 'squared this circle' by thinking that there was no pain without gain and, because of being in chronic pain anyway, just expected that this was normal and accepted it without undue care or question. In addition, it appears that I might have (at times) been overworked, which was not helpful and therefore added to my pain and fatigue. Again, I was so used to feeling this way, I had begun to accept this as 'my lot' and as normal for me. Conversely, my physiotherapy exercises seldom caused me anything other than an acceptable level of training pain and did not contribute unduly to fatigue. There is no doubt that attempting new movement patterns in physiotherapy initially caused flare-up, but these were usually explainable situations. What was going on in Pilates was some overwork, overuse and systemic global fatigue and pain.

Initially there was a period of time where I was doing some physio exercises – but nothing really new – and then ballet, as I had always done. Between September 2010 and very early November 2010 I had no Pilates, and at this point my physio was working on her own with me. However, I soon realised that because of stopping Pilates I would lose any strength I had gleaned from doing Pilates-based work and that I would further deteriorate. I mentioned this to my physio so that we could seek an alternative approach, which I defined as 'physiolates'.

Reflections about Pilates

I often end up in more pain after Pilates. It is interesting that I do not end up in as much pain after physio exercises. I do get training pain, but I don't end up in Global Widespread Pain. After Pilates, I was often in pain. The reason I am having a better time with physio exercises is that I make quick progress, and they are enough for me to manage and understand what you want me to do and I know what the outcome of the exercise is meant to be. I understand what I am doing it for and it translates incredibly quickly.

Physiotherapy, 24.11.2011

I think you need a huge amount of experience to pick up on what people are cheating at (in a movement capacity). You are the only person who knows your body well enough – I thought [Pilates] was helping – because I thought I needed it to get strong. I didn't understand the fact the deep muscles underwork and the superficial ones overwork. It is supposed to be the philosophy of Pilates. Talked to X about pelvic floor – if I wasn't accessing that – what good was I doing?

Physiotherapy, 5.1.2011

HMSA forum members make the following comments about Pilates:

I've done Pilates for a number of years now. The first class I went to was 'pure' Pilates, e.g. naval to spine, Abs 100, rolling down etc. I found this class very hard and the teacher had to modify the exercises a lot for me. Sometimes I wondered whether I was getting any benefit from it. I stuck it out as I thought any exercise was better than nothing. However, for the last five years I have been going to a class called Chek Pilates. It is a modified version of the pure Pilates and I find it a lot less painful than the pure Pilates and I actually feel as though my posture has improved.

I've been going to a 'Body Balance' class for the last three years and find it really helps. I was diagnosed about four years ago, and was looking for something to strengthen my core muscles, when my friend suggested this class. It's an hour long combination of Pilates, yoga and Tai Chi, once a week, and it has definitely improved my strength and the stability of my joints. If I miss a couple of weeks, I can tell the difference – I get more stiffness and aching, particularly in my lower back and legs. It also helps me to relax, and I come out feeling refreshed, full of energy and generally happy...which also improves my sleep!

My instructor is very good, and everyone works at their own level, so if I'm having a bad day I just do as much as I feel able to, then have a rest. I do have to be careful though, as some of the moves can cause me to overextend. For example, lying on the floor with one leg raised – we were told to lower the leg out to the side and back up again, only as far as we could get without the other hip starting to lift. But being Bendy, I could lower my leg right to the floor with my hips still facing the ceiling!!

After a couple of weeks I spoke to the instructor, and was quite surprised that she had actually heard of hypermobility syndrome! She told me that with moves like that, I should concentrate on using my core muscles to control and stabilise the movement, rather than extending as far as possible. The routine is changed every 12 weeks to keep it interesting, and she is always giving special instructions for pregnant women, about which moves should be modified or avoided – but unfortunately there isn't any such guidance for hypermobile people.

Although HMSA forum patients feel Pilates can be helpful, there are some threads in overuse and overwork similar to what I experienced.

Probably what would be ideal for all EDSIII patients would be specific physiotherapy exercises, many of which are Pilates-based anyway – but it is the quality/concentration or accuracy of movement and the number of repetitions which is most crucial to the EDSIII patient in avoiding fatigue, overuse and pain. Pilates sessions for EDSIII, chronic complex patients need to be conducted in either a one-to-one context, or a very small group session, with very experienced Pilates teachers, as Jessica Moolenaar, a very experienced Pilates teacher and teacher trainer (Pilates Foundation), explains.

PILATES AND HYPERMOBILITY
Jessica Moolenaar

Introduction
The Pilates Method is a holistic movement programme originally designed by Joe Pilates (1880–1967). Pilates was a sickly child but was determined to overcome his frailties and engaged in gymnastics, boxing, body-building and dance. He was interned in England during the First World War and created exercise programmes for himself and fellow internees during confinement. He also invented a system of exercises for those needing rehabilitation with the use of springs for resistance; the Pilates Method was born.

Nowadays we can distinguish 'classic' Pilates, exercises on the mat and on Pilates equipment – closely resembling Pilates' hardcore conditioning regime – from 'evolved' Pilates, a form of Pilates that has developed into a more person-centred form of movement education, taking into consideration the personal needs of the student and modifying the classic movement repertoire somewhat. In my opinion the Pilates Method as it is mostly practised in the UK is usually evolved, that is, an intelligent holistic series of movement sequences on mat and equipment, that allow the body–mind to repattern movement habits and that allow for a balancing of strength and mobility in the soft tissues. I therefore also believe that Pilates is inherently 'rehabilitative' in that it rebalances anybody, whether it is a body trained in dance and unbalanced by an injury or a body with a physical condition like hypermobility. The key is always the person-centred nature of the movement education: everybody needs a different set of movement sequences with a different teaching approach.

Joe Pilates originally coined his technique Contrology (Pilates and Miller 1998) and left us with a body of work, consisting of two books, in which he set out the philosophy behind his regime with descriptions of the movements themselves. As Pilates was not aware at the time of the way in which the sensory motor system acquires new movement patterns, he has given us little instruction in *how* to perform (or teach) his system. However, he uses language that might give us an idea of his philosophy: 'our muscles obeying our will... and our will not being dominated by the reflex action of our muscles' (Pilates and Miller 1998, p.10). These phrases imply a programme based on a body–mind connection, whereby our mind is *in control* of our body. In my opinion the 'body–mind' is a whole and functions as such. The more we listen to the body, that is, the more we are *in* the body with the mind, the more we will discover about ourselves and how best to develop. One could say that the body as part of the body–mind is a container of memory and is manifesting that which we need to uncover and develop, through making a conscious connection with it through our mind.

Pilates principles

Friedman and Eisen outlined the principles that are at work in modern Pilates: breathing, control, precision, flowing movement and centring (Friedman and Eisen 1980). Brooke Siler, 20 years later, named the principles as follows: concentration, control, centring, fluidity, precision, breathing, imagination, intuition and integration (Siler 2000). I have renamed these principles yet again for them to become a reflection of the inherent *holistic* nature of Pilates practice, in which the body–mind connection is central to the efficacy of sensory motor learning and which reflects the learning taking place through movement and embodiment rather than mindless and often boring bio-mechanical 'exercise'.

- *Concentration* I have renamed 'being present'. It is when we are in the moment, sensing and feeling what is going on in our body–mind, that we can facilitate change and allow for a greater range of choices in movement. We can also call this being present, this becoming aware, 'embodying'.

- *Control* I have renamed 'directing movement'. It is our present will that directs movement, but rather than having an emphasis on just using blunt muscle power, which 'control' implies, I would like to add that we direct movement in release. We are releasing faulty sensory motor patterns as we initiate new, more functional patterns by being mindful of making new body–mind connections. We are overriding old brain patterns, we are reorganising our body. If we use functional movement patterns we stabilise as well as mobilise in the right places.

- *Centring* becomes 'moving from the inside out'. We feel movement being connected to and initiated from our core; we can then make a choice to bring our awareness in other parts of the body simultaneously.

- *Fluidity* becomes 'moving with equanimity'. Movement never ceases, but is an ongoing flow from moment to moment, sustained and smooth.

- *Precision* I have renamed as 'moving through inner alignment'. We feel our body alignment internally and do not try to represent an outer alignment or form that does not support the opening and range of movement of our joints and soft tissues. Feeling this inner alignment is probably the most poignant aspect of Pilates that sets it apart from most other Western therapeutic movement modalities.

- *Breathing* I describe as 'moving with a natural rhythm'. We learn to listen to our breath, which can show us where it can soften and release our body, and it infuses us with energy. It can also show us patterns of contraction and release in the tissues and patterns of fluid flexion and extension, or the lack of them.

- *Visualisation* becomes 'using visual, kinaesthetic, tactile and proprioceptive imagery'. We use this imagery to help us increase our awareness and to increase our proprioception in order to change our habitual way of moving.

- *Intuition* I have translated into 'learning to perceive clearly what is going on in the body and learning to act upon what we perceive by being responsible for oneself'. We learn to mindfully listen to our own body–mind to empower ourselves to act upon our health and wellbeing.

- *Integration* in this context I would explain as 'using the body–mind approach to our body work in our daily life'. By becoming aware that our mind and emotions are interrelated with how our body moves and feels and vice versa, we are becoming aware of those connections in ourselves and in the world around us and we start integrating those insights, not just in our Pilates practice but into our day-to-day lives.

These renamed principles are not different from the principles as Siler described them in her book (2000). They just reflect a more scientific approach to the acquirement of new movement patterns and an acknowledgement of the holistic nature of mind–body exercise.

Dissociation

Thomas Hanna in his book *Somatics* talks about 'sensory motor amnesia', which is the ability of our body–mind to 'forget' or dissociate from parts of our body and its movements (Hanna 1988). It consists of a memory loss of proprioception and the ability to direct our muscles. Because this occurs within the central nervous system we are not aware of it, yet it affects our every movement. Hanna posits that during our lives our sensory motor system responds to daily stresses and traumas with specific muscular reflexes. These reflexes create involuntary habitual muscular contractions which we cannot voluntary relax as they are deeply involuntary and unconscious. Our main task then is to first become aware and feel what we are doing, before we set out to 'repattern' and strengthen. If we do not experience our faulty movement patterns or reflexes we will actually strengthen them. So we need to unlearn or release the faulty patterns and remember what has been forgotten. This will make us aware of how our minds and bodies interrelate and how we hold the key to our own feeling of health and wellbeing. We attempt to do this by being mindful and moving slowly, scanning our body positions and sensations from moment to moment, making different movement choices as we are moving and imprinting these new neural pathways by repeating sequences mindfully again and again.

Proprioception

Pilates seems to be a very efficacious form of movement for any musculoskeletal repatterning, as it deals with an enormous amount of proprioceptive information in our system as a whole, connecting movement, body structure, nervous system, sensations and feelings. As somatic movement modalities go, Pilates forms a bridge between structure and energy, between complementary and biomechanical approaches to body work. In my opinion it is the strength of the technique that it speaks many languages, that of body structure and that of somatics. It is not only what we do, but how we do it and how we experience it, that brings the greatest results. Proprioception is essential.

The becoming aware of where we are in space and where we are internally *and* of what connects to what and where our weight is in different postures and in movement, in other words our sense of proprioception, is something we acquire automatically in play when we grow up. When certain musculoskeletal patterns evolve that are less than helpful or even painful, our body will respond by giving off warning signals, however faint, in the form of numbness, pain or unease. We usually respond by first seeking treatment, such as osteopathy or massage. Treatment will not, however, necessarily change the local or global movement patterns that we have unconsciously acquired. When our proprioception is distorted as it is in hypermobility syndrome, it can happen that we do not hear the faint warning signals at first and seemingly suddenly become trapped in strong bracing patterns.

What is going on here? As the web of connective tissue in which the muscles and bones are embedded is overly lax in hypermobility syndrome, the body will organise itself by protecting unstable joints in movement by bracing local and superficial muscles, thereby inhibiting postural and deeper local muscles to recruit. The joint instability is therefore perpetuated. Fascia and embedded muscle both contract painfully over time and nerves can become impinged. When these patterns become symptomatic, the brain and autonomous nervous system will act to contract in familiar bracing patterns over and over again in times of 'danger' like perceived (emotional) stress and fatigue and sometimes just by sensitisation of particular (trigger) points in the body (Foster 2004). The bracing patterns 'learn' to act in a similar way each and every time until they become a pain syndrome that is hard to break.

What can Pilates practice do?

Before a stable, upright, aligned, dynamic and resilient posture against the pull of gravity and collapse will be possible, a balancing of the soft tissues needs to occur. When viewing the body as a 'tensegrity model', images of juicy, resilient, alive and aware fascia come to mind which moves the skeleton efficiently without buckling, jerking or immobilising (Myers 2001). Hypermobility syndrome by lack of biofeedback and by lack of joint stability, with joints operating out of a healthy range of movement (ROM), causes the myofascial structure to become unbalanced and to pull tissues into patterns of strain and tension and hyperlaxity. Hypermobile people literally 'hang' in their joints, or as I call it they 'park' in their joints. It is a position in which they do not sense where they are in space most of the time, as their proprioception is poor. We can balance the tissues by both mobilisation and stabilisation, first locally then globally.

Mobilisation

A release is needed of the areas in spasm. Gentle breathing into the braced areas can release fascia and muscles and release trapped nerves and restore a sense of proprioception, especially with the aid of the hands on guidance of a teacher. Gentle slow stretching (gentle!) of the braced areas and gentle local micromovement restoring coordination of musculoskeletal movement patterns can also help break the pain-cycle (Foster 2004). A little and often is recommended for the body not to feel threatened by a release that seems too long and too destabilising, which can trigger bracing again (Foster 2004).

Stabilisation

Secondly, a restoring of the underlying lack of postural stability is needed. The deep local postural stabilising muscles need to be strengthened. Most of those are so deep and close to our spine or other joints that we cannot sense them, let alone innervate them separately. Pilates practice takes us through a set of coordinated and gentle movements to strengthen the stabilising muscles locally at first and then globally in bigger movement patterns so that the body starts coordinating fluidly. The conscious use of the movement patterns restores strength and coordination on a deep level, first unconsciously and with each repetition more consciously, overriding neural patterns that were less useful. In time postural muscles strengthen sufficiently for the body not to have to brace to feel 'safe'. Using all the Pilates principles, we learn to breathe, moving in gentle, smooth, coordinated recruitment patterns of contraction and in patterns of release, all the way sensing and feeling the quality of our movement and body sensations. Pilates practice creates the feedback loops if done slowly enough to allow the local stabilisers in static contractions and then global stabilisers in movement to act before the local and global mobilisers threaten to take over as stabilisers in jerky contractions. The segmental stiffness of the stable single joints can then be built into smooth sequencing in more complex movement patterns. The local and global mobilising muscles often recruit in eccentric contraction in Pilates practice, to build slow, sustained control against gravity. This in turn develops movement patterns that both allow release and the building of strength simultaneously. Especially in lumbopelvic stability and articulation of the spine, Pilates practice has a myriad of movement sequences against gentle resistance that work length, strength, awareness, coordination, flow and a deep sense of embodiment simultaneously.

As I have outlined, the healthy coordination and balancing of tissues occurs first unconsciously, then consciously. In Pilates practice proprioceptive feedback loops are restored or improved with the help of the use of mirrors, wobble-boards, balls and thera-bands – Pilates equipment which offers gentle resistance in different positions and movement sequences – and not in the least by having a good teacher. Of utmost importance in restoring an upright resilient system that is able to respond in the moment, we need an experienced teacher to work in a safe range of movement with our joints, especially if we cannot feel where that safe range is. Proper alignment also restores the information pathways of our nervous system and the biochemical pathways, including the flow of blood and oxygen into every cell of the body. The teacher guides us with their own presence and proprioception, with the use of imagery and with hands on feedback to engage our reptilian brain, and with verbal corrections to engage our neocortex, so our nervous system calms and learns to trust this new way of being.

Obviously practice needs to be done with a very experienced (Pilates Foundation) teacher, and with HMS clients in a one-to-one setting, so a therapeutic relationship and a sense of safety can slowly be built. Pilates practice in small groups can be beneficial much later when deep skills are learnt and presence in the body can be maintained, even in an environment full of distractions. The danger of doing movement programmes by oneself without a well-trained eye of a teacher cannot be underestimated. As the central nervous system cannot give the feedback at first, slow, gentle and sustained practice, little and often, with a good teacher is the only way to restore healthy joint stability, improve proprioception and build a calm and happy nervous system that feels safe and therefore open to receive new information.

In my substantial teaching experience, and as a Pilates Teacher Trainer provider for the Pilates Foundation, I believe that some of the problems that both Isobel and other HMSA members were describing were caused by a lack of embodiment, a lack of sensation in the body, and therefore causing a lack of segmental control of joints moving in smooth coordination. The result of this lack of embodied quality of movement is not only manifesting in pain, instability and bracing but also causes sufferers to 'push' into extreme patterns of movement to release oneself or to enable them to feel any sensation at all. It becomes a matter of all or nothing in terms of muscle recruitment, resulting in hypertonicity or hypotonicity. As pain becomes a normal sensation in some parts of the body, it takes away further ability to perceive body sensation in other parts. The ability to restore a sense of embodiment, an ability to slowly feel the recruitment of muscles, to stabilise joints and to move from a centre in fluidity, would be addressed by slow Pilates practice using the principles as described above, regularly working in one-to-one settings led by teachers who have experience of working holistically and somatically and have experience with hypermobility syndrome. Additional calming of the nervous system caused by the slow movement with the conscious use of breath is very empowering for HMS sufferers and takes away the erroneous belief that only other people can take them out of their predicament. (For more information, contact the Pilates Foundation – see Appendix 3.)

Physiolates

Although I stopped doing Pilates studio sessions for a time, I eventually coined the term 'physiolates' which was almost in jest, but it was a term that I came up with to combine the approaches of both physiotherapy and Pilates. This happened after I had stopped Pilates for a while and realised that if I was not intercepted again with an appropriate rehabilitative exercise plan my progress was going to plateau or, worse still, deteriorate.

My physio met the concept with some amusement ('I think the term is hilarious!' – *Physiotherapy, 17.11.2011*), but I think she knew what I meant.

> I have coined the term 'Physiolates' which may yet catch on and is a made up term really for a session of physiotherapy exercises with a Pilates slant. I have got some old exercises 're-visited', for

example the good old clam for gluteals – and adductor exercises and hamstrings, so my new plan is as follows:

- Gluteals – going for quality and before I start to spasm too much.

- Clams – going for quality and control.

- Adductors – starting for one or two and aiming for quality, especially at the end of the movement and on descent and before I give up!

- Sitting – just practising sitting up but not into extension and allowing lower back to support me in extension. Initially I just do this for a minute or until fatigue sets in. My temptation thus far is to collapse into flexion and I am not sitting on my sits-bones.

- Hamstrings – standing curls against wall, going for quality and completing the movement before spasms kick in.

- Pelvic tilt on a block with leg raised – only one or two to the right where right abdominal is strong, but as many as can cope with on the left to allow for a training effect.

- Thoracic spine flexion keeping shoulders out of the equation and aiming for greater control on the ascent, which is far more difficult for me at the moment.

The session was interesting because my physio and I know that these movements are being done with far greater control than when I was given them 1–2 years ago. I had realised that left was weaker in abs and this now needs strengthening in order to allow the left calf to finally release.

The work made me spasm a lot and my left leg especially felt weak and very strange at the end of the session and it now feels (several hours later) like there is a change of balance and power in my legs and that my right leg is doing more. I can suddenly feel my right hamstrings and my right calf is fatigued – but the right leg is actually doing something!!!!! I really need this to happen so the left leg gets relaxed and gets a break.

Blog, 3.11.2011

Lumbar spine and core stability

Much of my rehabilitation in stage one was centred around obtaining more global muscular strength. My physio was limited in terms of what I would permit in terms of manual therapy and I had made it clear (owing to fear) that I would not allow her to work on my lumbar spine because it was 'stable' at the time. This resulted in a delay in her ability to access the area she believed was essential to stabilise before any of my calf symptoms would subside. We had, in stage one of physio (see Chapter 28), managed to gain some strength in gluteals, hamstrings, adductors and abdominals. In addition I was doing Pilates, so I was also working on abdominals and core stability. However, my physio did not begin working on my lumbar spine until stage two of physio (see Chapter 28), and it was a great challenge for her because, once manual therapy started, there was an increase in my pain and symptoms. Upon reflection and with my understanding as a therapist, if one is going to disturb the tissues and try and persuade change, there is going to be a reaction. All the while I continued my strengthening work whilst the crucial changes to offload my lumbar spine at L4/5, and hopefully my calves, also continued.

The next chapter explores the concepts of muscular repatterning, overuse and muscle stiffness.

CHAPTER 31

Movement patterns

Overuse and muscle stiffness

Reaction to new movement patterns and overuse

The introduction of new movement patterns has often caused me to go into crisis – possibly just because the body has been asked to do something new which was too much for it at the time, or that it couldn't cope with – or it is simply just a big reorganisation. Eventually the body accepts it, but there is very often a period of crisis and increased pain and fatigue whilst this goes on. The following two blog entries explain this type of situation:

> I went into my fourth physiotherapy session on the verge of crisis, which has today gone into full-blown crisis. Potential theories for the crisis are the right arm reaching exercise on transference of weight, given to me by my physio last week. She explains it is a spastic patterning and that my body doesn't like it. Clearly not! I ache all over, feel incredibly fatigued and have neck and shoulder pain and a splitting headache.
>
> *Blog, 12.5.2010*

> My physio asked me to start looking at walking in a different way – e.g. in doing a new hip exercise for walking and the backwards lunge/steps had caused me to go into a muscle spasm chaos with my sacral, lumbar spine and lower thoracic being in complete grid-lock. Additionally I have suffered extreme fatigue and then fibromyalgic nodules of pain all over thoracic spine, knee and elsewhere. The pain was terrible and only diazepam and codeine come anywhere near relieving the pain. I was unable to do my

physiotherapy exercises; ballet caused immense pain the only day I did it.

Blog, 2.3.2011

Overuse can also cause huge flare-ups in the EDSIII patient group and can certainly lead to chaos and crisis. I write that:

> I did too much Pilates and I am now paying for it. Last night I did a variation on a theme of physio exercises, only it was done too many times and as a result today I cannot do three of physio exercises because the whole area is far too fatigued. This is not good. I sort of knew at the time, but it was difficult to stop in a class, and then I thought I would 'get through it' – well, I have, but there is a pay-back. It is also less good as the exercise involved neck, which I can ill-afford to 'mess up' – anyway, I think the motto of the story is that very often, less is more and I should have stopped before I got to the point I was questioning myself. I should have stopped.

Blog, 19.4.2011

Rosemary Keer explains the implications behind physical repatterning and correcting faulty movement patterns.

PHYSICAL REPATTERNING AND CORRECTING FAULTY MOVEMENT PATTERNS[AQ]
Rosemary Keer

Joint motion and stability

Hypermobile individuals have a tendency to rest at the end of their range of joint movement. It is not known why this is so, but there are a few possible explanations.

Hypermobiles have more joint movement to control, so resting at the end of the range and letting the ligaments take the strain requires less effort and feels more secure. This is particularly so in static postures sustained for a period of time.

Within the range of joint motion a 'neutral zone' has been described (Panjabi 1992). This is a portion of a joint's motion, close to the neutral position, where there is minimal internal resistance to movement. It is in contrast to the end of the range of movement where there is an increase in internal resistance as soft tissues (ligaments and capsule) tighten to prevent further movement between the joint surfaces. The neutral zone is thought to be enlarged in hypermobile or unstable joints due to increased elasticity of soft tissues, and/or decreased muscle tone and function, and/or defective movement control strategies. Failure to maintain a joint's neutral zone within physiological limits, either during static postures or movement, will lead to pain and damage. The elasticity of the soft tissues cannot be changed significantly, but muscle function and motor control can be improved to keep joints stable and healthy.

Panjabi (1992) found in laboratory experiments that simulated muscle force was capable of reducing the neutral zone and hypothesised that muscles were capable of restoring stability after injury. This hypothesis has been validated in clinical research into exercises to improve knee joint stability following ligament damage (Keays *et al.* 2006) as well as in joint hypermobility syndrome in children (Kerr *et al.* 2000) and adults (Ferrell *et al.* 2004).

Optimising muscular control of stability

It is not always as simple as just building muscle strength. Exercise to build (hypertrophy) and strengthen muscle can provide support for the joint it surrounds by becoming stiffer and more toned. However, excessive exercising can lead to the muscle(s) shortening and tightening. If this occurs in the majority of muscles surrounding a joint there is the potential for increasing the stiffness of the joint beyond a beneficial level and producing compressive forces through the joint, which increases the load on the cartilage, which over time may produce symptoms. If excessive exercising leads to shortening and tightening of muscles on one side of a joint, that is, the pectoral muscle on the front of the shoulder, this can lead to increased stiffness on one side of the joint such that during movement there is a tendency for forces to be directed into an area of less stiffness, as movement generally takes the path of least resistance (Sahrmann and Associates 2011). In the case of the shoulder, this can lead to overuse or stress of the more flexible part of the joint, which in this example, in some instances, can produce a posterior subluxation.

This effect can be seen in the absence of an excessive strengthening exercise regime. It can also occur in muscles that are in a state of increased activation or spasm due to repeated activity, learned movement pattern or protective function in response to pain. An example here would be a ballet dancer being told to 'pull her shoulder blades down' because they are resting too high. The repeated, learned movement pattern can result in overactivity of the latissimus dorsi muscle, which in a hypermobile person with increased flexibility leads to excessive depression of the shoulder joint. This produces strain in the upper trapezius muscle which is insufficient to counter the force of the LD and results in pain over the top of the shoulder. In addition, if the LD remains active and cannot lengthen during movement of the shoulder into elevation, an impingement of the humerus on the acromion can result, or in more severe cases an inferior subluxation of the head of the humerus can occur. So what is needed is balanced, largely effortless muscle action to produce efficient movement patterns with effective joint control.

To date there has been very little research into movement patterns and muscle imbalance in hypermobile individuals, and much that is written is based on anecdotal evidence. However, a recent paper by Greenwood *et al.* (2011) has started to address this. The authors looked at the muscle activity of the pelvis and lower limbs during quiet standing and one-leg standing (eyes open and eyes closed) in a group of non-symptomatic hypermobile individuals compared to a control group. Results showed that hypermobiles used significantly more hamstring muscle work in all positions than controls and in addition used significantly more co-contraction of hamstrings and quadriceps in the least challenging task of quiet standing. Hypermobiles showed a significantly greater co-contraction of hamstrings and quadriceps than non-hypermobiles in less challenging tasks. Non-hypermobiles use co-contraction of hamstrings and quadriceps to stabilise the knee in more challenging balance tasks (one-leg standing), so the hypermobiles used a high-level strategy during low-level tasks. It is suggested that this may put hypermobiles at risk of increased compression through the joint and subsequently higher risk of cartilage degeneration. There was also less gluteus medius and erector spinae muscle contraction in one-leg standing in hypermobiles compared to controls. This suggests that hypermobiles have decreased ability to stabilise the pelvis and may be due to the tendency to hang or sag on the hip joint. It is also possible that hypermobiles are using the hamstring muscles to aid stabilisation, showing a less efficient strategy. Muscles work because they are given commands by a higher centre. How do we get the higher centre to work well?

Control of normal movement

Normal movement relies on a complex integration of proprioception, kinaesthesia and motor control.

Proprioception

Proprioception is the ability to sense the position of a joint and kinaesthesia the ability to detect movement of a joint. These skills are vital in order to prepare for activity, that is, ensuring correct joint position and muscle tone for the task in hand. Joint hypermobility syndrome (JHS) individuals have been found to have a deficit in position sense at the finger (Mallik *et al.* 1994) and movement awareness at the knee (Hall *et al.* 1995; Sahin *et al.* 2008). More recently, research by Rombaut *et al.* (2010) has confirmed similar deficits in the knee in EDS-HT individuals, but no significant differences at the shoulder.

The mechanism for these changes is unclear, but research suggests that the proprioceptive deficiency in JHS is at least in some cases peripherally mediated. Ferrell *et al.* (2007) found the quadriceps reflex was absent in almost 50 per cent of JHS patients, and when it was present it decreased in amplitude into hyperextension in contrast to non-hypermobiles. This may be part of the explanation for the common sensation among hypermobile individuals of the knee 'giving way'. Normally the reflex would facilitate the quadriceps muscle to extend and brace the knee during walking in preparation for heel strike and weightbearing. If the reflex is absent or diminishes into hyperextension the knee is less prepared for weightbearing and increases the risk of the joint giving way.

Skin plays an important part in proprioception, and because skin laxity is often present in JHS individuals movement can be improved by enhancing skin sensation through the use of tape (with care), tight-fitting clothing and 'hands on' muscle facilitation.

Exercise programmes to enhance proprioception have been shown to improve joint stability (at the knee), increase muscle strength, decrease pain and improve balance and proprioception (Ferrell *et al.* 2007; Sahin *et al.* 2008). In addition, the eight-week programme of Ferrell *et al.* (2007) found that the reflex which was absent in almost 50 per cent of JHS patients reappeared following the rehabilitation programme and is thought to be due to improved motor neurone activation and suggests peripheral nervous system plasticity.

Rehabilitation

Closed chain exercises are recommended to enhance proprioception and joint stability. A closed chain exercise requires the extremity (hand or foot) to be constantly in contact with a surface (wall, floor or piece of equipment). They are considered more functional and involve some compressive forces, which facilitates more co-contraction of muscles around a joint, so increasing stability. Examples are standing, standing knee bend, heel raises, standing on one leg, mini squats, single-leg knee bend, lunging and four-point kneeling. These can be progressed onto more dynamic postures and activities on an unstable surface such as a balance board, gym ball or foam roller.

Timing of muscle contraction has been shown to be very important. Deep postural muscle activation to support the spine should occur prior to any perturbation or movement which may load the spine. Pain has been shown to significantly delay this activation, leading to increased loading of the spine and subsequent increase in pain. This mechanism is mediated by the central nervous system and could be a factor in fear avoidance or kinaesiophobia shown in JHS.

Motor skill training or functional rehabilitation can reverse these changes. Specific focused exercise targeting a specific component of movement is essential for correcting faulty movement patterns. Exercises should be *painfree*, as pain alters the excitability of the motor cortex (the higher control centre) and contributes to a protective strategy which hinders learning (Boudreau, Farina and Falla 2010). They should also be *cognitive* to facilitate higher centres and focused on *quality* rather than quantity, to prevent fatigue and pain interfering with improvement of task performance. Research has shown that specific low-level, isolated, skilled stabilisation training improves the timing of activation of postural muscles to near normal levels. These changes can occur rapidly and can lead to cortical (higher centre) reorganisation showing motor learning. The specific exercise can be transferred to normal functional activities, and improvement has been shown to still be maintained at six months.

Muscle stiffness: implications of reduced ROM

There are real problems for hypermobiles when they lose their normal range of movement (ROM) and report feeling stiff or restricted. The following extracts are from a discussion with my physio during treatment:

My hamstrings are so tight and this is a real problem. I seem to have lost so much of my flexibility, although I now have more strength. I understand that if my hamstrings become stronger, I know that increasing their strength is a good thing, and if my core stability improves they will hopefully loosen again. It is good if you do release some of the tension in my sacral area because that seems to have helped... On [release of hamstrings] that feels so much better.

Physiotherapy, 3.2.2011

I still feel horribly stiff and I wondered if this is why hypermobiles give up with exercise. It seems that I strengthen my muscles, but I do keep needing physiotherapy to release off the muscular tension. It is hard going through this process of strengthening, whilst I lose some of my flexibility.

Physiotherapy, 8.2.2011

Rosemary Keer explains the rationale behind 'muscle stiffness'

SOFT TISSUE/MUSCLE STIFFNESS
Rosemary Keer

Many hypermobiles complain of stiffness. This would appear to be a contradiction in someone who is supposed to have an increased range of movement but is a complaint that is frequently experienced. It is generally thought to be a description of the resistance produced by the muscles and soft tissues crossing a joint. The effects can be felt when the joint is at rest if the resistance is great enough, or more likely on movement. There are a number of processes which may be responsible for this feeling.

1. *Soft tissue stiffness due to disuse:* This can occur when recovering from injury. In the early stages of injury, pain and swelling will encourage rest and decreased movement to reduce further damage to tissues and allow healing to commence. Later, collagen fibres are produced by the body and laid down to form a robust repair. This causes tightening of the tissue, in a similar way to how a scar tightens in the skin, and may restrict movement at one or more associated joints. This can happen to any of the body tissues, such as capsule, ligament, tendon,

muscle, blood vessels, nerves or their surrounding supporting tissues. However, there is often a fear that moving the injured joint or part of the body will damage it further and so the individual continues to protect or overprotect the area. There is a risk then at this stage that the area will remain stiff and never regain its former mobility or strength. The final part of the healing process involves maturation of the collagen fibres and final remodelling of the scar tissue. It is important that movement and controlled stretching occur at this stage to help orientate collagen fibres along lines of stress, and progressive loading through normal movement and activities occurs to prevent the de-conditioning effect of immobilisation.

In many cases an injury will damage more than one tissue, and during the repair layers of tissues may become effectively 'stuck together', affecting range of movement but also affecting the *ease* of movement. Healthy tissues should glide easily over one another during movement, and this ability may be affected by blood in the form of bruising, and/or tissue fluid in the form of swelling leaking out into the surrounding area following an injury. Normal movement and stretching will help to loosen these bonds and restore normal gliding. Massage and myofascial release can be a useful adjunct here.

Healing is thought to take slightly longer in the hypermobile individual and scar tissue may be less robust, so it is sensible to progress the loading of tissue more slowly and with more care. Nevertheless, gradual stretching and loading should still be done to prevent the injured area remaining weaker and more vulnerable, as this will almost certainly have a deleterious effect on other, more distant areas of the body.

2. *Muscle stiffness due to overuse:* Overuse occurs when an activity or movement is repeated for a period of time which is beyond the capabilities of the individual's tissues to accomplish without damage or to the point of fatigue or exhaustion. This point may be reached sooner in a hypermobile person. The worked tissues become tight, tense and tender and pain ensues. The pain is likely to be due to ischaemia, a lack of blood to the tissues, depriving them of the oxygen necessary for muscle work. Common areas to be affected are the upper trapezius and/or forearm muscles due to excessive computer keyboard use. Fear of making the pain worse may inhibit movement, but

once muscles have been irritated in this way, it is essential to improve the circulation to them through stretching, relaxation and large-range movements. Massage, heat and general exercise are all helpful. There is an accumulative element to this type of injury, and if the activity is repeated within a short period of time without relaxing the muscles and restoring good circulation the problem and pain will worsen.

3. *Soft tissue stiffness due to misuse:* Human bodies are built for movement. This is in contrast to how many of us live our lives today as technology and labour-saving devices have allowed us to become more sedentary. This has detrimental effects on our bodies. Our bodies are shaped by what we do, or put another way, use it or lose it! We all live in a world shaped by gravity. This natural force is constantly having an effect on us and it requires a certain amount of muscular effort to resist it, that is, to support our bodies in an upright position. From the moment we get up in the morning to the moment we go to bed our musculoskeletal system is working to keep us upright, whether we are walking, standing or sitting or being more energetic. It requires fairly constant, low-level, endurance muscle work from our slow twitch or postural muscles. But these muscles have often become lazy as we sit with support, adopt poor postural alignment or the muscles have been switched off due to injury. It is possible that with the extra range of movement available at hypermobile joints these muscles need to work harder and fatigue sooner than they otherwise would do. Whatever the reason, hypermobile individuals frequently show a tendency to poor posture and rest at the end of their range of movement. They 'lock' their joints because this is easier, more stable and requires less muscular effort. The hyperextending knee is a good example. It effectively means 'hanging' on ligaments which, if sustained for a while, will cause creep, where the ligament is effectively lengthened and deprived of oxygen. Pain is produced on release as blood rushes back into the ligament. Repeated resting at end of range will gradually stretch and weaken the ligamentous support of the joint.

Everyday activities, particularly in our more sedentary lifestyle, do not put our joints through their normal range of movement. This is especially true of the hypermobile individual. Good joint health requires adequate nutrition of the tissues and joints, and this is reliant on good circulation. Good cardiovascular fitness will ensure the heart and lungs are supplying the body with a good blood supply, rich in oxygen. But the cartilage in our joints does not have its own blood supply; it relies on movement to move synovial fluid around the joint bathing the cartilage. But if we do not move our joints through their full range of movement there will be areas of cartilage that do not get an adequate blood supply and therefore inadequate nutrition.

Stiffness is a characteristic of muscle and is felt as the resistance encountered when a muscle is passively stretched. This resistance is thought to be due to the elastic components of muscle which are joined in series, the main contributor being a large connective tissue protein (titin) (Sahrmann 2002, p.29). Increasing muscle bulk (or hypertrophy) through exercising increases the number of contractile and connective tissue proteins, which increases the stiffness of the muscle. Muscle atrophy reduces both contractile and connective tissue proteins and so muscle stiffness decreases (Sahrmann 2002, p.30). On the face of it this would not appear to be the explanation of why hypermobiles complain of stiffness, because many are in a de-conditioned state, but in some it could be that overuse of some of the global muscles causes hypertrophy and resultant stiffness.

Another source of resistance to passive stretching and therefore a potential contributor to muscle stiffness, albeit a minor one, is a process of thixotrophy, whereby a substance that has been static for a while becomes stiff and resists movement (Sahrmann 2002, p.29). It is usually applied to gels which become liquid when moved or agitated, as in shaking (think of the difference in consistency of honey between the first stir and after several brisk stirs). Thixotrophy is the process which contributes to the increased flexibility which occurs through repeated stretching or warming-up prior to exercising.

To understand the effect that muscular stiffness has on movement it is helpful to think of muscles having similar properties to springs. A spring when elongated will display resistance to lengthening in a similar way to that of a muscle being passively lengthened. If two springs of different stiffness are attached together in series and then lengthened, the less stiff spring will lengthen sooner and much further than the stiffer spring. To give an example in the body, this may be a hypermobile lumbar spine (loose spring) and a stiff hip due to a tight hamstring or gluteal muscle (stiffer spring). During forward bending, where movement should occur at both joints, the lumbar spine will move earlier and more easily into flexion than the hip. The body, following the laws of physics, will take the path of least resistance (Sahrmann and Associates 2011), and over time or with repeated motion the lumbar spine will potentially increase its flexibility into flexion and compensate for the lack of flexion at the hip. This may be the explanation for the instances of back pain experienced by hypermobiles during yoga or with repeated bending movements where increased flexibility into flexion leads to overstretching or overuse of the lumbar spine into flexion due to a lack of control.

Muscle or soft tissue stiffness and shortness can also lead to increased compression through a joint, both at rest and on movement. Muscle may shorten through not being taken through its full range of movement. Examples here would be tightening of hamstrings through repeated and prolonged sitting, or a muscle which is shortened because it is in a state of increased activity or spasm due to repetitive activities or switched on in response to injury or pain in a protective mode. This will restrict the movements at the joint(s) and decrease blood flow to the tissues (both joint surface and muscle) which may potentially accelerate degeneration.

Propriospinal myoclonus

One of the things that neither my physio or I had considered was that all this change in my body was going to expose these strange muscular spasms, twitches or propriospinal myoclonus, which are described and discussed in the next chapter.

CHAPTER 32

Neurology and movement disorders

During treatment

If I am lying prone or supine (or even in bed at home) 'spasms' or 'propriospinal myoclonus' seem to initiate almost immediately in physiotherapy, prior to the commencement of any manual body work. The movement is in a vertical shape and is predominantly to the left of the spine and occurs in the lumbar-thorax region. The spasm is triggered with cranio-work, cervical spinal work and thoracic spinal work. The greater the stimulus or pain and 'fear', the more pronounced the spasm becomes. This mimics the behaviour of a person with a stutter. I do not instigate the fear, but this is definitely going on subconsciously. I think that the spasms that are emerging are undetected and, as yet, unresolved traumas of either a biomechanical, physiological or psychological nature, or likely a combination of all three. The spasms are a warning that there is a perceived hidden danger or threat, hence unresolved trauma. The body is voicing 'back off', although the spasms do not cause me physical pain. I cannot make them stop on their own, but equally I do not trigger them consciously. I can sense when they are going to start at certain times though, owing to a sudden surge or 'charge' that I feel. Maybe I need to try to articulate this if possible and see whether talking about what is happening will stop the spasm. Mostly though, I don't know why or how it is happening. I haven't 'decided' at a subconscious level that I don't want a certain area of my body being palpated – although it would suggest this is a possibility given that I am sitting here and thinking about my left calf and my body is 'twitching'. Until physiotherapy has systematically exposed all these spasms in whatever form they are triggered, I don't believe that complete recovery is possible from all related syndrome phenomena.

During exercise

During physiolates exercises, I have now discovered that spasms occur when an area of unnecessary overuse is abruptly knocked out. For example, when doing pelvic tilts with the left leg raised in order to facilitate left abdominals, I began to realise after doing the exercise for a few days that my ribs and diaphragm were 'overused' and 'held'. Knowing what I do about my body, Pilates and this work, I knew that this was incorrect. I then applied pressure to my ribs and left abs so as to focus my attention on releasing my ribs. At this point I went into spasm and lost control completely. In this situation the spasm was exposing a faulty movement pattern, and removing excessive muscular control exposed the weakness. I rested for a few minutes before attempting to do the work without using the ribs unnecessarily, and the spasm continued, but the force of my mind and concentration were greater, and although the spasm continued it did diminish.

When I was lying prone and doing hamstring curls, I noticed that when working my left side (again) that my right upper thoracic was working more than it probably should be and I was using it as a counterweight to stabilise myself. When I put my right limb down by my side (it had been up by my head) I started to spasm, presumably because yet again I had exposed a movement pattern flaw, trunk instability and an area (upper right thoracic) of overuse. Again I knew that this was going to cause me difficulty in continuing with the exercise, but I carried on in order to re-educate my body in an alternative movement pattern.

It was becoming extremely apparent now that the weaknesses are all on the left trunk and that when the dominant right side (trunk, but not lower limb) is removed, or the accessory muscles, the spasms occur because the body cannot cope without all these extra muscles and has to 'warn' of instability. Given this enlightenment, I am going to have to keep playing my body at its own game so that the weaker side starts to take over. The amount of extra muscle I am using in order to do simple but gross movement is ridiculous, and is hugely inefficient. It is abundantly clear why my energy is constantly 'drained' through my existing movement patterns and why in effect I had to 'start again' from scratch. I think that in terms of exercise patterns the spasms might now be a useful tool to expose continuing weakness so that new and more efficient patterns can be learned. It will be hard work and frustrating, but the long-term outcome is likely to be extremely rewarding, energy efficient and with much clearer motor patterning, function, strength and control.

Eccentric muscle contractions

Part of my new 'physiolates' work has involved focusing on eccentric muscle contractions and 'completing' the muscular movement, then disengaging the muscles involved completely before repeating the repetition. After now doing this work for ten days I am beginning to understand how radically inefficiently my muscles have been functioning in eccentric muscular work. The coordination and control have been extremely poor, and previously the muscles have fatigued in the last 20 degrees of the movement on descent, highlighting a lack of strength and control. Muscle spasms have interfered at this level and woven their way into the movement – particularly in hamstring curls, which has obviously made the work very challenging, but fortunately I am also very stubborn, and pure determination is meaning that I am regaining control of movement patterns which 'normal-mobiles' must take for granted.

I have used imagery to help me in this work, notably imagining a glass ball (Christmas decoration) is balancing on my foot and must not fall when doing hamstring curls. Making the effort to 'switch off' the muscles at the end of the rep has been a crucial part of this work because this just never happened in the past, but at the moment is still taking an enormous amount of mental energy. However, I can now feel the muscles working in a new way in their correct and opposing forces. At the moment my proprioception does not allow me to accurately sense the last 20 degrees of movement, so I have to keep going until my leg has very gently closed against the floor. I look forward to having a greater sense of proprioception eventually so I have to work less hard to sense what most people must already innately sense – for example, where they are in space. I often have no idea at all! The effort to work in this new way is presently superhuman, and I am aware of how 'charged' my muscles feel after my physiolates work. The work is paying off because there is already a change in the balance of working power between my right and left lower limbs, with the right leg finally taking on more of the load. Calf girth difference is now 2cm – but should now be verified by an independent tester.

Neurology

I had an appointment with my neurologist to review the headaches and neck pain situation. I was happily able to report an improvement in these owing to physiotherapy and to the Bowen therapy release that had subsequently had such a dramatic outcome (described later in this book). Mr T was still interested in my 'propriospinal myoclonus' and that these were still going on. To that end he requested a spinal and brain MRI scan which I had, the results being that apart from minor wear and tear arthritis (as was expected) there were no other significant findings other than the original disc bulge at L4/5. He also sent me to a 'movement disorders' specialist. I blogged the following:

> I saw the lovely Dr M today at the Neurology Hospital. I was able to show him and his team of three colleagues the benefit of some of my movement patterns (see below). We talked about whether I did any of these things as a child (no). He tried unsuccessfully to stop me doing this movement pattern, so was able to determine that it wasn't a movement tic that could be suppressed with a combination of CBT + medication. I was offered medication but have declined it – although could have a stronger version of a drug like diazepam for severe episodes of these twitches (e.g. like I had on a long-haul flight). The other option would be injections – but again I feel I will wait and see what happens. Dr M is aware that I have a newer twitch in my left shoulder, but thought that my eyelid twitches might be due to a thyroid imbalance, so has suggested that this is tested. I suspect that will be normal as am sure that has been tested before.
>
> Moreover, Dr M thinks that this is all linked into my Hypermobility Syndrome and Chronic Pain syndromes and the way that the nervous system has been wired up. He certainly didn't think it was psychosomatic or 'put on'. He is aware that it started just over two years ago during physiotherapy. He has suggested I carry on with my Bowen treatment and Physio and keep exercising and all the good things I have been doing. As the myoclonus don't hurt me I said I am not too bothered by them as they mainly happen during treatment or when I lie flat. After my appt I was asked to take part in some research as my hands aren't affected by the movement disorder and the experiment showed that those with movement disorders are much more accurate at assessing repetitive finger pressures than normals/controls. Although the trials are in their early stages, I thought this was fascinating – but obviously I have a heightened awareness of my sensorial feedback – perhaps because of my history of chronic pain and EDSIII. Anyway, all very interesting, and I have offered to help them with other research.

Blog, 5.4.2012

Extract of a report by my neurologist

An extract of a letter to me from my consultant neurologist explains my movement disorder (snake-like movements in my spine and other twitches – e.g. shoulders):

> I think [her] movements are best characterised as a functional movement disorder. This is a rather poorly defined term, and one where synonyms like psychogenic imply very clearly a psychological explanation (typically based on the idea of an underlying emotional trauma). While this may be a cause in some people, the vast majority of people I see have physical triggers (physical illness, injury and pain), and I think this is a much more important and understandable way in which such learned patterns of abnormal movement can emerge. This is not to minimise the importance of psychological factors such as anxiety or depression – these can be important too, just as they are in more traditionally accepted neurological problems such as Parkinson's disease or tic disorders.
>
> I have now seen a number of people with joint hypermobility syndrome who additionally have movement problems that seem to me to best fit within the 'functional' category. I think that the common experience of people with hypermobility of chronic pain, abnormal problems that occur in HMS (e.g. bowel, autonomic bladder problems, anxiety and depressive disorders) act together to increase vulnerability to development of these abnormal movement patterns.
>
> *Consultant neurologist*

In the next chapter, and despite the ongoing 'spasms' as I referred to them, we look at my subjective and objective progress in physiotherapy between a particular time span running from December 2010 until June 2011 (30 weeks, or six months). This corresponds with phase three of my rehabilitation (see Chapter 28), which was a very challenging time during treatment with many POTS symptoms and spasms.

CHAPTER 33

Measuring treatment outcomes and assessing progress

Subjective reports

I always found myself with so much to say at each physiotherapy appointment. There was always a great deal happening, and with so many body systems affected it could potentially take one third of the consultation time in simply reporting back to my physio what was going on. In the first two years of treatment I did this verbally, often emailing my physio in between sessions (which is generally unusual practice) and also blogging my progress. From the summer of 2010 I came up with a 'subjective table' (see Table 33.1). This gave me the scope to provide my physio with a succinct summary of what was going on, and was certainly useful, but not measurable.

From December 2010, I decided to think of another way in which to measure and track my symptoms and came up with a graphical plot giving my various symptoms or bodily areas a score from 0 to 10, with 0 being asymptomatic or pain-free and 10 being severe pain or disruption (see Table 33.2). The graphs proved a useful way in which to monitor progress and to identify continuing problem areas. The outcome of the graphs also enabled us to be able to correlate various symptoms, for example neck and neurological symptoms.

TABLE 33.1: Subjective table 8.2.2011		
Acute summary	**Musculoskeletal**	**Sleep**
Stressed and distressed – so psychological issues predominate over physical ones. If I was calmer, happier and more relaxed we might find that I could have had a very good physical week. As things stand things are generally good on this front.	Hamstrings – ongoing. Lumbar spine/sacrum very sore. Abdominals in huge fixation spasm and having an effect on digestion as a result. Sore!!!	Sleep – just woefully inadequate and waking all the time. Stress and anxiety. Bladder – irritated again and overactive.
POTS/asthma	**Skin/harm**	**Chronic**
Fine.	Severe again and very stressed and anxious and not managing other coping strategies this week.	Anxious. Globally body sore owing to training pain.
Exercise	**Ballet**	**Digestive**
Hamstrings still an issue and very tight and sore – also left knee clicks persistently so exercise is very hard. Hamstrings still not engaged in ballet! Abdominal – severe burn and lower back sore. Thoracic spine exercises showing an improvement. ☺	Hamstrings – still tight, but slightly better after last physio. Did petit jetés in a big series and jetés ordinaire in a big series. Getting braver with allegro and calves accepting. ☺ However last night very tight again and calves sore – DOMS?	Poor – linked to anxiety and stress and abdominal exercises and fixating them in ballet because I am feeling fat. Guts terrible after class and IBS is poor.
Other	**Psychology**	**Support**
Was very hypermobile and chaotic in body on Saturday – especially in knees. It is the funeral of my neighbour on Wednesday 9th.	High levels of stress and anxiety (mainly work-related) which is having a very negative knock-on effect on sleep, digestion and mood. Hopefully this will improve over the next few weeks.	ITB. Left knee. Hamstrings. Stomach muscles. Lumbar spine.

TABLE 33.2: Physiotherapy: subjective graph

Scale measurement

0 = no pain, no symptoms; 10 = severe symptoms and pain; NA = not available

Comment:

Spasm	0 1 2 3 4 5 6 7 8 9 10 N/A
Neck pain	0 1 2 3 4 5 6 7 8 9 10 N/A
Headaches	0 1 2 3 4 5 6 7 8 9 10 N/A
Neurological	0 1 2 3 4 5 6 7 8 9 10 N/A
Thoracic spine	0 1 2 3 4 5 6 7 8 9 10 N/A
Lumbar spine	0 1 2 3 4 5 6 7 8 9 10 N/A
Hip/groin	0 1 2 3 4 5 6 7 8 9 10 N/A
Knee(s)	0 1 2 3 4 5 6 7 8 9 10 N/A
Sleep	0 1 2 3 4 5 6 7 8 9 10 N/A
Fatigue	0 1 2 3 4 5 6 7 8 9 10 N/A
Bladder	0 1 2 3 4 5 6 7 8 9 10 N/A
Asthma	0 1 2 3 4 5 6 7 8 9 10 N/A
POTS	0 1 2 3 4 5 6 7 8 9 10 N/A
IBS	0 1 2 3 4 5 6 7 8 9 10 N/A
Gynae/endo	0 1 2 3 4 5 6 7 8 9 10 N/A
Ballet	0 1 2 3 4 5 6 7 8 9 10 N/A
Physiolates	0 1 2 3 4 5 6 7 8 9 10 N/A
Self-harm	0 1 2 3 4 5 6 7 8 9 10 N/A
Mood	0 1 2 3 4 5 6 7 8 9 10 N/A
Psychology/other	0 1 2 3 4 5 6 7 8 9 10 N/A
_____	0 1 2 3 4 5 6 7 8 9 10 N/A
_____	0 1 2 3 4 5 6 7 8 9 10 N/A

The data was collected for a six-month period from December 2010 (30 weeks), with the last subjective cut-off on 30 June 2011. Occasionally I completed the form even though I wasn't having treatment – the last two weeks of June fall into this category as I was on holiday. However, this was an interesting thing to do because it allowed me to see what treatment would have been required and also how I coped with no treatment – or to allow for a placebo effect.

A decision was made to omit 'Gynae/endo', 'Ballet' and 'Physiolates' from the score sheet and miscellaneous symptoms (space left for these at the bottom of the chart); they were omitted because the score was very often zero and because they were not providing any new information.

Results

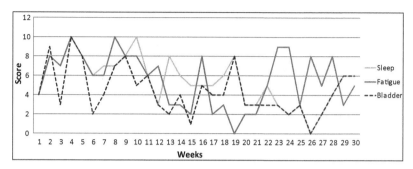

FIGURE 33.1: SLEEP, FATIGUE AND BLADDER

The results of the variables of sleep, fatigue and bladder highly correlate, especially sleep and bladder. The results show that these decline in score over time (30 weeks). The rise in the last two weeks reflects an unexpected period of difficulty with both symptoms whilst on holiday. Anecdotally, both symptoms settled again upon return from holiday. The results show an improvement across time, indicating that treatment was effective for both sleep and bladder.

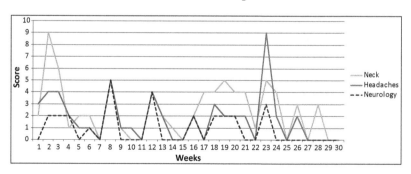

FIGURE 33.2: NECK, HEADACHES AND NEUROLOGICAL SYMPTOMS

Again, there is a clear correlation with all three symptoms across time apart from a time when there were severe headaches around weeks 23–25, which coincided with some Pilates exercises that I took part in during a ballet class which caused symptoms (mainly in resultant headache, with some increase to neck pain and neurology). The graph shows that by the end of the 30-week time period blips in symptoms were brief and short-lived and that symptoms were virtually non-existent by the end of the 30 weeks.

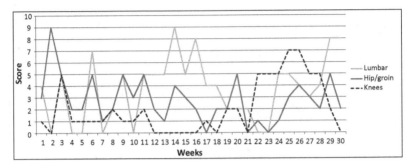

FIGURE 33.3: LUMBAR SPINE PAIN, HIP/GROIN AND KNEES

It was expected that this group of symptoms would correlate, and there is some relationship, particularly at the beginning of the time period when far more attention was being paid to my neck and neurological problems. Two-thirds of the way into the experimental time-measure, my ITB was regularly becoming a problem and was pulling my left knee out of alignment. Since one of my goals was to be able to cycle normally (ideally in parallel rather than knees protruding laterally), there were several weeks of treatment focusing on knees and hips (and sacral). Whilst the knee and hip pain did decrease, lumbar spine pain rocketed at the end, but this was largely owing to training pain as the muscles in the area had to work to support a new and functional parallel alignment.

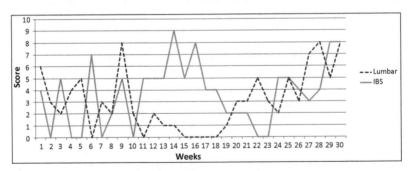

FIGURE 33.4: LUMBAR SPINE PAIN AND IBS

Since it is known that IBS can cause back pain (Azpiroz *et al.* 2000) it was expected that these two symptoms would correlate. There is correlation both at the beginning and the end of the time period, but a period in the middle where lumbar remains high and IBS low. What the graph cannot reflect was that I was not accurately reporting IBS symptoms all the time as I was going through a period of denial about my own symptoms and was not reflecting them to score as highly as they should have done. I had come to accept my (abnormal) symptoms as normal, which might explain the partial lack of relationship in these figures. At the end of the time period it does indeed show that both symptoms do relate, and had not been addressed adequately in treatment. This is a point of knowing when an ongoing referral is required, and I was sent to hospital for further testing and investigation of bowel symptoms.

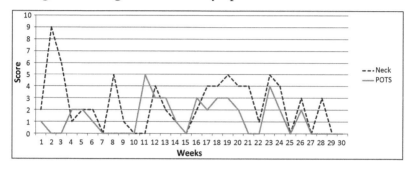

FIGURE 33.5: NECK AND POTS

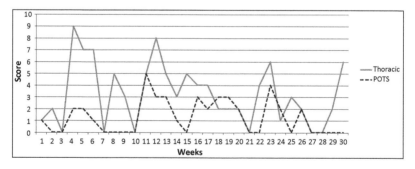

FIGURE 33.6: THORACIC SPINE AND POTS

Figures 33.5 and 33.6 look at neck and postural orthostatic tachycardia syndrome (POTS) and thoracic spine and POTS across time. There is a very clear correlation between neck and POTS symptoms; this might be because my neck function improved and strengthened considerably during this time. In fact it was an overriding treatment objective that the affective relationship with POTS is clear. Thoracic spine and POTS is more interesting and less clear. There is a relationship but thoracic spine had still not been addressed in rehabilitation, which shows it is still unrehabilitated and still subject to flare-ups. The thoracic spine is where the autonomic nervous system (ANS) is situated, so as thoracic spine was rehabilitated we could hypothesise that both POTS and thoracic spine symptoms would entirely correlate and reduce to very minimal scoring.

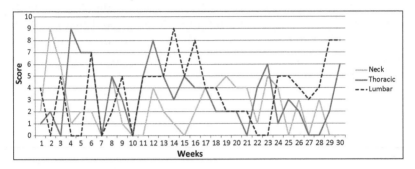

FIGURE 33.7: NECK, THORACIC AND LUMBAR SPINE

This graph shows the true impact and intention of rehabilitation during this time period, which was primarily aimed at cervical spine or neck and regaining essential control and stability. The results clearly show that neck is virtually asymptomatic by the end of this time period whilst lumbar and thoracic are still symptomatic and not fully rehabilitated. Thoracic spine, as previously mentioned, was not particularly addressed during this rehabilitation period and lumbar had exacerbated owing to increase of training pain relating to hip and knee function. Lumbar spine was always a difficult area for me as a patient owing to chronic insidious pain in this area and is still highly sensitised. Thoracic spine was the area yet to be addressed at the end of this 30-week time period.

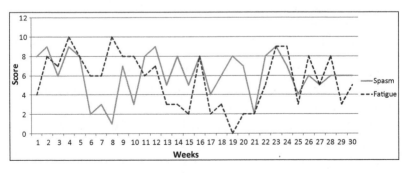

FIGURE 33.8: MUSCLE SPASM AND FATIGUE

Spasm and fatigue seem to have a relationship and there is a correlation between them, and although not yet resolved (especially spasm), it can be shown that treatment does affect and improve them across the 30-week time period.

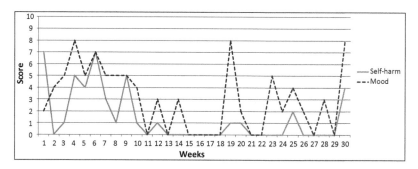

FIGURE 33.9: SELF-HARM AND MOOD

There is a relationship between mood and self-harm, which indicates that when one was bad the other was also affected. We would have predicted this to be the case. During this 30-week time period I had eight weeks of cognitive analytical therapy that started in week 8 and finished in week 15. There is a huge deceleration of symptoms during that time period, and apart from a major blip around week 20, which related to upsetting news about my bowel symptoms (and GP visit), symptoms remain low again until I am on holiday where I have some bad anxiety and depressive episodes, mainly relating to being alone for too long. Nevertheless, the intervention of CAT highly supports the psychological aspect of treatment and is clear on the graphs.

Discussion

It was extremely useful to complete the subjective forms each week in a more numerical fashion. I did not keep them, so I could not be influenced about what I had done the week before, and the results were stored in my patient notes file.

The graphs show clearly where symptoms had improved – especially in neck since that was a major goal of treatment from the end of December once we knew how unstable neck was. The relationship between neck and POTS shows a high correlation, although this is less clear with thoracic spine for the reason that thoracic spine is still undergoing rehabilitation.

The results show how clear and essential outgoing referral is necessary at times to support my physio's work. For example, it is clear that the intervention of CAT improves my mood and self-harm and was a critical intervention by an expert in that area. It was entirely appropriate for this to be conducted by an external medical expert. Similarly, the graphs indicate a need for support with IBS and bowel-related problems, and at the end of the time period of these graphs, we were still waiting for a more formal surgical intervention, the initial and conservative intervention not showing any benefit. Knowing when to seek external advice and support is very important, and these referrals were particularly important and also supportive to my physio who couldn't be expected to manage absolutely everything.

The graphs showed the areas that are rehabilitated against those where rehabilitation was still ongoing – for example, neck is considerably better than thoracic by the end of the time period, but that is because thoracic spine was still in rehabilitation. Neck is much improved. The graphs also provide an indication of flare-ups amongst symptom groups – for example, hip and knee. The graphs also show what symptoms/body areas work well against those that don't. The graphs are subjective measures and therefore do not show any obvious objective measures – for example changes in calf measurement over time or that by the end of the 30-week time period I was able to walk in a completely normal and 'true' parallel. However, what we charted here are symptoms and how they felt for me on a weekly basis. If this had been conducted over a further six months it would be hoped that most symptoms would have an average score of three or below, showing the effectiveness of rehabilitation 'in the end'. A decision was made to cut off the measures after a six-month time period for the purposes of analysis for this book. Nevertheless, it has been an invaluable tool to assess progress of symptoms both from a patient's point of view and from the point of view of the treating therapist.

CHAPTER 34

Returning to normal life

My core stability improved, and particularly when I was able to retain a neutral hip alignment it was time to start considering the concept of improving my physical conditioning and endurance. The blog entry below describes my early attempts:

> I have just been swimming for the first time since pre-physio, not long after I started this blog in March 2008. I really have come a long way since then. Although I am still lacking in confidence in the water and still need floats, the session highlighted a few things:
>
> - Cardiovascular fitness is still very poor and overall endurance. I fatigued after six laps of ten metres. I kept on doing laps of six throughout the hour I was there, and by the end of the hour probably managed 8–10 laps with one rather than two floats!
>
> - My left-sided weakness was exposed in the water with the right side being more dominant and wanting to pull me over to the right. I got around this by stopping kicking with the right leg from time to time.
>
> - Weakness in the upper body – I did some work with foam weights pushing into the water, starting from my arms out to the side at 90 degrees.
>
> - I tried some one-sided float work, but freaked out when trying with the left arm working.
>
> - I did some walking in the water and feel my trunk is now working really well.
>
> - Overall my abs and trunk are working well in swimming, and the only thing stopping me swimming unaided is me!

- I did some floating and a little bit of going underwater and it is just a matter of confidence.

- I had fun…

- I came out feeling taller, stronger, fitter, that I had worked hard and…I had fun!!

Blog, 30.7.2011

Building endurance in corrected alignment

It was not really possible for me to contemplate endurance or the concept of endurance and building on other cardiovascular fitness until I had deep core control of pelvis and lower back and indeed until I was able to maintain a true parallel alignment. This had been a challenge for me all the time because of my preference for lateral rotation at the helm of classical ballet and because I innately lacked control of my hypermobile hips. However, my hypermobility is a wonderful asset and therefore makes lateral rotation easy for me. Nevertheless, as I finally gained control of both my hips and pelvis, I was able to walk in a natural parallel and also cycle without my knees protruding laterally as had previously been the case. The true parallel finally materialised some time in June 2011 when my physio had been working on my left ITB which had frequently been pulling my left patella out of alignment and causing pain. Additionally, it was very evident that my left side was weaker, and so we had to wait for the left side to catch up in strength before I was able to maintain control in parallel.

Several things speeded up this final process. These included a kneeling exercise that my physio gave me where I had my hands on the wall in front of me and had to transfer weight between the knees. This helped to reinforce the hip alignment which fed down through the kinetic chain. I had to bias all movements to the left. Cycling in France in June 2011 was the final breakthrough I had in being able to maintain control of my hips and knee alignment and to retain a parallel alignment in cycling. Once I had achieved this through cycling, I was able to transfer the movement very naturally to walking.

Here I describe the time I first realise I am finally cycling in total parallel:

After my 90 minute cycling stint I realised I was tracking my knee really nicely and on walking to a cafe, I realised that my left leg was in total parallel.

I got back just after 6.30pm and then did my physio and ballet exercises. I am finding this being in a really 'true' parallel really strange. I would say that we are now 'pre-broken leg' – it is great shame it has taken 30 years to correct what would have been a six week job during the summer that I broke my leg in 1982. All these very recent changes are also beginning to highlight that calves and Achilles are both tight, but I am still anxious about letting my physio treat there.

Diary, June 2011

The road to recovery

As my musculoskeletal system and movement patterning improved, particularly in the lower limb, I was able to start thinking about doing more 'normal' exercise again rather than just rehabilitative physiotherapy exercises. This was possible to start to consider particularly when I finally had control of my hips in a neutral and more normal parallel alignment. I had been doing ballet classes throughout this whole time, but unfortunately ballet was continuing to reinforce former movement patterns with my preferred positioning of hips in lateral rotation, which is my natural alignment, given a choice. It was now necessary to start to do exercises that used a more corrected movement pattern. It was also important now to start to develop my endurance and then cardiovascular fitness. However, it wasn't possible for me to consider myself better 'recovered' until I had total resolve of my neck problem, which eventually came about through physiotherapy and ultimately through doing Bowen work on myself. Temporomandibular joint (TMJ), eyes and speech also needed addressing.

CHAPTER 35

Speech, swallowing and hearing difficulties, TMJ and eye problems

Yes, I have [swallowing/voice problems] all the time. When my jaw is bad or my neck, shoulder muscles are in spasm (which is basically all the time at the moment!). It affects my throat quite badly. I am in a singing group and it is making life very difficult! I can feel the tight/knotty muscles in my neck with my fingers and it's basically like having tight hard bands of something around my neck so it's no surprise it causes trouble really!

EDS patient, Facebook

I have problems talking but not because I've dislocated my jaw, I had grommets as a kid and got a speech impediment as a result so when my mouth is dry I can't get words out! I'm a singer so my jaw affects my singing more than anything. Can't open my mouth wide so it changes the sound and volume. And my over bite affects my soft palate!

EDS patient, Facebook

New research is starting to link EDSIII with speech, swallowing and hearing difficulties (Hunter 2011; Zarate *et al.* 2010). Hunter, who is a speech and language therapist (SLT), conducted a survey in 2010 involving both patients from Enlers-Danlos Support UK (EDS-UK) and HMSA, where she had formerly surveyed EDS patients in 1996. This is relevant because of HMS now being known as EDSIII. Hunter analysed 136 returned surveys, 28 being seen by SLT.

Respondents reported a range of symptoms including frequent ear infections, hearing loss and difficulties with maintaining clear voicing. Hunter reports that half of respondents frequently repeat themselves and have difficulty with vocal volume, articulation and stamina (2011). Respondents also have difficulties with swallowing, coordination and clearing of the pharynx and coughing (Hunter 2011). It is also no surprise to find that there were problems with the temporomandibular joint (TMJ) in this patient group with jaw joint pain, difficulties in biting, sustained chewing and TMJ 'fixing', which Hunter relates to fatigue of joints, just like other joints in the EDSIII patient. Hunter recommends that SLTs working with the EDSIII patient group are aware of fatigue and stamina issues and overstrain in the case of excessive exercises and intensity (Hunter 2011). She writes that 'it seems that the effects of generalised ligamentous laxity, perhaps coupled with fatigue, take a toll on the vocal health and ability of this population' (Hunter 2011, p.20).

TMJ

In addition to problems with my bowels and digestion, I had a long history of problems with my tempromandibular joint (TMJ). I came up with the following thoughts and hypothesis (16.5.2011). I suggested that:

> If the patient has TMJ pain, clicking or popping of jaw, dislocation, hypermobility and misalignment of TMJ this will result in poor mastication and the initiation of production of saliva and the other important hormonal and chemical signals which inform the digestive system about what is about to be eaten. This would then have a domino effect about what the stomach expects to receive and other digestive enzymes etc such as bile will not be produced properly, or, conversely, too much hydrochloric acid would be produced if the wrong signals are being sent (e.g. chewing gum for ages on an empty stomach). If the patient does then not chew food properly and is then swallowing unchewed food and probably air-gulping, owing to difficulties in swallowing which are also linked to EDSIII, the digestive system already has to work very hard before it has barely started.

Digestion

Food arrives in the stomach in a semi-chewed state, and if there is a lot of gas swallowed as well, will cause heartburn or indigestion and feeling overfull quickly. This is further enhanced if the patient overeats, or eats too quickly before the brain signals that the stomach is full. If there is a delay in vascular response because of tissue laxity, why not a delay in other systems?

If, as I predict, the other chemicals involved in digestion are similarly out of balance because they have been badly informed by the brain and how the patient masticates, by the time the food leaves the stomach and into the small bowel, things become more compounded. An imbalance in bile will mean that fats are not adequately broken down and other essential nutrients may well not be absorbed quite as well and the laxity of the tissues will compound upon the tone of the bowel in general, coupled with the general potential that the deep core muscles are not working adequately to support the bowel. Therefore it is hardly a surprise that patients with EDSIII are likely to have IBS and or related symptoms.

Posture

The poor posture and lack of functioning deep core and postural muscles has a resultant impact on the large bowel and at the other end of the digestive system in terms of emptying the bowel. The 'toilet' posture of patients with EDSIII was commented upon generally at the Hypermobility Club lecture I attended on bowels last year. In terms of myself I don't 'normally' sit on my bottom, but tuck under, therefore sitting more on my sacrum. Have a little think about what this alignment has done in the long-term to my digestive system and you can probably see that the result is in straining to evacuate, haemorrhoids and eventually anal fissures and tears. Furthermore in EDSIII patients there is a tendency for anal prolapse and for retrocile pouches to develop and 'pockets' in the bowel and rectum. For many patients, taking high doses of codeine and a poor diet, lack of exercise and water will contribute to very poor digestive function and constipation. Lack of abdominal tone and poor posture will impact upon effective bowel evacuation. Normal toilets do not help with the process of evacuation, whereas the squat toilets found in some parts of the world are actually far more conducive to bowel evacuation.

It then occurred to me that the tucking under I do in squat has had a lasting impact upon my posture in sitting and therefore a resultant change most probably in my bowel alignment. Now, in order to evacuate properly, I have to make changes in my posture just to be able to go to the bathroom. Sometimes I take laxatives to make things easier, but I haven't been able to empty

my bowels probably for a 'long time' but would not class myself
as constipated either, yet I potentially am. I have been bleeding
from my bowels for ages, but when I had endometriosis as well,
this was worse.

Back pain

It is only by thinking all this through that I have realised why I
have ended up in [a] mess. I would suggest my bowel symptoms
started at 18 and then there is a beautiful correlation with lower
back pain starting, and a worsening of menstrual pain, as per
timeline. What happened at 18? – I went to university = diet
change, poor diet, smoking and doing much less exercise for
a while all contribute to bowel changes across time which
although I am given a vague diagnosis of IBS in 2001 (whereby
I was already diagnosed with haemorrhoids, but did not seek
further treatment for them) and I continue to 'manage' until
finally sitting at the proper angle is just too painful, coupled
with increasing left abdominal pain despite improved muscular
control, coupled with bleeding and severe pain on defecation
= need to get help, but very delayed help (not uncommon,
unfortunately, owing to high embarrassment factor).

Conclusion

In conclusion then I believe that if the TMJ problems are resolved
that digestive problems could also be significantly improved
in the EDSIII patient alongside developing endurance and
postural control and the correct abdominal support. Evacuation
would also significantly improve if digestion and postural
support were improved in conjunction with adequate diet, fluid
intake and exercise. My bowel needs to be sorted out, but so
does my TMJ problem.

Whilst there has been treatment for my bowel, as seen in Chapter 7,
things are still not entirely resolved with my TMJ.

Isobel's TMJ symptoms

I am not quite sure when my TMJ became 'symptomatic' but it was
probably in my mid-twenties, although I can find no significant event
to correlate with the appearance of symptoms. In my adolescence I had
to undergo four extractions of premolars owing to overcrowding and
subsequent orthodontic treatment for realignment and treatment of a
cross-bite. I had train-track braces which frequently broke, although

we don't know whether this was owing to a diet of very chewy foods (probably unsuitable for braces), and my braces were thus removed before my lower jaw was completed in treatment because they broke so often. I had a retainer for the upper jaw, and as a result the teeth in my upper jaw are straighter. Whether because my orthodontics were incomplete can be said to have contributed to a temporomandibular disorder (TMD) is unknown.

I saw a private orthodontist in 2007 who said that the approach to orthodontics had moved on significantly since I had treatment in 1987. He said that nowadays my teeth would not have been removed and that they would have made space for them by moving the teeth more laterally in the jaw. Premolars weren't my only extractions either, and I had all four of my wisdom teeth removed separately, two in hospital on separate occasions. The bottom teeth were growing horizontally and had to be 'cut out'. One had to be removed with the root left behind as it was so awkward to extract. The orthodontist who saw me in 2007 arranged for a Michigan splint to be made to help both with bruxism and to relieve the pressure of the TMJ and to rest my facial muscles. This appliance was for night use. There was also an option of taking my treatment much further and to improve the alignment of my TMJ and facial/neck appearance, but unfortunately this treatment is very costly and so far I have not been able to manage this. Nevertheless the Michigan splint (see Figure 35.1) has made an enormous difference to the amount of pain I was experiencing in the TMJ joints and made speech and chewing of food easier as my TMJ and facial muscles were less fatigued. I hope to be able to consider the possibility of completing treatment, although because of my hypermobility it is possible the teeth may not remain in position. An MRI scan showed no disc abnormalities and normal condylar movement, so treatment has been addressed through Bowen and physiotherapy.

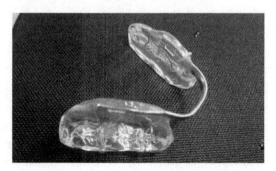

FIGURE 35.1: ISOBEL'S MICHIGAN SPLINT: APPLIED TO THE LOWER JAW AND WORN AT NIGHT

Although Bowen work has been helpful in relieving some of the pressure in my TMJ area and possibly giving some temporary tracking improvements, physiotherapy has partly helped my bite and alignment of my TMJ:

> My physio has recently started treatment to my TMJ (Jaw). I have probably had about 3–4 sessions where she has worked on TMJ and already there are significant improvements. For a start I have now got significantly more range of movement (ROM) on opening my mouth, and prior to the intervention, there was significant deviation to the left. The right side was the stronger side and I chewed predominantly on the right side. Since my physio has started work on my TMJ I am now chewing much more on the left side – but am actually deliberately biasing this for time being to build up the muscles on that side and to give the right side a rest. This is also resulting in improved articulation of the masseter and facial muscles when I talked – because prior to treatment, there was little movement on the left side of my face and jaw.
>
> *Blog, 21.5.2011*

During a much later physiotherapy session, my physio explains why I started to experience ringing in my ears:

> My physio did a lot of work on my T-Spine and C-Spine and TMJ. He said this could explain some of my symptoms and that my recent problems with ringing ears could also be explained in terms of the blood vessels in the area all being squashed. My physio has given me an exercise to do for my TMJ, in order to loosen my jaw but also some pressure release points to press at the back of my mouth.
>
> *Blog, 1.5.2012*

TMJ appointment

I had an appointment with a Maxillofacial surgeon who said that my occlusion was good, but that my jaw deviated to the left upon opening. Although my MRI scan was completely normal, ongoing management will involve trying a new type of night-time splint which will cover all teeth in the lower jaw, and an arthroscopy remains a possibility if Bowen therapy and/or physiotherapy are unable to resolve remaining clicking and 'stickiness' of my left TMJ. My consultant said to me 'absolutely no surgery' to the TMJ because it is (in this patient group) only likely to worsen my symptoms. I remain under review.

TMJ dysfunction

There is a relationship between cervical spine functional issues including pain and the TMJ. Baptistella Ferão and Traebert (2008) suggest a 90 per cent prevalence of temporomandibular disorder (TMD) in physiotherapy patients presenting with unresolved cervical spine pain (Baptistella Ferão and Traebert 2008). Other writers and researchers also postulate that there is a relationship between cervical pain, postural alterations and TMD (Baptistella and Traebert 2008; Bryden 2010; Nicolakis *et al.* 2001). Nicolakis *et al.* suggest that anterior head posture increases tension in the masticatory muscles, increasing the upward pressure on the mandibular. They further suggest that cervical spine and other postural faults, such as difference in leg length and having flat feet, might also affect the TMJ (2001). Baptistella Ferão and Traebert write that 'disturbances in the TMJ can affect the positioning of the skull over the cervical region and can determine the postural balance through a common neuromuscular system' (2008, p.63). Given that a weakened posture is related to EDSIII, it is not surprising that TMD can result. The TMJ is a joint and is also predisposed to joint laxity in this patient group, resulting in excessive joint opening, but equally muscle spasm might prevent excessive movement in hypermobile patients, and impaired proprioception (which is well known in this patient group) and excessive mobility could lead to ligament and joint capsule trauma (Bryden 2010; Kavuncu *et al.* 2006). Indeed, Kavuncu *et al.* (2006) suggest that the risk of TMJ problems is great if hypermobility and condylar hypermobility co-exist.

The definition of a 'normal' mouth opening is 35mm–50mm. A person who has less than 35mm of mouth opening might be considered to be hypomobile, whereas an excess of 50mm would be considered hypermobile (Smekal *et al.* 2008). It is curious to learn that some patients develop TMD symptoms after excessive dental work such as tooth extractions and orthodontic treatment, where the mouth is held open for prolonged periods (Smekal *et al.* 2008). Women are more commonly affected (Bryden 2010; Knezevic *et al.* 2008). As many as 70 per cent of the randomised population might be affected with TMD; only about one quarter are aware of it, and then only about 5 per cent actually seek treatment (Smekal *et al.* 2008).

Baptistella and Traebert (2008 p.65) suggest the following to discuss upon patient referral, including questions such as:

difficulties with joint mobility and with opening and closing movements of the mandible, lateralisation movements of the mandible, tiredness, or muscular pain on chewing, headache, pain in the cervical spine, ears or TMJ, presence of joint sounds; presence of trismus of teeth grinding as well as factors of emotional tension; disturbances of vision and balance problems.

Bartley (2011) writes that TMD is a risk factor for migraine and tension headache. He writes that 'anxiety, depression and muscle tenderness are common factors in jaw joint pain, tension headache and migraine' (Bartley 2011, p.295). There is a significant similarity in the general 'other' joint pain and symptoms that EDSIII patients will experience along with the associated psychological overlaps of anxiety and depression, and physiotherapists are reminded to be aware of TMJ symptoms in this patient group (Bryden 2010).

In terms of the management of TMJ symptoms, Bryden (2010) suggests using heat or ice, avoiding excessively chewy foods and chewing gum. Bryden also suggests the use of a night splint to rest the masticatory muscles. Such patients are also advised to refrain from excessive mouth opening (e.g. wide yawning) and to remind patients to request breaks during dental treatment to rest the TMJ (2010). Specific TMJ exercise therapy might also be beneficial to symptomatic patients as it is suggested that this (as indeed other exercise for this patient group) will reduce pain and muscle spasm, aid relaxation and improve joint mobility (Bryden 2010; Nicolakis et al. 2001). Nicolakis et al. (2001) suggest that exercises for active and passive jaw movement, correction of body posture and exercises to strengthen the muscles of mastication and correct jaw closure resulted in a 75 per cent excellent or distinctive improvement in jaw function in a study of 18 patients. Again, it is important for physiotherapists and other medical professionals working with the EDSIII patient group to consider the treatment and management of TMD symptoms and factor the necessary rehabilitation into treatment plans (Bryden 2010; Nicolakis et al. 2001).

Eyes and TMJ

At times there were some 'interesting' things that went on when treating my TMJ. This involved my eyes (which is perhaps more explainable), but perhaps more extraordinary was the iliotibial band

(ITB). ITB was often implicated. This is an example of when my physio did some work on my superior left tibia and fibula and my eyes went crossed and I couldn't open my jaw:

> You have gone cross-eyed, and now you can't open your mouth? So releasing ITB, and going into superior tib/fib and now we have got eyes crossing and jaw doing strange things! How can moving your leg and working on your ITB make your eyes cross and stop you opening your mouth? It is no wonder you are a challenging patient!
>
> *Physiotherapy, 13.1.2011*

This is just one extract of some interesting physiological phenomena that used to occur during some of my physiotherapy treatments.

Vision abnormalities in patients with FM and EDSIII

An EDS patient writes on Facebook:

> My eyesight seems to be worst when my jaw and neck pain is worst.

Patients with FM are more likely to have vision abnormalities encompassing strabismus, the medical term for being cross-eyed (Berne 2002), including other problems such as dry eyes, latency and intermittent blurred vision (Berne 2002).

Myopia is part of a measure of the assessment of EDSIII via the Brighton Criteria.[1] I had often wondered why this was, and received the following email answer from Professor Howard Bird:

> The evidence for an association (probably through genetic linkage on the same chromosome) is strongest for Marfans though also reasonable for EDSIII though here there is the suspicion that this may be an acquired secondary overuse phenomenon in compensation for the lax ligaments that support the lens. The evidence for a genetic link becomes stronger, however, in the Stickler area of the HM syndromes probably because these conditions affect a different collagen.
>
> *Email from Professor Howard Bird, 19.4.2012,*
> *reproduced with kind permission*

In Chapter 36 we look at the cervical spine.

---

1   For more discussion about diagnostic criteria see Beighton *et al.* (2012); Hakim *et al.* (2010); Keer and Grahame (2003); Knight (2011). Also see Appendix 1.

Cervical spine

I get a really tense cramped up neck and sometimes feel a bit lightheaded because of it.

EDSIII patient, Facebook

There is a very good reason the phrase 'pain in the neck' became the idiom that it is. There are few more annoying places to get a pain. I can't even begin to think straight when my neck flares up. It's the kind of pain that makes me nostalgic for labour pains.

EDSIII patient, Facebook

Until December 2011 I still had huge problems with my neck or cervical spine. I was still experiencing POTS symptoms of dizziness, nausea and temperature changes. I was still getting left-sided headaches and severe muscular spasm and pull to the left. I blogged the following:

My physio has explained to me that my neck is in severe muscular spasm because the deep muscles do not work properly and the superficial ones (e.g. upper traps and SCM) overwork. The deep ones do not work because they are trying to control such a large range of movement, but they do not manage it and then therefore fatigue or go into a muscle spasm which is protective and locking. This is happening to my hip flexors as well and they are also 'locked up'.

The pain would be tolerable if it ever responded to pain medication, but it is not – other than diazepam, which is not recommended as a long course of treatment. I am using my neck collar, having periods without it, but if I go too far with this, I just end up in more pain, so I need to find the right balance. The pain is not the only problem. I am experiencing sickness, dizziness and visual disturbance which are neurological symptoms and what my physio required me to be checked out for in hospital. I am now waiting for an MRI scan to see if there are any other clues as to what is causing my neck to remain in this state of spasm – but it might be that the MRI scan does not show this and it is just another very difficult feature of the Ehlers-Danlos Syndrome (Hypermobility, Type 3).

Blog, 27.12.2010

When my neck became symptomatic again my physio treated my neck again as the overall plan was to begin to reduce physiotherapy for some things as I develop strength and stamina doing other activities – for example, swimming and walking. I have to say that I felt 'worse' after the session, but my physio had done over half an hour on my neck. I got back from physio and had to go to bed for a few hours, and got up and had this almighty pull to the left. I took diezepam and ibruprofen for tension headaches. I recall sleeping well, possibly because of the painkillers, but I did not wake up feeling any better.

I was asked to go for a coffee with a friend, but couldn't manage it. I felt dizzy and nauseous. I felt 'out of myself'. I decided to go for a walk and drop something off locally to me, but didn't really know where I was and felt a million miles from myself. I felt angry in the shop and very impatient and like shouting at people. I felt distressed because the pain was so severe in my head and I felt completely out of balance (physically and mentally). With (literally) the last bit of common sense and intelligence I had, I recalled there was a 24-hour GP surgery very local to me and went there. It was a Saturday afternoon and there was going to be a long wait and I wanted to go home and keep my eyes closed. The receptionist said I needed to come back – but said to go and wait at home for a while. I returned, and there was still a long wait and I kept my eyes shut. I had sharp pains into my left temple, centrally at C3(ish), and otherwise this huge pull around the occiput and to the left side. There was sharp pain into my left ear and temporomandibular joint (TMJ).

When I was called to be seen, it was a nurse practitioner who saw me, who was obviously going to be out of her depth with me. My BP was high – one reading was approximately 150/105, but was also quite normal at 131/76. It was random and fluctuating. Temperature was normal – but not if you palpated my hands, which were freezing. The nurse asked the doctor to review me and also tested my urine, which had raised white blood cells and blood in it, suggesting possible infection. He wanted me seen at A&E – for blood tests if need be, and so I went there.

A&E were less than thrilled to see me, and eventually gave me all the painkillers I had anyway – for example, oramorph, codeine and diazepam and anti-sickness medication. My pain did not change significantly and the doctor conducted some neurological tests – only reflexes and pupils – and then said I needed reviewing, and sent me on my way. Again, no one seemed in the least bit interested about what was going on here – but there was a huge and sudden neurological response, hugely biased to the left, and my head did not want to go into flexion and was quite blocked. Ten days later this was still the case, although the neurological symptoms abated after about 48 hours. Things still felt slightly 'on the brink'.

Things appeared to settle down for a while and then there was another set of episodes:

Following last Monday's treatment, I started to get headaches on the Tuesday afternoon. I had partly put this down to the potential stress of having my appraisal in the morning (that had gone very well), but after Tuesday, things massively escalated. On Wednesday I had to leave work early owing to nausea and POTS symptoms. I then felt neck had completely restricted at its same level of problem – not quite sure which level this is – but I have ended up with Eczema on the left side, a sore throat, both on Wednesday and then a very severe sore throat (now possibly cold) on Saturday. Bladder has been very, very affected and last night (Saturday) went to the bathroom approximately 15 times at night. Sleep has been very poor for the past few nights, and there is pain and spasm in neck and upper traps/T-Spine. Additionally arms are affected and weak. Fatigue is very much around and a very big one feels in the offering, which I am trying to fight off. Mood is affected. I am quite depressive and 'flat' and there has been skin irritation in the area. My behaviour is on the border and I have already hugely annoyed my physio by emailing her too much in the past week – so behaviour is very child-like and demanding and manic, but also cognitively 'fuzzy' headed and very slow as extremely tired. I have to say that as much as my physio has had enough of this and suggested I found someone else – partly as a result of a lack of support for her from other medics – I too am utterly fed up with this situation as it does not make me feel at all well. We truly seem to be up against it, and I do feel for my physio, as I am sure she has had enough.

Blog, 30.10.2011

Rosemary Keer writes about the importance of the cervical spine along with explanations for some of the neurological symptoms I (and many others) experience.

CERVICAL SPINE
Rosemary Keer

The cervical spine is a very important part of the vertebral column. It supports the head, which weighs approximately 5kg, from the moment we get up in the morning to the moment we lie down again in the evening. In addition it protects and transports the vital neural tissue to the rest of the body. It is the most mobile part of the spinal column, and this mobility comes at the expense of stability, making the cervical spine more vulnerable to injury (Magee 2008, p.130) and potentially even more so in a hypermobile individual. It has been estimated that the bone and ligamentous structures of the cervical spine only support 20–25 per cent of the weight of the head and the remaining 75–80 per cent is reliant on the efficiency of the cervical musculature (Panjabi *et al.* 1998).

There is a tendency to adopt a forward head posture, particularly with prolonged sitting. This is partly due to the weight of the head and partly due to muscle insufficiency, weakness or injury. In this posture the deep neck flexors and infrahyoid muscle lengthen and become weak and the opposing suprahyoids and neck extensors become shortened. This produces increased extension of the upper cervical spine with potentially an increase in load and compression through the joints of the neck, which can lead to head and neck pain. But it can also lead to a change in the position of the mandible (downwards and backwards), which can affect the temporomandibular joint (TMJ) and produce symptoms (Bryden 2010). In some individuals there may be laxity in the upper cervical ligaments connecting the occiput to C1 and C2 (the occiputoatlantalaxial complex), allowing the head or atlas to shift forward slightly on the vertebral level below. This can produce pain and other symptoms such as nausea, difficulty swallowing, throat tightness, dizziness and feeling unwell. Symptoms in this case may be relieved by lying or gliding the head backwards on the neck.

The posture of the shoulder girdle also has an effect on the cervical spine as muscles such as trapezius and levator scapulae connect the shoulder blade to the neck. Shoulders held in a forward and downwardly rotated position (often due to overactivity and tightening of the pectoral muscles) can lead to lengthening and weakening of the upper fibres of trapezius which then exerts a pull on the cervical spine. This is exacerbated further if the muscles supporting the shoulder blade (scapula) on the chest wall are insufficient for the job and the weight of the arms is then transmitted to the cervical spine, restricting movement and producing muscle tension and pain which may extend up to the base of the skull.

A few, rare syndromes have been identified which can occur in the cervical spine, which can be responsible for a variety of unpleasant symptoms. Weakness or insufficiency of the cervical muscles may lead to minor clinical instability (MCI), which can be diagnosed if there is a history of major cervical trauma, neck catching or locking, giving way, poor muscular control, hypermobility on X-ray and on movement testing by palpation and unpredictability of symptoms (Niere and Torney 2004). It is thought that major trauma is not necessary for MCI to develop in a hypermobile individual who may be more prone to instability due to ligamentous laxity.

Cervical cord compression may occur with hypermobility of the mid cervical spine (C5/6), the most mobile segment of the cervical spine. Poor muscular control of this spinal segment, particularly during extension, may lead to functional or intermittent compression of the spinal cord. This may produce symptoms of pain, fatigue, cognitive impairment, instability of gait, pins and needles, dizziness and numbness (Heffez et al. 2004). To date it has been associated with the diagnosis of fibromyalgia, but as there is considerable overlap between this and JHS, it is possible that hypermobility and poor segmental control during extension may lead to irritation of the spinal cord, producing symptoms in some hypermobile individuals.

Treatment for the cervical spine is normally concerned with improving postural control and endurance. Stability of the cervical spine is achieved through efficient co-contraction of the deep flexors (longus capitis and longus colli) and extensors (multifidus) of the neck. This can be achieved through isometric exercises maintaining the neck in a neutral position and non-weightbearing (if necessary) and progressing into range and weightbearing. The craniocervical flexion test (CCFT) (Jull, O'Leary and Falla 2008) is useful to assess the performance of the deep neck flexors and can be used in association with neck flexor endurance strength training to reduce neck pain and disability and improve upright posture (Falla *et al.* 2007). However, it is important to progress rehabilitation onto postural and movement control in functional activities and also to integrate this with good movement control of the thoracic spine and shoulder girdle. Improving strength and stability around the shoulder girdle can be particularly important to ensure the weight and activity of the upper limbs is evenly supported across the shoulder girdles and upper back (Keer 2010).

Use of splinting and taping
Cervical neck collar

One thing that particularly helped me to recover if I had excessive C-spine symptoms or migraines was use of a (hard) cervical neck collar. Normally this would go against the grain in terms of a neck with no acute injury, but in the patient with ligamentous laxity and muscles that have completely fatigued it could be seen how this strategy which was recommended by my consultant rheumatologist, Professor Howard Bird, makes much sense. Although I hated wearing it, and found it very embarrassing, it gave me 'increased battery life' whilst the muscles had a rest. I even managed to do a ballet class using it and ended up feeling less dizzy. The use of a protective collar definitely 'sped up' my fatigues or improved neck symptoms when these flared up. It would be worth physiotherapists considering usage of this or other splints (e.g. for patients with weak wrists) as a triage whilst continuing to build the 'deep' underlying muscles, which are so important, as Keer previously explained.

Not long after this my physio and I met with Professor Howard Bird who kindly wrote to my GP requesting a further X-ray of my cervical spine at the C1/2 level, amongst other things. The requested X-ray came back as normal, which was no surprise in the end given the outcome of the Bowen session I had, and is described in the next chapter. However, the strengthening work that Keer emphasises and other stability work remained ongoing.

Kinesic taping

The use of kinesio taping has become very popular in recent years. It was commented upon in the 2012 Olympics as many athletes were seen with this brightly coloured and sometimes interestingly patterned tape on various parts of their body. The tape, which can be applied anywhere on the body (see Figures 36.1 and 36.2), offers potential proprioceptive feedback to the body and helps to support and assist with rehabilitation following injury (Keer and Butler 2010). It might provide 'information' to certain muscle groups to reduce effort, whilst subtly encouraging other muscles to engage a little more. Care should be taken to avoid overdependency (Keer and Butler 2010).

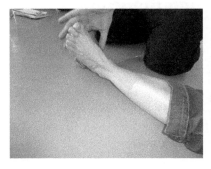 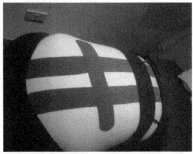

FIGURE 36.1: TAPING ANKLE/FOOT   FIGURE 36.2: TAPING OF THE SPINE

Hypermobile people like it – especially those who are prone to subluxation (partial dislocation) or even for those who dislocate. Others like it for the reasons described above – to provide support and perhaps proprioceptive guidance. There is no doubt that the tape has advantages providing there is not an overdependency, and in the EDSIII population there needs to be some caution in usage of this tape as it can anecdotally cause skin allergies. Early experiments involving me and my physiotherapist have started to show that reducing the tension of the tape applied can minimise allergic reaction, but more research needs to be carried out. EDSIII patients comment on Facebook:

> I use it in my shoulder when I'm going through particularly intense phases of instability. It feels like a second layer of tendons holding my shoulder in place.

> I find it really helps – I always feel extra stable when taped and more aware of my body in space but as with all of us, our Hypermobile skin doesn't like the tape much and after a day I have to remove [it] due to redness and [being] itchy.

CHAPTER 37

The trauma of birth and post-traumatic stress disorder

Mind Body Bowen

Although it is certainly possible to treat oneself using Bowen, it is not conventional, and certainly not when doing an approach called Mind Body Bowen (MBB) developed by Margaret Spicer and Anne Schubert under the close jurisdiction of Oswald Rentsch, Director of the Bowen Association. I qualified as a Bowen therapist in 2003 and attended a 'Mind Body Bowen' course in London in 2008. I had experienced a few sessions of this work with my own Bowen instructor, and had two very contrasting outcomes from the work, as can be expected. The way in which one uses MBB differs from 'normal' Bowen work in that one sets up the patient in a different way so that they track and follow different sensations in the body as they occur (or not) once the therapist puts the Bowen moves into the body. The other difference is that the breaks during treatment (normal for Bowen therapy) are much longer than the minimal two-minute waiting time. During one session I had, I experienced the release of a memory about being 'dunked' in a swimming pool when I had not yet inhaled any air before I was pushed under. The other experience resulted in a huge improvement to my shoulder range of movement, and the word 'patience' was strongly associated with this experience. After an MBB treatment it is usual practice to issue the patient with some kind of homework. After the swimming pool experience, I wrote the experience in ink so that I could then wash away afterwards to properly get rid of the memory. I did this, and the next day went punting in Cambridge, which was amazing considering I cannot swim!

When I attended Anne and Margaret's course in 2008, I had the most amazing traumatic release witnessed by 34 people. It took two separate attempts, but I incredibly went through my own birth. I experienced this both as my mother and as myself. Since that huge release I felt calmer and more in my body than I had felt before until that time. I have conducted the work with varying degrees of success on a few patients, but have experimented with the work on my own body at various times. The potential danger of this is if the release is huge and there is no one around to talk to, or if there is no story reached in conclusion. I decided to do some Bowen work on myself purely because I was feeling very anxious and couldn't sleep. Here is what happened:

> Last night I was feeling very anxious and couldn't sleep. I decided to do MBB on me. Did Moves one and two and not 'very much' happened, so thought it was going to be a very quiet session (sometimes I fall asleep). After Moves three and four it all kicked off. Left hand was flapping about. Left little finger very twitchy. Spasms on left side of the body, particularly in T-spine. I was often either breathing very deeply, very fast, or not at all! Pulse rate was fast. Eyes fixated and staring. This must have gone on for about half an hour. I then moved slightly and was then at an odd angle. Right little finger was twitching, but spasms on left continued and I started making strange sounds. As I was being pulled further around to the right, so left pulled around, I started breathing more strangely again, with deep breaths, fast breathing, or none. I was making more strange noises as if gasping. Then, I felt a huge pull around my left neck and was completely gasping. I was choking and being strangled. This happened twice. I was very scared (in myself at the time), but managed to free myself and pull myself away. I was trying to get my hand to move the object. The realisation was immediate and obvious. The umbilical cord was caught around my windpipe and left side of my neck. I managed to move it myself (possibly hence the hand flapping). I was near to death twice. My neck felt sore (SCM) but I was going through this whole experience for about an hour. There is no doubt in my mind what I went through. I am sitting here now having no problem doing forward flexion. If I am right about what I have experienced and document, it might mean that things improve.

> Today I feel much calmer in myself and completely 'connected'. I have got normal neck flexion, no dizziness, no pain, no headaches,

no temperature or pulse rate changes. My head looks straight and not rotated or in lateral flexion. Only my physio would be able to verify the change so will see if she notices. I will obviously have to see if this holds for at least a week with no repercussions, but if so, it could explain why physiotherapy had not ultimately managed to rehabilitate this aspect of my neck. I am hopeful this could be the final end of the matter.

It looks like the fact I almost died twice during my birth has contributed ongoing to held trauma. If I have really successfully released this my neck symptoms should now improve. I managed another jog this morning – Onwards and upwards!

Blog, 12.12.2011

John Wilks, Bowen instructor and author, explains in the following.

THE EFFECT OF BIRTH ON LATER HEALTH ISSUES
John Wilks

The potential impact of how we are born on our long-term health prospects has been studied for many years by the French doctor and author Michel Odent amongst others (Gluckman *et al.* 2008). Although the conclusions of many of the research papers in Odent's extensive database (www.primalhealthresearch.com) are considered controversial by some (he calls them 'cul-de-sac' research because many of their conclusions are too difficult to integrate into mainstream medicine because they would involve too radical a rethink of birthing practice), they nevertheless show overwhelmingly that the birth experience has a major imprinting on the physical, emotional and psychological wellbeing of the adult to be (Odent 1986).

Even if we look solely from the point of view of how birth affects the baby on a physical level, it is not difficult to see why this is so. We are the only mammals that rotate as we come down the birth canal. In evolutionary terms this is because our heads are rather too large for the mother's pelvis so that we are essentially born nine months early compared to other mammals. Ask a mother how she would feel about an 18-month pregnancy and then giving birth to a baby double the normal weight and see what response you get. This need for rotation causes torsion in the various articulations of the baby's cranium and the neck, which has additional sutures and fontanels compared to the adult. Osteopaths and chiropractors have observed that the majority of us have a degree of imbalance (termed subluxation by chiropractors) at the junction between the axis, atlas and the occiput (the top of the neck) resulting from this anomaly of rotation. Rotational forces from birth also affect the jaw and the temporomandibular joint (TMJ). In the opinion of many health professionals, imbalance in either of these two relationships (the occipito-atlanteal joint or the TMJ) can lead to distortions elsewhere in the body and specifically have a marked effect on posture (Sakaguchi *et al.* 2007), with a more general knock-on effect on efficient functioning of the organism (Cuccia and Caradonna 2009). Indeed, some paediatric dentists work extensively with the relationship between posture and bite (Levinkind 2008), helping conditions such as scoliosis and kyphosis by adjusting a child's bite. The rotational effect of descent down the birth canal can be more pronounced with posterior births (back-to-back position, common with first-time mothers), which either leads to a longer rotation or, in some cases, interventions such as epidurals or caesarians. Midwives have commented that this position appears to be more and more prevalent nowadays, possibly as a result of extended periods of sitting and lack of exercise during pregnancy.

If you add into this evolutionary mix the effect of obstetric interventions, it is clear that the potential for further pressures on the baby's head and body is extreme. Many health visitors will say that minor distortions in the cranium will subside over the days following birth. This is often true of the cranial vault, which is quite soft. However, many interventions put a strain on areas of the head and neck which are not visible, particularly the cranial base. This is an area of the cranium formed by the more solid parts of the occiput, sphenoid and temporal bones, that derive embryologically from cartilage. For example, the area around the foramen magnum (at the top of the spinal cord) is formed partly by the condyles of the occiput, which sit in the concave superior facets of the atlas, allowing for easy flexion and extension of the head. However, in the baby, the occiput is formed by four bones (not just one as in the adult), and more specifically the condyles, which articulate with the atlas, are not fused at birth. This means that forces such as traction and/or torsion (inevitable in births that involve caesarian section, forceps or ventouse, but often also occurring in normal vaginal births) will create an imbalance here, with potential effects such as restricted blood flow to the cranium (Flanagan 2010), a pulling up of the brain stem, as well as stress on the short suboccipital muscles, dural membranes, venous sinuses and ventricles (particularly the fourth ventricle). As a protective reflex, you will often notice that babies born this way will have a tendency to contract through their psoas muscles, thereby putting undue pressure on the diaphragm and abdominal cavity. This can result in symptoms such as colic and also the kind of long-term neck issues that Isobel describes.

This brief focus on the physical ramifications of birth has so far not considered the psychological effect of interventions such as ventouse (used in around 10% of births in the UK), forceps or even such routine procedures as induction. Few mothers realise that research shows a clear potential link between a baby's exposure to synthetic oxytocin (as used in induction) and long-term emotional and psychological health, for example an increased risk of developing ADHD (Kurth and Haussmann 2011) and the ability to maintain stable relationships (Carter 2003). It also used to be generally accepted until recently that babies did not experience pain in the adult sense of the word, and that even if they did, they would not remember it. This resulted in practices such as operations being performed on neonates and even on babies as old as four without anesthetics. Even today babies are routinely subjected to circumcision with little or no anaesthetic. This has been shown to affect a baby's ability to create secure attachment (Laibow 1991). Common sense would suggest that being subjected to a trauma of this kind might have a life-long effect on a child, and indeed this is borne out by research (Chamberlain 1998; Van der Kolk 1994). When I started lecturing on birth I used to take around a small disposable ventouse suction cap, which I used to apply to the arm of poor unsuspecting members of the audience to give them a taste of the forces involved. I never encountered a single adult who was able to endure the suction cap being brought up to pressure, let alone any traction being applied. One has to ask, if this is the kind of welcome that we give to a baby as it enters this world, is it not surprising that it might feel a little upset and angry later in life?

The body tends to hold physical patterns it experiences at birth, which manifest later in life when the person is stressed or anxious. These might be compressive patterns, which to some extent the baby's body is designed for, or the opposite, which it is not. Patterns can be held in the tissues for many years unless resolved (possibly by a skilled therapist). There are some common patterns that tend to show up in clinical practice; for example, the temporal bones can suffer medial compression from the tight fit in the birth canal or from external forces such as forceps. This can (and often does) result in symptoms such as headaches or even torticollis (due to the pressure on the accessory nerve as it exits the cranium through the jugular foramen).

I remember many years ago, when I first started in clinical practice as a craniosacral therapist, working on a young woman with severe regular headaches and migraines, which she had suffered from since she was a child. Whilst palpating her temporal bones it became clear that there was an unusual pattern being manifested that involved medial compression, rotation and a pull inferiorly. I worked with this over a couple of sessions and the patterns eased off to the point that it was hardly noticeable. Her migraines and headaches also improved dramatically. Because this was such an unusual pattern, I questioned her about what might have caused this. It turned out that she had been born breech but with forceps, and the temporal area was still manifesting this unusual pattern some 35 years later.

There are various mechanisms by which the body might hold 'memories' of birth apart from the purely mechanical (e.g. inter-osseous or intra-osseous patterns). For example, the actions of proprioception and interoception involving the myriad of receptors in the joints, skin, muscles and fascia are well developed and very sensitive in the newborn. Research by Professor Stephen Porges (2001) has also shown that a baby is born with a highly developed 'social' nervous system, able to pick up on the emotional nuances of all around it. Hameroff, Rasmussen and Mansson (1988) describe other mechanisms that might be at play whereby memories can be held on a tissue level in the cellular microtubules. This is sometimes referred to as 'tissue memory'. Oschman and Oshman (1995) pose the questions:

> Can 'memories' encoded in connective tissue and cytoskeletal structures lead to a conscious mental image of past events? How might such information be 'released' during massage or other kinds of bodywork? And how is such information communicated from the tissue being worked upon to the consciousness of both the client and the practitioner?
>
> *Oschman and Oschman 1995, p.60–74*

Many early feelings and emotions are experienced by the adult as a 'felt sense' of the kind described by Damasio (2000). Perhaps because these felt sensations derive from powerful but pre-verbal experiences they are more difficult for adults to conceptualise and rationalise later in life. This is why early experience can have such a dominating effect on our unconscious desires and emotional outlook throughout our adult life.

The good news is that there are a lot of therapeutic interventions such as Bowen, craniosacral therapy and other body-based psychotherapeutic approaches like somatic experiencing out there that can help to address issues arising from pregnancy and birth as well as many organisations that help address the long-term consequences of how we are born (see Appendix 3). The bad news is that despite the large body of evidence and some vocal campaigners, little has been done over the last 30 years to improve the potentially negative impact of the birthing experience on both mums and babies. There is so much information in the public domain (e.g. the link between acquired immunity and psychological and developmental problems in children [Campbell-McBride 2010]), which for some reason is not promoted in mainstream practice, but which could, with a little effort, make a huge difference to the lives of so many.

As Wilks describes, there is no doubt that my experience instigated enormous relief. I blogged the following:

> Since the spectacular traumatic release that I got through Bowen Technique, I have had an extraordinary week. I have slept right through the night, every night more or less, so this is a huge improvement. I feel energetic and totally 'in my body'. I have coped with a very emotionally challenging week, and managed very successfully a big event at work. I look quite different, alive and sparkly. I have had lots of energy to go out. I have done lots of exercise. I am a new person!
>
> *Blog, 16.12.2012*

Trauma work

Janov (1990) writes that:

> trauma is not registered simply as an idea, but an experience, and must be dealt with as an experience – not simply discussed... It is a powerful notion that one can travel back decades to recapture one's personal history and undo aspects of that history. But it is so. It is possible to release the suffering component of early trauma into consciousness along with the specific memory and to discharge the energy and the pressure

of that memory forever. When this has been done, as we have seen, there are significant permanent changes in important physiologic parameters including growth, stress and sex hormones, cholesterol levels and immune functioning. The same thing that makes us sick – pain – makes us well. The difference is only a matter of integration. No integration means illness; integration means health. Hope abandoned becomes despair and hope is essential for survival. Even unreal hope.

Janov 1990, p.288

The notion and concept that hidden trauma continues to exacerbate symptoms is a very powerful message that these symptoms need addressing and then releasing. There is no doubt in my mind about the improvement of my symptoms since my traumatic release. Yet, many others are continuing to harbour hidden and unreleased trauma that is perpetuating their symptoms, that stem from their birth as Wilks suggests, or their symptoms show little or no improvement with most medical interventions. I had negative test after negative test result for my amelioration of neck symptoms, when all along the underlying reason for them was hidden birth trauma. The trouble is that some conventional medical doctors might have great difficulty in understanding the rationale behind people like Janov's work, and yet the qualitative outcome, improvement and relief for the patients is both profound and self-evident. Since research has shown that there are links with chronic pain and post-traumatic stress disorder (PTSD) (Lew *et al.* 2009; Roy-Byrne *et al.* 2004; Sharp 2004; Sharp and Harvey 2001), it would surely be worthy of research, if only it would be funded, to provide treatment sessions of work like Mind Body Bowen to see if it indeed uncovers hidden trauma and then results in the improved health and wellbeing of EDSIII/FM patients. In the end, who is to argue if there is an improvement in health and wellbeing?

Trauma

Research might be inconclusive in terms of self-harm and traumatic events, but it is a risk factor in terms of the development of personality disorders (Golier *et al.* 2003; Paris 2005; Sansone *et al.* 2001, 2006; Zittel Conklin and Westen 2005). Freud defined trauma as 'a breach in the protective barrier against stimuli leading to feelings overwhelming helplessness' (Levine 1997, p.197). If one already had a propensity towards a disordered way of coping, then to add trauma in whatever form it manifests itself would suggest the risk of self-harm increases alongside the development of post-traumatic stress disorder (PTSD), frequently found in war veterans for example, which more typically occurs in adulthood (Martin-Santos *et al.* 2010).

Post-traumatic stress disorder (PTSD)

'Post Traumatic Stress Disorder (PTSD) is more likely to be a reaction to experiencing or witnessing type 1 traumatic events, which are single, catastrophic, unanticipated experiences' (Williams and Poijula 2002, p.10). We know that there is a high prevalence of PTSD in war veterans (Lew *et al.* 2009) because of the traumas they have witnessed. Other examples might include the death of a parent, experiencing abuse or being in a traffic accident.

Symptoms of PTSD and trauma

Symptoms might include:

- hyperarousal
- constriction
- dissociation (including denial)
- hypervigilance
- intrusive memory or flashbacks
- extreme sensitivity to light and sound
- hyperactivity
- exaggerated emotional and startle responses
- nightmares and night terrors
- abrupt mood swings (e.g. rage, temper tantrums, shame)
- reduced ability to deal with stress
- difficulty sleeping
- frequent crying
- inability to make commitments
- feelings of detachment, alienation and isolation ('living dead')
- chronic fatigue or very low physical energy

- psychosomatic illnesses – particularly headaches, neck and back pain, asthma, digestive spastic colon, asthma, severe PMT
- inability to love, nurture or bond with individuals
- amnesia and forgetfulness
- feelings and behaviours of helplessness

Levine 1997, pp.148–149

Fear response and altered behaviours in EDSIII and other chronic conditions

Research has shown that individuals with chronic conditions such as hypermobility and fibromyalgia are linked to psychosomatic disorders such as IBS and other 'stress-sensitive' medical disorders (Eccles *et al.* 2012). Owing to POTS symptoms (described in Chapter 6) patients are more likely to be diagnosed with anxiety (see Chapter 23), because the symptoms also make them behave in this way (Eccles *et al.* 2012). Hypermobility has also been associated with intense fears and phobias. Research documented in Martin-Santos *et al.* (2010) suggests that 'men had more fears related to social-phobia, whilst women had fears related to death and being rejected.' (Martin-Santos *et al.* 2010, p.55). Furthermore, Montpetit (2012) writes that 'when we are suffering from post-traumatic stress, we become hyper-alert on a sensory level, which tends to overstimulate our ANS... Other factors that exist will accentuate hypersensitivity' (Montpetit 2012, p.163). Although not all patients will experience all or even any of these listed symptoms, when examined there appears to be an interesting overlap in symptoms endured by those with chronic complex pain conditions such as EDSIII and fibromyalgia, and symptoms associated with PTSD. Rothschild (2000) writes:

> People with PTSD live with a chronic state of Autonomic Nervous System – ANS activation – hyper-arousal – in their bodies, leading to physical symptoms that are the basis of anxiety, panic, weakness, exhaustion, muscle stiffness, concentration problems and sleep disturbance... It is a vicious cycle... Symptoms can become chronic or can be triggered acutely. Breaking this cycle is an important step in the treatment of PTSD.

Rothschild, B, 2000, p.47

It is therefore easy to see how patients with any of these conditions are often labelled as hypochondriacs or as suffering from 'psychosomatic illnesses'. This is unhelpful to the patient as a stigma is attached to this and they are then frequently dismissed by other medical professionals who read their previous history (see Chapters 15, 19 and 27). What is very much required is a multidisciplinary team of medical experts in working with patients with chronic complex conditions who may well be experiencing psychological trauma or undiagnosed PTSD, let alone other potential personality disorders or self-harm. The insurmountable problem is costing and resourcing in an already over stretched health care system and a lack of sufficient centres able to cope with the true complexity of such patients. There is no one magic bullet or drug to cope with such a myriad of symptoms. Good communication between patient and medical professionals is a vital starting point, as Lucas and Keer both document. Ideally, mental health conditions such as self-harm, PTSD and hidden trauma need to be brought further into the medical and public domains, and patients given early psychological intervention to improve coping skills. However, patients could find (as I did) that treatments such as Bowen therapy or craniosacral therapy might benefit some of their symptoms and safely release hidden traumas (such as those endured during birth). They might also benefit from counselling and psychotherapy to support any traumatic lifetime incidents as well as the process of managing a chronic health condition.

In Chapter 38 the Bowen technique is described by Wilks in great detail to explain how Bowen works, both medically and scientifically.

The Bowen technique and working on fascia and connective tissue disorders

John Wilks, Bowen therapist, instructor and author, explains how Bowen technique works, including exceptional and fascinating detail about fascia and connective tissues.

THE BOWEN TECHNIQUE AND EDSIII
John Wilks

Introduction
The Bowen technique was developed in Australia in the middle of the last century by Thomas A. Bowen (1916–1982). The technique is unusual in that it involves very gentle but direct manipulation of a wide variety of connective tissues (muscles, tendons, ligaments and fascia, etc.) as well as joints, nerves and skin. One reason for the beneficial effect of Bowen treatments on people with EDSIII may be because the treatment simultaneously affects muscles, joints and fascia as well as having a powerful effect on the autonomic nervous system.

When we refer to 'connective tissue diseases' (which might include fibromyalgia, EDSIII, HMS, etc.) it is important to differentiate how any therapeutic body work might affect muscle contraction (or lack of tonus) as opposed to connective tissue contracture (or in the case of EDSIII and HMS, a potential lack of contractile properties). Muscle contraction is a high-energy shortening of tissues, whereas contracture of connective tissue is a 'slow, (semi-) permanent, low-energy, shortening process, which involves matrix-dispersed cells and is dominated by extracellular events such as matrix remodelling' (Tomasek *et al*. 2002, p.357).

Because the Bowen technique works primarily on the connective tissue, it is important to understand the physiological changes involved in conditions such as EDSIII so that treatment can be tailored specifically. This is primarily concerned with increasing tonus in the core muscles and contractile strength within the fascia, as well as initiating a lowering of sympathetic tone in the autonomic nervous system (ANS).

In EDSIII (and HMS generally) there are a number of observations that have been made concerning the effect of the condition on connective tissues, in particular the superficial and deep fascia. Various researchers have identified changes in both the composition and the way the connective tissue responds to physiological changes. Amongst others, these include the following:

1. A change in the ratio of type I to type III collagen in the body. Collagen is the most abundant protein in the body and the building block of the fascial network. Type I collagen is the most common collagen in the body with high tensile strength whereas type III is more extensible. This might explain the inherent laxity in the tissues in hypermobility syndromes (HMS) (Simmonds 2012).

2. A general thinning of the diameter of collagen fibrils that make up the bulk of fascia (Simmonds 2012).

3. Less expression of Tenascin-X (TNX) (Voermans et al. 2007). TNX helps to produce stiffness in tissues and acts as a bridge between the collagen fibrils.

4. A change in the function and possibly density (Remvig et al. 2007) of myofibroblasts. These combine the function of fibroblasts and smooth muscle cells and as such bring strong contractile properties to the fascia (Schleip et al. 2012).

5. A change in the expression of transforming growth factor (TGF β1), a protein that is secreted by many kinds of cell and plays a crucial role in many cellular functions including cell division and proliferation. In fact TGF β1 has a key role in the creation of the extracellular matrix (ECM) that is critical in determining tissue characteristics in general. In the fascia, TGF β1 is released from the ECM in response to contraction in myofibroblasts (Wipff et al. 2007). This is significant therapeutically, as changes in myofibroblasts (i.e. contracture or otherwise) are initiated by a variety of different factors, including body work (such as the Bowen technique), exercise, diet, stress and inflammatory conditions. The level of

expression and effective dispersion of TGF β1 would appear to be critical in fascial health and therefore the management of HMS, particularly as its expression can be influenced in a variety of ways. TGF β1 has been used experimentally in wound healing and is key in the formation of scar tissue and, in excess, fibrosis (Li *et al.* 2004).

6. A change in the expression of smooth muscle α-actin (SMAA), critical for the function and formation of myofibroblasts (Tomasek *et al.* 2002).

Symptoms and mechanisms in EDSIII and HMS

Because fascia is ubiquitous in the body (it surrounds and forms an intricate network with every structure in the body) EDSIII symptoms are inevitably varied and variable. Symptoms might include the following, with some occurring independently and others in conjunction:

- muscle tiredness
- gastro-intestinal (GI) disorders
- tissue fragility
- hyperextensibility of the skin
- tiredness
- joint pain
- headaches and migraines.

To understand why symptoms might appear diffuse but are in fact connected, we have to understand the important and varied role of the so-called 'connective tissue' in the body, a tissue which according to Dr Guimberteau (2010) plays a much more important function than just connecting one structure to another, and one that 'has been largely ignored in most textbooks of anatomy'. For example, one of the crucial functions of fascia in efficient locomotion is its property of 'recoil'. This can be seen clearly in the thoraco-lumbar aponeurosis and other aponeuroses (areas of thick tendon-like fascia in the body). In walking and running, the lumbar fascia acts as a kind of 'bungee' and greatly reduces the amount of effort that one needs to exert via the muscular system. This is demonstrated in the movement of animals such as kangaroos, lemurs and gazelles (Kram and Dawson 1998). Humans have been shown to use this property of the fascia in 'effortless running' (Sawicki, Lewis and Ferris 2009). Where this 'recoil' property is compromised through a lack of reciprocal tension in the fascia, certain movements like running and walking require more exertion through the muscular system. This may be why some people with muscle tiredness find it easier to walk faster rather than slowly. Changes in the quality of the lumbar aponeurosis may well also explain the propensity for lower back pain in EDSIII patients, as this area is also highly innervated with sensory receptors.

Looking at GI symptoms that are so common in HMS, there is undoubtedly a link between digestive problems and the changed function of the myofibroblasts in the gut wall. Myofibroblasts appear to serve an important role in the whole digestive tract from the stomach to the colon and have been linked to conditions such as Crohn's disease (Powell *et al.* 1999).

Because fascia is the most richly innervated tissue in the body it is actually the largest sense organ in the body with the highest density of proprioceptors (Schleip 2009). Due to a potential decrease in proprioception in EDSIII, it has been suggested (Remvig 2007) that there may be a causal link with joint instability. This decrease in proprioception has also been noted in reference to vibratory stimuli in people with HMS, possibly as a result of altered functioning of Pacini receptors (involved in proprioception, important in EDSIII).

Contractile properties in connective tissue

For efficient functioning of the human system, connective tissues need to hold certain contractive patterns to maintain stability. In dissection you can see clearly that all connective tissues are under stress – for example, dissected nerves and blood vessels have a length of around 25–30 per cent less than their *in situ* length (Tomasek *et al.* 2002). Contracture is also important in wound healing (which is mostly mediated by type I and type III collagen, which is probably why it occurs differently in many EDSIII patients).

Myofibroblasts play a crucial role in maintaining constructive tension within the connective tissue, and their structure and function are affected in many kinds of connective tissue disorders. On the one hand, fibrotic contracture in conditions such as Dupuytrens reveal an imbalance in myofibroblast density and function (Naylor 2012). It would also appear that there is some mechanism involved where fibroblasts are encouraged in certain areas of the body to transform excessively into myofibroblasts (Hinz and Phan 2007). In the case of Dupuytrens this happens in the palmar aponeurosis of the hand. The mechanism by which this occurs is not sufficiently understood. Could it be that in EDSIII the reverse is the case, where function and density are affected, resulting in laxity in the myofibroblasts rather than contracture (Remvig *et al.* 2007)?

One of the ramifications of a lack of contractile strength in myofibroblasts is joint hypermobility, a common symptom of many types of HMS. Apart from the possible role of changed proprioception, the reason for this is that joint stability is dependent on reciprocal tension in the connective tissue. This is referred to as a 'tensegrity system', a term coined by the celebrated American architect Buckminster Fuller. In applying the ideas of tensegrity to the human body, various authors use the term 'biotensegrity' to explain the relationship between rigid structures such as bones, and the reciprocal tension in the connective tissue (Levin and Martin 2012). Biotensegrity can be used to explain the complex interaction that maintains structural homeostasis in gross anatomical structures like the spine and joints, to more subtle interrelationships in the myofascial system (Guimberteau 2010; Guimberteau *et al.* 2007) and even in the cytoskeleton of the cell (Oschman 2003). Biotensegrity offers an elegant explanation as to how space is held in the joints of the body and how when the delicate balance of reciprocal forces that are held by the connective tissue begin to break down, all kinds of musculoskeletal symptoms can begin to emerge (Turvey 2007). Beautiful artistic representations of this are found in the magnificent sculptures of the Canadian artist Kenneth Snelson, where none of the rigid structures (i.e. struts, but in the case of the human body, bones) touch each other. The anatomist Tom Flemons (www. intensiondesigns.com) has also made elegant models demonstrating the principles of tensegrity when applied to the human body (www. biotensegrity.com) which give a clear visual representation of why joints are so often affected in the range of HMS conditions.

Soft-tissue techniques such as the Bowen technique rely on effecting structural change by directly influencing this tensegrity aspect of the connective tissue, which is why it is one of the most effective therapeutic tools in the treatment of EDSIII.

Myofibroblasts and TGF β1

When it comes to the way that myofibroblasts operate to maintain structural integrity it is important to understand the difference between muscle function and connective tissue function:

> Viewing connective-tissue contracture simply as a result of muscle-like contraction of myofibroblasts is an oversimplification, and leads to the misconception that myofibroblast function is simple and muscle-like. From our present understanding, it is reasonable to conclude that myofibroblasts are predominantly responsible for contracture, whereas smooth (and skeletal) muscle cells act by contraction. Although some mechanical contraction is an inevitable part of the process of contracture, the reverse is not necessarily true.
>
> *Tomasek et al. 2002, p.357*

Tissue laxity and fragility are determined by the action and composition of collagen fibres (particularly the ratio of type I to type III) and factors such as TNX and TGF β1 production. It is known for example that TGF β1 promotes changes in myofibroblast function and morphology as well as promoting the formation of stress fibres. This has been shown to correlate with an increased generation of contractile force within myofibroblasts (Vaughan, Howard and Tomasek 2000). From the point of view of HMS, an increase in myofibroblast contractile quality would seem logically to be beneficial in encouraging joint and tissue stability.

There are mechanisms for the way TGF β1 is dispersed in the fascia, which have ramifications for therapies such as the Bowen technique, as well as the choice of exercise regimes, specifically in what would potentially help or hinder recovery. This is partly to do with what is called myofascial force transmission, which is the complex interaction of stress on the various components of fascia, muscles and tendons, which could potentially influence the expression of TGF β1. Wipff *et al.* (2007) show that contraction of myofibroblasts encourages expression of TGF β1 into the extracellular matrix (ECM). Conversely, mechanical loading that might occur with some types of exercise or deep manual therapy may interact with cytokines such as TGF β1, thereby activating an inflammatory response resulting from tissue microinjury (Masi *et al.* 2011). This could be why too much stimulation of the myofascia (by excessive pressure, too much work in a treatment or, in the case of exercise, too strong a regime) tends to have an adverse effect on EDSIII patients.

It would be valuable to know how therapeutic approaches such as the Bowen technique affect TGF β1 and/or TNX expression. A simple research project would involve measuring levels of TGF β1 and/or TNX before and after a series of treatments. It is known, for example, that excessive production of TGF β1 (e.g. after surgery or prolonged inflammation) creates fibrosis as it has a powerful effect on cells to encourage the deposition of the ECM. Could it be that the opposite is true in HMS?

Fascial fitness

Addressing the key issue of fascial fitness (Muller and Schleip 2012) in terms of tissue hydration, balance and composition of collagen fibres must be the overriding concern for anyone involved in treating or self-managing the range of HMS conditions. Fascial health is influenced by a number of factors including diet (pH and inflammatory markers), hydration, exercise (including stretching (Myers and Frederick 2012)), gentle therapeutic approaches (such as the Bowen technique) and managing stress levels. Prolonged inflammation has been shown to have a deleterious effect on many structures and mechanisms in the body and may derive from a variety of causes, for example old injuries, operations and inflammatory conditions such as endometriosis (common in HMS patients). It is well known, for example, that inflammation in the gums (gingivitis) or in the jaw after root canal fillings can affect organs such as the heart and cause joint and muscle pain. Frequently the original site of the inflammation is asymptomatic but will have effects elsewhere in the body. Diet also has a profound effect on inflammatory markers, which can be increased by eating pro-inflammatory foods (such as grain-fed animals and fish) and reduced by adopting a low-inflammatory diet (Hankinson 2012; Reinagel 2007). Long-term inflammation and tissue damage can also have an activating effect on the sympathetic nervous system (SNS), leading to symptoms that are common in HMS such as panic attacks, anxiety, lowering of vagal tone and a racing mind.

Gentle therapeutic approaches that directly affect the myofascial system would appear to be the most obvious choice for EDSIII. Some therapies such as Rolfing and myofascial release involve direct manipulation of fascia, but many patients experience these techniques as too strong and painful due to their inherent tissue sensitivity.

Interestingly, one very gentle approach used in craniosacral therapy (CST) relates directly to the rhythmic oscillations that myofibroblasts exhibit (Follonier Castella *et al.* 2010). This rhythm has a period length of 99 seconds, which correlates to the 'long tide' oscillations that Dr Sutherland, the founder of cranial osteopathy, described. Because myofibroblasts are in close proximity in the body, they tend to express this rhythm globally, so it is possible to palpate this tide-like rhythm with sensitive hands anywhere in the body.

The Bowen technique

The Bowen technique has a very specific effect on the myofascia. Primarily, Bowen moves are made directly on muscles (although some moves are also performed on tendons, ligaments, joints and nerves). Because all these structures are surrounded by a network of fascia, it is inevitable that whatever structure is activated, the fascia that surrounds it (and is integral to it) is affected at the same time, albeit with slightly different physiological effects.

There is a large range of mechanoreceptors and other types of sensory nerves that are stimulated during a Bowen treatment, as well as a direct effect on fascia and the extracellular matrix itself. Apart from the sensory receptors in the skin such as Merkel's discs, Meissner's corpuscles and free nerve endings, there are key intra-fascial mechanoreceptors activated during a Bowen treatment. These are largely Golgi, Ruffini and interstitial receptors. Occasionally, Bowen moves involve a fast release of pressure, which affects the Pacini receptors, but these types of move are rare. Mostly, Bowen moves involve taking skin slack, applying a challenge (or gentle push) for a few seconds, and making a slow steady move over the structure being addressed. Bowen moves mostly consist of a type described by Schleip (2009) as 'slow melting pressure'. These types of move strongly affect the numerous Ruffini receptors, which are found in the skin and in many deep tissues of the body, including the lumbar fascia, dural membranes, ligaments and joint capsules, etc. Slow moves over these structures have a lowering effect on the sympathetic nervous system (SNS) (Schleip 2003) and induce a profound sense of relaxation in the client. Other receptors that induce a decrease in the SNS and corresponding increase in vagal tone are the interstitial receptors, which are found nearly everywhere in the body. Some of these receptors (particularly the nociceptors) are high-threshold, and known to be involved in chronic conditions, but interestingly about

50 per cent of these receptors are low-threshold fibres and are sensitive to the kind of very light touch (similar to skin brushing) that is used in some Bowen moves. This mechanism explains the deep relaxing effect of Bowen treatments and the crucial healing effect of increased vagal tone (Gellhorn 1967).

On a more structural level, Bowen moves affect the Golgi receptors (found in myotendinous junctions, ligaments and the deep fascia) by using slightly more pressure, longer holding times and working close to origins and insertions. It has been suggested that manipulation of these receptors causes the firing of alpha motor neurons, resulting in a softening of related tissues. This process also seems to happen via gentle stretching of the tissues such as in yoga (Schleip 2003).

Muscles themselves are stimulated by the 'challenge' in a Bowen move, which activates the muscle spindles in response to the stretch on the muscle fibres. Much of this response is mediated at the level of the spinal cord, but some impulses do make their way to various areas of the brain like the cerebellum, the basal ganglia, the reticular formation and the brain stem, before being coordinated in the thalamus and sent back down the various motor nerve tracts to the muscles or organs.

It takes around 90 seconds for muscles to respond, so it is interesting that it is normal practice for Bowen therapists to leave a two-minute break (and sometimes longer) between the various activations or moves. Other key elements in a Bowen treatment are relaxation and comfort. Whilst awake and moving around, large amounts of interoceptive and proprioceptive information from the muscles, tendons, joints, skin and fascia are being processed at any one time. However, when lying down, there is very little activity happening in the self-corrective feedback mechanism. It would appear therefore that inputting targeted but minimal sensory stimulus during a Bowen session without extraneous interference allows the body to recalibrate. For example, Dietz *et al.* (1992) have shown that the CNS can reset Golgi tendon receptors and related reflex arcs so that they function as delicate antigravity receptors (Schleip 2003). One thing students of the Bowen technique are taught is always to get clients up so that both feet land on the ground at the same time, thereby stimulating a response in the many Golgi receptors in the plantar fascia of the feet at the end of a treatment.

Certain factors are important for a successful Bowen treatment – critically that there is not excessive stimulation of the CNS by an unnecessary number of moves. This is particularly important when there is a general sensitisation of nerve pathways and tissues, as is the case in EDSIII, which is why a favourite Bowen maxim is 'less is more'. Second, if the person is not relaxed or comfortable, the key areas of the brain that are involved with the coordination of movement would not be able to 'hear' and process this distinct information to their benefit. Specifically there are certain situations that tend to activate specific areas of the cortex, so these are best avoided during a treatment:

1. speaking to the patient, particularly if the conversation refers to something that is not in the patient's current field of sensation (e.g. asking where they went on holiday or what they are going to have for supper)

2. feeling cold

3. feeling unsafe

4. bright lights.

Bowen also affects the fascia directly through encouraging hydration, as this is assisted by gentle stretching, repetitive squeezing and release with pauses (i.e. pressure applied and then waiting) – all elements of a Bowen treatment. The waiting time would appear to be essential as there is a significant increase in hydration after half an hour (Schleip and Klingler 2007).

Myofibroblasts contract and expand slowly in response to factors such as tissue pH and stress (Schleip 2009). This occurs over a period of minutes or hours and will certainly occur to some extent during the length of a Bowen treatment (normally around 45 minutes) as the person relaxes.

Fascia as a communication network

There is considerable interest amongst therapists in the concept of fascia as a communication medium in the body (Oschman 2012). It has been known for many years that piezoelectric effects initiated by stressing collagen fibres have a strong healing effect on tissues (Becker 1985). There is no doubt that something of this kind is occurring during a Bowen treatment as the impulses created by stressing collagen fibres in the challenge and roll of a Bowen move can be felt clearly with sensitive palpation. These impulses seem to have the effect on the tissues of freeing areas of fascia that are 'stuck', a process Deane Juhan (2002) refers to as thixotrophy. Ho and Knight have studied these effects in reference to acupuncture meridians (Ho and Knight 1998). In relation to Bowen, the findings may be summarised like this:

1. Impulses are created in the collagen fibres by very light pressure. The type of stretching that is used in Bowen creates a stronger piezoelectric current than just pressing on it (such as might be used in Rolfing) or going along the length of it (as might be used in massage). The fact that impulses can be generated by heat might give a clue as to why clients are asked to avoid exposing the area treated to extremes of hot or cold after a session.

2. The conductivity of collagen is strongly dependent on how hydrated it is. This means that the impulses created during a treatment will travel much more effectively if the fascia is hydrated. This is probably why some people respond better to treatment than others – babies, animals and those who practise yoga all tend to have a much more hydrated and fluid system. Hydration of the fascia generally decreases with age and under-use.

3. Impulses created in the fascia are amplified via the action of proteins in liquid crystals. Ho and Knight (1998) describe fascia as essentially liquid crystalline in nature – in other words, highly responsive to electrical charge and able to carry electrical impulses very fast (much faster than the central nervous system).

4. Fascia responds as a single coherent system, rather like the liquid crystal display that is used in computer monitors. In other words, the fascia will respond as a whole to stimulation, not just locally, and it will respond in large part directionally, determined by how the impulses travel through it. This in turn is determined by the orientation of the collagen fibres, which in turn is determined by use.

In terms of why Bowen may be helpful with EDSIII, my own clinical experience of using Bowen on scar tissue has been enlightening. Scar tissue that is raised and red responds to Bowen moves by becoming visibly less fibrotic and less inflamed quite quickly. This means that there is some physiological change in the tissues, specifically in the ratio of type I and type III collagen. This is significant in relation to EDSIII as this ratio is a crucial element in the make-up of fascia in terms of laxity. Because scar tissue can also cause restrictions through the tissue field (not only structurally but also in terms of communication), it can be very useful to work directly on it (Wilks 2007).

The exquisite images in the various 'living fascia' DVDs produced by Dr J-C. Guimberteau show clearly why techniques that encourage more fluidity in the fascia, such as Bowen, would have a profound effect on vascular and nerve supply by freeing up the connective tissues that surround capillaries, veins, arteries and nerves. Vascular supply is one area that can be compromised in EDSIII, and it would be interesting to find out if slightly longer rest times between Bowen moves would assist in the process of revascularisation.

The ability of the Bowen technique to help patients with EDSIII is borne out by clinical experience, and although more research needs to be done in this area, it is clear that there are mechanisms by which the Bowen technique can assist in terms of fascial fitness, reducing stress levels, increasing vascular supply and improving mobility and posture.

CHAPTER 39

The Feldenkrais Method®

Another form of work that I have found invaluable throughout my ongoing rehabilitation has been the Feldenkrais Method®.

The Feldenkrais Method®

I first came across the Feldenkrais Method® when studying for my MSc in Dance Science at Trinity Laban Conservatoire of Music and Dance. The Feldenkrais Method® was created by the late Moshe Feldenkrais, a scientist, engineer and well-respected Judo instructor. He developed his work in response to a long-standing knee injury that threatened to leave him disabled in his forties. Feldenkrais refused surgery and instead used his knowledge of physiology, anatomy, psychology and engineering to develop a way to interact directly with the nervous system in order to regain his mobility. He realised that it was vital to improve his whole self-organisation if he was going to make these improvements permanent. His method focuses on using experiential movement patterns to improve sensory-motor awareness and thus the efficiency and functioning of the skeleton and the nervous system. Feldenkrais' work is included under the banner of somatic education. Thomas Hanna (originally a Feldenkrais practitioner) coined the term somatics as a way of working in a bodily holistic manner. A simplified definition of somatics might be '"bodily based access to information about the whole system and its interactive patterns" or very simply, knowing oneself from the inside out' (Fitt 1996, p.304). The holistic nature of working somatically, or somatic repatterning, very much appealed to me, and Feldenkrais appeared to leap out at me from other distinctive and well-known somatic practices which include yoga, the Alexander technique and body–mind centring. Feldenkrais had an enormous impact on me from the beginning when I tried it for the very first time and now, four years later, I have done two (separate) week-long courses on Feldenkrais, a range of other shorter workshops and one-to-one sessions, and I have also been taught by a range of teachers.

My earliest experience was possibly my most profound in terms of my hypermobility. We were doing a lesson that was centred around the pelvis and knees. Feldenkrais work involves a series of gentle experiential moves under (often) beautiful instruction by a teacher. The teacher's explanation of what they require has to be explicitly clear so that you are able to interpret the movement instructions and experiment with them yourself. As a dancer always being told what to do by a teacher, I found the fact that there is no 'right' way to conduct a movement very refreshing, and in fact most liberating that I had the choice about how I moved my knee, or whatever it was. In between each set of instructions (offering alternative explorations), there are critical rest breaks so the body has time to process the new information or way of moving, and so that concentration does not wander. I fully understood the application of the rest breaks through my own work as a Bowen therapist where the work is regularly punctuated by breaks for a similar reason and to allow the body to process and rest. The 'lesson' then continues and frequently concludes with a request to stand and then walk about the room, noticing anything that has changed since the lesson commenced. It was during one of my first ever Feldenkrais lessons, when I thought 'not much' had happened, that I realised that I was actually walking with my legs in a neutral alignment and out of their hyperextension for the first time ever.

I remembered feeling extremely tired after the session and also very hungry – but my body had gone through a huge change. I felt wobbly in my 'out of hyperextension' posture and so all sorts of other adjustments were having to be made, including to my balance and proprioception. I recall 'dying' to be able to show my new-found alignment to my physio and ballet teacher. I blogged:

> Since this is my first class with my knees behaving freely, it felt almost like learning again – and in some ways I am; since I am re-educating my body to work in a new way… In the centre, things felt different again – I felt my calves were less tight and knotted than normal, and everything felt more fluid. I just felt more relaxed in myself, but also a bit uncertain. I need to learn to trust my body in this new state, and accept how good the relaxation feels in my legs. Hopefully this will follow on through the upper body also, in due course. I am just so thrilled to feel how a 'normal' dancer feels. The only snag is

that I might lose some of my extension in higher lines such as grand battement and arabesque. My legs were tired after class, but not in a negative way.

Blog, 23.1.2009

Although my legs didn't remain out of hyperextension forever (perhaps for a week), it did allow me a very useful opportunity to understand that I didn't need to remain locked into hyperextension and how I could try and move a little more freely.

I have had further enlightenments in Feldenkrais including how doing 'less is more' and that it is possible to gain much from the work even if one is listening and not doing. I had to particularly take this on board when I became very fatigued during a one-week Feldenkrais course. This was a significant learning moment for me in how to try to accept my fatigues and not fight them. Fatigue is something nearly all EDSIII patients are familiar with. In Feldenkrais, you are in control and in charge of how much movement you do, which means that if you have a very mobile joint you can make the movement much smaller. Conversely, if you are able to, you can also stretch out a tighter area. From this point of view, I believe Feldenkrais is entirely safe for EDSIII patients, especially as there are many rest points in the classes (and you can even image movement if you are too fatigued).

Feldenkrais is also about efficient movement. Most hypermobile people move in an incredibly inefficient and energy-wasting manner. I nearly always fix muscle groups or use many extra muscles to move when fewer would do. Feldenkrais has allowed me to explore much greater movement patterning and efficiency, and because the premise of the work is on bone and joint movement (movement leading from bone) rather than muscle, I use much less effort than I would in Pilates, but am still getting an extremely deep core musculature workout, with much less pain and fatigue. For this reason I highly recommend it to all EDSIII patients and for medical professionals to become informed about the value of this amazing work. I am now doing Feldenkrais regularly and I am finding it is really enhancing my wellbeing as well as reminding me about how to work my body much more efficiently and with less effort. Sometimes I do experience fatigue following new work, but learning something is hard work and the body has to respond. I no longer fight any fatigues, but accept them as a way of moving forwards.

One of my Feldenkrais teachers, Maggy Burrowes, explains the work in more technical detail.

THE FELDENKRAIS METHOD®
AND HYPERMOBILITY

Maggy Burrowes

Hypermobility presents Feldenkrais teachers with an interesting and distinctive challenge. Throughout our four-year training we spend a significant proportion of the time immersed in the Awareness Through Movement® (ATM) process we will be teaching when we graduate – and much of that time is spent experiencing directly the functional range of motion of our joints and how they interconnect as we organise ourselves to move. The Feldenkrais Method® (FM) uses movement as a way of developing greater self-awareness: Moshe Feldenkrais was as interested in helping people to free themselves from habitual thinking as he was to free them from habitual action. He designed his work with the intention of integrating thinking, feeling, sensation and action in order to restore and improve proprioception in children and adults. He combined his experience of engineering and judo teaching with his knowledge of child development and came up with a process designed to give people strategies that would enable them to help themselves, through greater sensory-motor (kinaesthetic) awareness and the direct experience of new possibilities.

Of course hypermobility creates an excess of possibilities in the joints affected – some adults stand with locked knees, which is not efficient and over time may lead to pain and postural issues, but with hypermobility the knees lock into positions that are much less supportive and the individual has to organise themselves in relation to gravity without the vital structural feedback the rest of us take for granted. Usually an arm only goes back so far and then it stops. In an ATM lesson we experiment with all the possible positions an arm can move into *with ease*, and for most people that is functional and healthy, but for hypermobile people the joint does not send the same clear signals and the person has got used to acting without this feedback. Feldenkrais work focuses on instilling a clear sense of the way a well-organised skeleton moves, and the lessons – many hundreds of them – have been carefully designed to make skeletal connections much clearer. In one-to-one Functional Integration® the teacher is able to tailor the lesson to the individual and recommend specific movement patterns as therapeutic homework.

Most physical techniques are founded on our natural range of motion – the golf swing, the way the wrist interacts with piano or guitar, avoiding injury when lifting something heavy – and so when these techniques are not supported by feedback from the skeleton the world must seem as unfamiliar as it does to the left-handed, and adaptation becomes a daily necessity. Adaptation is what FM teachers specialise in.

Isobel was an open and vivacious member of the class, who was easy to teach because she was already aware of her tendencies – overworking, losing clarity with some movement directions and replacing that clarity with determined physical effort. My general experience with hypermobile people in my classes is that they are aware of having unusual joints, but may need time and extra attention from the teacher to find the developmental movement patterns that come naturally to the rest of us. Once they can find this easily supported posture for themselves they instantly feel the difference.

Feldenkrais classes are gentle and slow, carefully designed to produce clear results in the students without causing injury, and to steadily develop a true skeletal awareness in moving. The long-term goal of self-awareness and discovery and freedom from habitual thinking makes it ideal for dealing with the issues caused by hypermobility syndrome.

In the next chapter the tone changes from somatic-based work such as the Feldenkrais Method® to looking at cardiovascular fitness and endurance work.

CHAPTER 40

Cardiovascular and endurance work

My physio gave me a pep talk and I managed to get back into some regular exercise and have been pushing through the pain to manage some gentle cardio and abdominals daily over the last two or three weeks. The first thing I noticed was obviously more energy and mobility and a better attitude (alas the pain is still bad) but I have now noticed that the heart racing is improved. I have also cut down coffee though, so that could also be relevant – but I suspect it's a combination of both. It's not gone away but it's noticeably improved. Anyway, to cut a long story short, I do think it got worse because of the inactivity and the increased daily exercise has helped.

EDS patient, Facebook

EDS expert physiotherapist and lecturer Dr Jane Simmonds writes the following about cardiovascular and muscular endurance reconditioning.

CARDIOVASCULAR AND MUSCULAR ENDURANCE RECONDITIONING
Dr Jane Simmonds

When considering the rehabilitation and reconditioning process, it is important for hypermobile individuals and therapists to implement an integrated approach. Normal movement and optimal performance relies on the integration of three core physiological systems: musculoskeletal, neurological and cardiovascular. These core systems work as a flexible functional interdependent unit (see Figure 40.1). For example, where there has been a primary impairment of the musculoskeletal system, such as an injury or dysfunction of the knee joint, the individual will tend to protect the knee, move it less and reduce their levels of physical activity. If reduced activity extends for more than a few days, muscles will become weaker, and connective tissues such as supporting ligaments, bones and cartilage will also gradually decondition in a process known as disuse atrophy. With the reduction in physical activity and in particular sustained cardiovascular activities, there will be both peripheral and central changes to the cardiovascular system, resulting in a less efficient exchange of essential oxygen and nutrients in the heart and lungs and also the working muscles and vital organs. A period of reduced activity results in the reversal of many of the physiological adaptations associated with training (Brawner, Keteyian and Saval 2010). These result in decreases in maximal oxygen uptake (VO2max), maximal ventilatory capacity, decreased cardiac output and reductions in total blood volume (Mujika and Padilla 2000; Raven, Welch-O'Connor and Shi 1998). Muscles are dependent on sufficient oxygen supply and other essential nutrients carried in the blood to function efficiently in terms of strength, power and endurance. Muscle strength and endurance are of key importance for joint stability, particularly in areas such as the spine and inherently less stable joints, such as the shoulder, hips and ankles. Cardiovascular changes during the deconditioning and reconditioning process are summarised in Table 40.1.

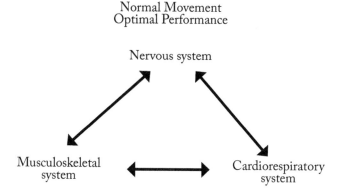

FIGURE 40.1: CORE PHYSIOLOGICAL SYSTEMS (DAVENPORT 2012)

TABLE 40.1: Summary of cardiovascular effects of deconditioning and reconditioning		
Component	Reconditioned	Deconditioned
Stroke volume	Increased	Decreased
Resting heart rate	Decreased	Increased
Resting blood pressure	Decreased	Increased
O_2 delivery	Improved	Reduced
Gas exchange	More efficient	Less efficient
Capillary density	Increased in myocardium and active muscles	Reduced in myocardium and active muscles
Fatty deposits	Cleared from vessels	Recurrence in vessels
Mitochondria in muscles	Increased	Decreased

Alongside the changes to the cardiovascular system, a period of reduced activity will impact on the neurological system. This may further impact on the individual's proprioception, balance and coordination and perceptions of pain. Research has demonstrated that activity and movement participation drive cortical mapping in the brain (Tyc, Boyadjian and Devanne 2005). The motor cortex is highly plastic and changes quickly in response to altered activity (Boudreau *et al.* 2007; Sanes and Donoghue 2000). Interestingly, the presence of dysfunction and changes in motor performance are proposed to be a factor in maintenance of pain (Boudreau *et al.* 2010). Various research has demonstrated cortical reorganisation and abnormal muscle sequencing within chronic pain populations (Falla, Jull and Hodges 2004; Tsao, Galea and Hodges 2008).

Therefore, when embarking on a reconditioning programme, it is important to consider all three systems and to strike a balance between motor control and stability exercises (which help to stabilise and strengthen local joints) and cardiovascular reconditioning (which works as the body's energy providing the fuel for core function and muscular endurance). With this concept in mind individuals are encouraged to progressively challenge and train the cardiovascular system as part of their reconditioning programme. This may begin with as little as just a few minutes of structured and planned land-based walking (assisted if necessary by walking aids), stationary bicycle riding, walking a few metres in a swimming pool or swimming. It is important to allow time for recovery, especially where chronic fatigue and pain are present, and therefore this planned exercise may initially be encouraged on an every-other-day basis. Individuals are encouraged to gradually increase the duration and frequency of exercise. In some cases pedometers are useful for monitoring step count, although these devices are not always reliable, and where possible pedometers which have been shown to be reliable should be selected.

Once a foundation for cardiovascular training has been established, intensity of cardiovascular training can be addressed, that is, monitoring heart rate in order to provoke a more optimal training effect. Individuals may also want to try other forms of cardiovascular activity, including use of the cross trainer, Nordic walking, rowing or dancing. Initially, training heart rates may start as low as 35–40 per cent of maximum heart rate. As fitness and general conditioning improve, the training heart rate may rise to 60–70 per cent of maximum heart rate. The Borg scale of perceived rate exertion is an easy-to-use scale to monitor intensity. Some individuals benefit from using heart rate monitoring devices, although it should be recognised that immersion in water impacts on cardiovascular function and adjustments need to be made to calculate training heart rate when exercising in water (Graef and Kruel 2006). The frequency of training is another important parameter. Pacing and carefully progressing the reconditioning training process is very important as there needs to be adequate time between sessions to allow for the training adaptation. Anecdotally, this very measured approach to reconditioning has resulted in an improvement in perceptions of pain, improved functional capacity and an enhanced quality of life.

Strong evidence suggests that adherence to treatment is an important factor influencing physiotherapy outcomes (Jack *et al.* 2010). In a general outpatient setting, factors such as low pre-morbid exercise levels (Rejeski *et al.* 1997; Stenström, Arge and Sundbom 1997), depression (Oliver and Cronan 2002) and perceived barriers to exercise (Alexandre *et al.* 2002) have been demonstrated as barriers to rehabilitation.

Improving patient engagement through identification of potential barriers to effective participation is therefore important. There are various theories of behaviour change, many of which involve the concept of facilitating moving the patient from a motivational phase, whereby intention to achieve an outcome is initiated, to the action phase, whereby goal-directed behaviour is maintained (Scobbie, Wyke and Dixon 2009).

Goal-setting has been found to improve self-efficacy in rehabilitation (Coppack, Kristensen and Karageorghis 2012). Goals should include a combination of short- and long-term targets, be individualised and involve patient participation (Baker *et al.* 2001). It is recommended that goals are challenging to improve motivation (Locke and Latham 2002). With this concept in mind, it is important to develop realistic and achievable short- and long-term goals for the cardiovascular aspect of reconditioning. For some, an initial goal may be to undertake a planned slow walk for five minutes on five days of the week, progressing by one minute per week, with a long-term goal of going on a supported five-day walking holiday in 18 months' time.

In their papers on the rehabilitation of EDSIII patients Simmonds and Keer have recommended a return to exercise and sport, but they suggest doing this very carefully and how strengthening exercises and stability are essential first (Keer and Simmonds 2011; Simmonds and Keer 2007, 2008). The research and medical literature is abundantly clear about EDSIII and the paramount importance of exercise in terms of both the prevention of deconditioning and the continued overall management of the condition itself (Simmonds 2010). One of the biggest overall problems for patients with chronic complex (pain) conditions such as FM and EDSIII is that they often reduce exercise in response to pain levels and fatigue or injury which has a resultant impact on fitness levels and tolerance to exercise (Simmonds 2010). However, the research does indicate that if all bodily tissues (e.g. muscle, nerve and bone) are better conditioned the tissues themselves receive improved nutrients, via improved cardiovascular function, which leads to improved health and functioning overall (Simmonds 2010). Frequently there are psychological barriers to re-starting more 'physical' exercise and sport again where there has been resultant injury and pain in the past, but if these can be overcome in a slow and gradual programme, the outcome should be improved performance, fitness and good general health throughout life (Simmonds 2010).

Rooks, Silverman and Kantrowitz's (2002) research into patients with FM (n=15) has shown how a progressive strengthening and cardiovascular training can be safe, tolerated and improve endurance without worsening symptoms and improve FM symptoms such as pain, fatigue, sleep, stiffness, anxiety and depression. Mannerkorpi and Daly (2003) report that low-intensity exercise such as walking can improve function and symptoms, but that caution is advised in high-intensity exercise initially as this can worsen some symptoms. Patients with POTS can report an initial worsening of symptoms in higher-intensity exercise, so have to be more gradually introduced into higher-intensity exercise; however, reconditioning is very important (Bravo et al. 2010). The psychological value of exercise is also crucial in the FM and complex patient group (EDSIII) as well as an improved feeling of wellbeing (Rooks 2008; Simmonds 2010). This particular patient group needs special encouragement with exercise and the importance of continuing with some daily exercise for maintenance. Research by Ang et al. (ND) suggests the value of 'telephone delivered motivational interviewing' to improve compliance. Research by Jentoft, Kvalvik and Mengshoel (2001) suggests that in participants (n=18 for pool exercise and n=16 for land exercise) there was an increase in the number of days that the pool exercise group participants felt good. There were significant improvements in cardiovascular fitness in both groups, although the pool group also improved some physical symptoms. Finally, Rombaut et al. (2010) suggest that people with EDSIII need appropriate treatment and management in health care in order to return to exercise, so it might be concluded that it is essential this patient group is given the right package of care to ensure this happens. The literature is extremely clear that patients with EDSIII/FM will only improve if they are reconditioned (Rombaut et al. 2010; Simmonds 2010). I documented the following in my blog:

> My endurance and cardiovascular fitness are both improving. I managed to jog for 15 minutes with very minimal walking breaks. Not so long ago I was still only managing about 6 minutes, with 1.30 continuous jogging. This is much better. I had some left anterial leg pain, but it is only because I am still not going through my feet enough – also I prefer running on grass to concrete.
>
> Anyway, it is clear that what with now occasionally sleeping right through the night and having less POTS symptoms and improved cervical spinal function, this aspect of my treatment

is now giving me improved endurance and hopefully I won't experience less frequent fatigue. I had back pain today, but I coped with doing some stretches and the exercise has made it all feel much better. There are no short-cuts in managing hypermobility syndrome, but I am considerably better since my release of last week.

Blog, 17.12.2011

I further wrote:

There is no doubt that since I have started to do a much more regular programme of cardiovascular exercise that my pain levels have reduced, my endurance has really improved, I am much less fatigued and I sleep much better. My mood is also improved, and I notice it if I haven't done some exercise for a day or two in that I feel 'flatter' and more restless and agitated.

I am now able to run for the bus when I see it and feel much more 'bright-eyed and bushy tailed'. I feel I have a much better battery life than I did before and more agile. I get about much faster and more efficiently and I am excited by the speed of my own improvements, as per blog.

Blog, 5.1.2012

In the next chapter I bring the reader up to date with my progress. There are never any shortcuts with this condition, and as the patient at the beginning of the chapter says, and I agree, inactivity makes pain and symptoms worse.

CHAPTER 41

Isobel 'now' and thoracic spine

Where I have come from

I have come a very long way over the last four years. It has taken a colossal amount of time, money, energy and determination to achieve this. It has been a very self-centred, some might think self-indulgent, study of myself in order to rehabilitate my body. A moderate tear of my right gastrocnemious on February 2008 changed my life completely. That very week I applied to do an MSc in Dance Science so I could understand (amongst other things) why I was always getting injured. I passed my MSc in 2009. I started to have physiotherapy from April 2008 and expected to require a few sessions of physiotherapy to 'repair' my calf and then expected to be on my way again. Until my formal diagnosis of EDSIII came through in the summer of 2009, I could not really start to piece together everything that had been bodily wrong with me for over 30 years. It is not just fundamentally 'physically' what was wrong, but there has also been a huge psychological impact, and this has also had a colossal effect. As Montpetit suggests, I needed to find meaning behind my 'illness' (Montpetit 2012).

Years went by and I stopped exercising because of pain, I gradually did less and less work, I became depressed and gained 20kg. By 2006, I started to reverse some of this and then the real rehabilitation started in 2008. I have had to work to strengthen all core muscle groups (e.g. abdominals, gluteals, hamstrings, adductors) whilst completely re-learning new movement patterns from scratch and undoing existing and incorrect movement patterns. This has been risky and difficult, and caused other compensatory problems. For example, whilst regaining hip and deep abdominal control, I had lower back pain again and problems and pain with ITB tracking. Attempting to rehabilitate my cervical spine has had a resultant effect on temporomandibular joint

(TMJ) symptoms and worsened POTS symptoms, but these have all been a part of the process of healing and a rehabilitative journey.

Specialists required

Even now there are still elements that are not complete – bladder, bowel and TMJ still require further treatment and management. In addition, I have received treatment for bowel symptoms, including surgical intervention and biofeedback treatment, whilst endometriosis remains medically managed. I have had psychological treatments such as cognitive analytical therapy and also medical treatment for mood swings and psychotherapy. Very recently I started to consider just how many specialists have been required to manage my case. This is a list of specialists I have seen since 2008:

- 2 rheumatologists
- 2 physiotherapists
- 1 psychologist
- 2 podiatrists
- 1 psychiatrist
- 1 cognitive analytical therapist
- 1 counsellor
- 2 gynaecologists
- 1 urologist
- 1 gastroenterologist
- 1 colorectal surgeon
- 3 neurosurgeons: 1 for migraines, 1 for POTS and 1 for movement disorders
- 1 orthodontist
- 1 maxillofacial/oral surgeon
- 1 Bowen therapist
- pain management team (2006)
- 4 visits to A&E.

In addition, I have not mentioned that I wear glasses (I am myopic, which is part of the Brighton Diagnostic Criteria for EDSIII/HMS – see Appendix 1) and that I also needed an echocardiogram done of my heart/aorta to rule out the more serious form of EDS (type IV) and any heart/vascular problems based upon my family medical history. This is an incredible amount of NHS resources – apart from the physiotherapy, orthodontics and Bowen, which have been privately funded. If one looks at the list it becomes clear how truly multisystemic EDSIII is and how many bodily systems are affected. There is a huge team of specialists required, but the real problem comes with communicating between this huge team and how referrals are conducted, and how one avoids becoming completely lost in the system. Most of my treatments have been across three central London hospitals, one predominantly. I have had numerous medical appointments and then follow-up investigations, for example ongoing MRI scans, X-rays, blood tests, etc. Some of my treatments have involved surgery – for example, for bladder (2012) and bowel (2011), and gynaecological (prior to 2007). It is hard work and time-consuming coordinating all of these appointments around my working life and there came a time when I was so worried about work that I stopped attending my medical appointments. It all just became too much, so I then started deferring appointments, some of which would have been helpful much sooner had I not delayed. Sometimes when I felt unwell I would also defer appointments, once on the day of treatment itself. I have had to devote myself 'to myself' in order to get this done, so it is understandable that people might see this as a very self-centred project. Perhaps it was – but also had my treatment begun much earlier on in my life and the condition recognised when I was very young I would not have required half the treatments I have had to have now as an adult in my late thirties. This is where the medical profession could have taken more responsibility, and better training of some of the doctors, GPs and physiotherapists I saw in my youth could have helped identify the condition and stopped it in its tracks.

Patient responsibility

The patient themselves also has a responsibility for their own treatment management. Much of the rehabilitation for EDSIII is focused around rehabilitation of the musculoskeletal system, and there is no doubt that mine is now functioning in a much more 'normal' capacity, so I now only require minimal physiotherapy, but it was required four years of intensive physiotherapy to achieve this. Hardly any other patients are going to be this fortunate. What is provided is generally going to be woefully inadequate, which is why some patients are likely to be 'bounced' around the system and why so many deteriorate so severely, as I was on my way to doing prior to 2006, when I received pain management support which started my own recovery.

Economics

Cost was an issue. As well as finding a physiotherapist I could trust because of their experience in working with dancers, and therefore help me to realise my goals, the physio I chose was private because I couldn't (at that time) find an NHS physiotherapist. Because I had no idea that my case was incredibly complicated at the time of meeting my physio, I just thought I would only need to see her a few times anyway, based upon my previous experience of physiotherapy. Unfortunately cost was an issue, so this did limit the number of sessions that I had initially until six months into treatment when I purchased an excellent health cash-back plan which reimbursed 75 per cent of each treatment session. There is no doubt at all that economics have a substantial effect on treatment (Potter *et al.* 2003a). I have been extremely fortunate with an excellent health plan which has allowed me to be able to continue with long-term treatment. I am very aware I might not have had that opportunity, or necessarily the fortune.

Remaining treatment required

I still have a lot of trouble with sleep and ongoing fatigues. There are still some problems with my ANS, which mainly relates to bladder, with some minor POTS episodes. TMJ requires ongoing treatment and management and my thoracic spine requires further rehabilitation. There are still some remaining problems with homeostasis (temperature, HR/BP changes – POTS), and Maslow's most basic physiological needs are still, at times, unmet – including sleep and excretion. Bowel still quite possibly requires further treatment for IBS and excretion. The rest I am now managing myself – for example, exercise, which is very much a part of the management of EDSIII. Come rain or shine, whether in pain or not, I have to take the responsibility to ensure I continue my exercise regime and to continue to work on my cardiovascular endurance. It is known that EDSIII patients lose muscle more quickly and fatigue more quickly (Simmonds and Keer 2008). This is why exercise will remains so vital.

However, I am much fitter in my late thirties than at any other point in my life. This is an amazing legacy for overall good health to take forward into future decades of my life. I should have a better and healthier quality of life and I intend to keep my weight normal whilst having a very much fitter and toned body. The exercise, including my beloved ballet, of course all feeds into an improved psychological state, releases endorphins, helps with relaxation and is fun. It also helps to reduce stress and anxiety and minimise depression.

Pain

In terms of pain – my pain will never be cured. I have chronic pain and a hypersensitised nervous system. The pain will not entirely go away, but it can be managed. I have a range of strategies including medications, treatments, exercise and other pain management strategies (e.g. hot baths, films, relaxation) which I can draw upon when the need arises (see Appendix 2). I have finally accepted my pain, but understanding it has been crucial to accepting it. The hardest thing is how invisible it is and what makes it so difficult for others to appreciate or comprehend. The best way I learned to accept and manage my pain was through education. Primarily this took place during the pain management programme I attended in 2006, documented in Knight (2011). Once I understood that pain didn't always equal damage (Knight 2011) I was well on my way. Additional conversations during physiotherapy have been invaluable in supporting my learning and understanding of a very difficult conceptual topic.

Life quality: exercise and physiotherapeutically

My life quality is now better than it was four years ago. I can manage much more and I am considerably fitter and better conditioned. My lower limbs are now very well conditioned and functioning normally. I am now doing exercises to stretch my ankles and Achilles tendons which are areas of tightness in my otherwise mobile body. After four years I have managed to conquer my fear of calf palpation and allowed my physio to work on them – several times. I have only recently discovered that in fact many EDS patients experience cramps in the leg muscles, which is worst at night and often resolves in adulthood. Beighton *et al.* (2012) write that 'the cause is as yet unknown, but it is thought to relate to overstretching of the muscles which is permitted by an abnormal range of movements at the lax joints... Limb pain is a major reason for referral to Hypermobility Clinics' (p.162). I was delighted to come across this as it finally validated my years of calf cramps as an adolescent. My calf musculature has also changed over time – left calf has decreased from 43cm (2008) to 40cm (2012). My right calf has also decreased, from 39cm (2008) to 38cm (2012), although my physio and I would like to increase the right calf to 39cm so that there is only a very acceptable difference of 1cm between each limb.

My hips have much greater control, meaning that I can sufficiently control parallel alignment as well as the lateral control required for classical ballet. I am still better at the latter. My lumbar spine is better and generally much less painful. I have strength to support my hinge and vastly improved deep abdominal musculature. My cervical spine is in a much better state and I am only occasionally symptomatic. TMJ still requires some further rehabilitation but is improving.

Thoracic spine

The most recent physical improvement related to thoracic spine. I am, for the first time, getting sensation in my thoracic spine, which has been stiffened and blocked for ages. This will mean that I can now strengthen the area, which will take pressure off my trapezius muscles which are so overworked and will also help with cervical spine and TMJ. My arms had experienced symptoms – coldness, tingling and hand pain – but I think that these will also improve as thoracic spine is strengthened and mobilised. I can see the end – or what that might look like. I recently blogged:

> Amongst the revelations of improved strength and control I noticed a new sensation in and around about T8 where I had feeling in that section of my spine for the first time, giving me extension at that level, but also greater functional support in that level for my arms. Actually the area felt sore – but I see that as an encouraging awakening of a new area of my body which will finally relieve pressure from C-spine and particularly traps.
>
> *Blog, 23.7.2012*

I am still very passionate about my ballet classes. I do ballet from home at least three times a week, and attend classes on average of two times a week (if not dancing from home). I consider my hypermobility a real asset in terms of ballet, and it is because of my hypermobility I am so able to dance. In terms of other exercise I go for a walk and run about two to three times per week – this involves a period of approximately 10–20 minutes running. I do physiotherapy exercises as and when required, depending upon what needs more work. I also do the Feldenkrais Method® and Pilates from time to time. Occasionally I go swimming, but my next challenge requires learning to swim (properly) again. When I am on holiday or out of London I might also cycle. I now have aspirations to try other sports again such as tennis, badminton and netball. It is now clear to me I couldn't play tennis as a child/adolescent because I couldn't even mange to hold the racket – equipment is definitely something schools and PE teachers need to consider with hypermobile children. I remembered playing badminton for a week (happened twice) but suffered appalling overuse. I was previously good at netball and a good 'goal shooter'. I see no reason why I cannot return to trying these sports again. I think that there is every chance I might be better at them now that I am so much better rehabilitated. All movement patterns have had to be re-learned over time and this has taken considerable energy and brain power, but my movement patterns are considerably more efficient than they were and I can now work my deep core muscles more effectively, thus resting the more superficial ones. Although I still get fatigues, these are generally becoming shorter and my endurance has improved over time. I am hopeful that this will continue to improve as I work at my cardiovascular fitness.

I do still suffer from severe muscle stiffness and, although exercise and stretching do help, I do require ongoing manual therapy to help with this, including both Bowen and physiotherapy. However, I now consider myself in the final stage of my rehabilitation and that treatment is now about maintenance and management. I blog that:

> I am feeling really positive at this stage in the treatment and can now see some kind of end stage when all remaining faulty patterns have been removed and final areas of rehabilitation (including TMJ) take place. Then I will just need physio for maintenance only. I am continuing with all cardiorespiratory work, carefully pacing up activity. I have come a very long way in my musculoskeletal rehabilitation over the past 4 years.

Blog, 30.7.2012

I have been very lucky in the quality of physiotherapy that I have had from both physios.

Life quality: psychological/behavioural – ongoing!

It is apparent to both my physiotherapist and I that some of my behaviour is continuing to fuel some of my physical symptoms. I seem to continue in an entrenched pattern of working in an adrenalin-fuelled capacity and then wonder why I experience catastrophic (albeit briefer) fatigues. Until I improve my goal-setting and pacing, I will impede my remaining physical and physiological progress. It might be that there are still unresolved traumas, and another birth-related trauma as this book was going to press suggests that I may be held in a 'freeze' trauma pattern that is perpetuating my behaviour. As these traumas are released and I can drop my guard and reduce my hypervigilance (see Chapter 37), it might be that we can start to change my overreaching, perfectionist, adrenalin-fuelled behaviour. This will be what we start to tap into during physio as well as continuing to even out my bilateral differences, strengthening and softening the left side, and allowing it to follow the nicer, more relaxed feeling that there is in the right side of my body. As this book goes to press I have chosen to temporarily stop physiotherapy whilst I reflect on some things and perhaps try other healing modalities. I am still a work in progress!

Life quality: work and social

My physiological and musculoskeletal rehabilitation have also affected and improved my psychological health and wellbeing. Although I still suffer from a tendency towards depression, I am more moderated than I was and less bodily preoccupied, because my body is now behaving better. I can understand it now and how to manage it (mostly).

In the past few years I have managed a full and varied life. I did my MSc and then worked as a Bowen therapist (ongoing) and started writing. I had my first book *Skin Collection* (poetry) published in 2009 and *A Guide to Living with Hypermobility Syndrome: Bending without Breaking* in 2011. I have plans to write a new book in 2013, on a new topic area. I am writing in journals and have now started lecturing on EDSIII. I have started to teach adult ballet classes. My life is interesting, active and varied. I have met many new people, especially as a result of the 2011 hypermobility book, which has proved to be unexpectedly successful. I would like to continue working within the EDSIII community and continue writing and research into the condition.

My social life is busy and varied. I am more reliable than I was in the past and I am now able to manage more. A new goal for me is to improve my work–life balance and look to stepping up to the next rung of the Maslow Hierarchy of Needs and look at my 'belonging and love needs'. One reviewer of my 2011 book was very disappointed that I was not in a relationship and living happily ever after. Whilst I might continue to disappoint the same person, this is life, and not everything has a fairy tale ending! However, perhaps it is also worth pointing out that because I have had no dependants in my life, in part this journey *has* been possible. It would have been significantly harder if I had children and other dependants to manage as well. I am otherwise lucky that my immediate family are very supportive and I have a good network of close friends and enjoy many varied pastimes including balletic and musical ones. I have also found a wonderful writer's retreat called 'Retreats for You' (see Appendix 3) in North Devon which I have now visited several times. I not only hit all my writing targets, I am fed delicious food, enjoy the company of lovely people and manage to rest and go on lots of walks. It is the nearest I seem to manage to having a rest! I am looking forward to taking the concept of rest and relaxation into my future lifestyle.

The future

The future looks full of optimism. My life quality is now infinitely better. I am heading up the Maslow Hierarchy of Needs (see Chapter 5). I still suffer flare-ups, but I am better at managing them and have the resources to do so (see Appendix 3). I have carved out an interesting career path and see writing, teaching and research work as my future career, whilst also continuing my work as a Bowen therapist. I am ambitious and determined in all that I do, and I look forward to continuing to extend my boundaries and to experience new things, meet new people and take on new challenges. I remain indebted to those who have helped me along the way and shown me a better quality of life, especially my physios, doctors and fellow patients. I remain dedicated to the pursuit of supporting other EDSIII and chronic complex patients to have an improved and better quality of life. I conclude with a blog quote that I am still pondering. I invite you to do the same.

> I wonder that if I conquer all my symptoms whether I just lose the status of EDSIII to 'Hypermobile'. I wonder with all my chronic pain and symptomatic overlap whether this is

possible...? I will always have faulty connective tissues, but can they be fully managed and tamed???!!! Not 'Taming the Tiger' so much as 'Taming the Tissue'!

Blog, 1.1.2012

Postscript

Just as I had finished this chapter in the summer of 2012, I went running and encountered some medial left knee pain. It was frustrating. I tried walking where my knee seemed alright and then tried running again. Not possible. So it is back home to do some Bowen, rest and do some core stability exercises and to ask my left ITB to be less bossy, thank you very much. I had lunch, read in the sun (one of the few sunny days in 2012) and crashed with fatigue in bed. My left hip is also 'out to lunch' and so I picked up my management plan. I have some choices to make: sleep, painkillers, bath, film, book... The motto of the postscript – management of EDSIII is ongoing. I am not, however, going to let this ruin my day.

CHAPTER 42

Conclusion

I think for me one of the advantages of having assumed everyone was like me until well into adulthood is that I just feel normal. I've lived a lot in the dance world where hypermobility is the norm anyway, so I tend to have to adjust myself to students who aren't hypermobile. For me, it's they who are different!

Jess Glenny, moving body teacher, facilitator and therapist

I now feel more 'normal' and finally no longer feel quite so subsumed by my condition. Rather than being a patient with a condition I think I have now moved on to being a person or dancer who happens to have EDSIII. As this book comes to a close I hope that you will have appreciated the challenge of my personal journey, the complexity of this insidious condition and that the book will have increased your awareness for all the other EDSIII/FM, chronic patients who still urgently require medical treatment. I hope that you will value the honest psychological insights I have provided, both via my treatment sessions and in general, and that you gain a real sense of the scale of suffering I have endured at the hands of delayed diagnosis and the effects of a multisystemic condition which has become huge compared to the presentation of a moderate calf tear. I hope that some of my resources will prove to be useful, including possible treatment measure outcomes. I understand that these are basic – but these are examples of measuring in a case study capacity the effects of physiotherapy on my own symptoms over a six-month time period (see Chapter 33 and Appendix 3). Moreover, I hope that you understand how lonely and tiresome the patient journey becomes in such a chronic complex condition and this opens your heart as you continue to provide support to future patients. There are so many patients who badly require support, and more doctors and physiotherapists (and also teachers and schools) need to recognise this rare condition. Far more education is required. I am hoping that this book will successfully reach a target audience of medical professionals so that we can truly convince any remaining sceptics that EDSIII really is the new 'rheumatological disability' (Grahame, 2011 EDS Conference) and therefore really deserves to be treated with more respect. If the book helps in this plight for my fellow EDSIII and FM patients, then I am pleased, and all the work involved in my recovery and in writing this book has been entirely worthwhile. Having said that, I would still very much see my hypermobility as a natural asset in terms of dance and would therefore see that as a positive aspect of being hypermobile, and agree with Jess's quote – as an adolescent and even now, being hypermobile is an essential aspect of my person, body and identity.

In terms of alternative treatments to manage symptoms, I do hope that more doctors will consider complementary alternative medicine (CAM). Although there are remaining issues with evidence-based research (not helped if said CAM therapists cannot obtain funding to treat and conduct evidence-based research), it can be seen from my experience with Bowen therapy and Feldenkrais how significant that work was in terms of my recovery. Please keep an open mind in your views of CAM. Most CAM practitioners would dearly love to be involved in the treatment of such a complex group of patients – I certainly would, but at the moment could only do so as a volunteer unless funding became available, as has been the case in past times. However, we are in very challenging economic times, so this might have to be one of my personal goals for the future.

There are a few centres of excellence in the treatment of EDSIII, but this is so inadequate in terms of the needs of this very complex patient group. In addition there needs to be a real overall coordination of treatment when so many bodily systems and experts are required. I am truly fortunate in that I am very articulate and have managed to obtain the treatment I required by being assertive and also by becoming very friendly with the consultants' secretaries. This has been very useful on a number of occasions and has even saved at least two of my consultants from having to see me again in the flesh as we worked out my needs by email. I have had a battle to 'save myself' and to ultimately try to get someone to help me understand what was going on and so I could make a true autoethnographical study of myself and my condition. I really hope that now I have done this I can move away from the ego to support and fight for improved treatment courses and more holistic care for EDSIII patients. Somehow there needs to be much more improved coordination of care for this group of complex patients who otherwise get completely lost in the system (see rare diseases information in Chapter 1). The rheumatologist and GP can act in this way, but at times someone must take an overarching view of what is going on and communicate this to everyone involved so that they are all on the same page. I would not say that this has always happened in my care, and the whole process of treatment could have been more streamlined. For example, it would be so much better to have several hospital appointments on the same day to save (already fatigued) patients from having to attend on so many separate occasions, before even factoring in that some patients are also still trying to hold down jobs.

The hypermobility centres of expertise – for example, the Glasgow Infirmary, the Royal National Orthopaedic Hospital, University College Hospital and the (private) Hospital of St John and St Elizabeth – have experts who focus on rehabilitation in pain management, physiotherapy and psychology. The doctors involved then refer on (as need be) to other specialists, and we are lucky that finally more doctors are beginning to be interested – for example, Professor Aziz, who is interested in EDSIII and gastrointestinal disorders. However, even stays at hospitals or centres where there is a much greater understanding of the condition can only do so much – and there frequently seem to be so many experts involved and then it all takes a long time – that ultimately we are looking at best possible management.

I want to continue working and supporting EDSIII and other patients with chronic complex conditions such as FM/chronic pain. I would like to keep writing and lecturing. I am so completely passionate about what I do because of the profundity of my health complaints and how totally they have affected me. Autoethnographical writing might be considered self-indulgent by some, but I do hope that it has taken rather less self-indulgence than courage at attempting my complicated story so that others hopefully benefit in the future. Other patient examples have been given as much as possible so that I have culturally represented this hidden and marginalised patient group. I want to keep researching and supporting organisations such as the HMSA and EDS-UK so that the patients of tomorrow have a better future ahead of them. There is still much research to do into this condition and I hope that it becomes a deserving medical funding priority in the future.

I am beginning to realise where I want my life to go and that I have come off the fighting-line in physiological needs with my EDSIII and now moving up a notch to a newer and higher quality of life. I can see all sorts of doors opening and new opportunities coming my way. Life feels good and it is now starting to feel good to be me.

Blog, 19.8.2012

Diagnostic criteria

Five diagnostic questions:
Do you have hypermobility syndrome?

Here is a five-part questionnaire to identify hypermobility. If you answer yes to at least two of the five questions then there is an 80–90 per cent chance you are hypermobile.

1. Can you now (or could you ever) place your hands flat on the floor without bending your knees?

2. Can you now (or could you ever) bend your thumb back to touch your forearm?

3. As a child did you amuse your friends by contorting your body into strange shapes or could you do the splits?

4. As a child or teenager did your shoulder or knee cap dislocate on more than one occasion?

5. Do you consider yourself to be double-jointed?

Source: Professor Rodney Grahame and Dr Alan Hakim,
Department of Rheumatology, University College Hospitals, London

The Beighton Score

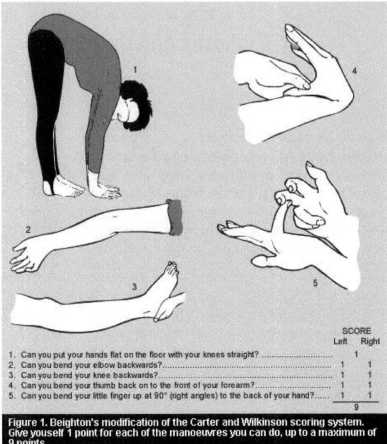

	SCORE	
	Left	Right
1. Can you put your hands flat on the floor with your knees straight?		1
2. Can you bend your elbow backwards?	1	1
3. Can you bend your knee backwards?	1	1
4. Can you bend your thumb back on to the front of your forearm?	1	1
5. Can you bend your little finger up at 90° (right angles) to the back of your hand?	1	1
		9

Figure 1. Beighton's modification of the Carter and Wilkinson scoring system. Give youself 1 point for each of the manoeuvres you can do, up to a maximum of 9 points.

Source: With kind permission from the Hypermobility Syndrome Association

Brighton Criteria
Revised diagnostic criteria for HMS
MAJOR CRITERIA

- A Beighton score of 4/9 or greater (either currently or historically).
- Arthralgia for longer than 3 months in 4 or more joints.

MINOR CRITERIA

- A Beighton score of 1, 2 or 3/9 (0, 1, 2 or 3 if aged 50+).

- Arthralgia (> 3 months) in one to three joints or back pain (> 3 months), spondylosis, spondylolysis/spondylolisthesis.

- Dislocation/subluxation in more than one joint, or in one joint on more than one occasion.

- Soft tissue rheumatism: > 3 lesions (e.g. epicondylitis, tenosynovitis, bursitis).

- Marfanoid habitus (tall, slim, span/height ratio > 1.03, upper/lower segment ratio less than 0.89, arachnodactily [positive Steinberg/wrist signs].

- Abnormal skin: striae, hyperextensibility, thin skin, papyraceous scarring.

- Eye signs: drooping eyelids or myopia or antimongoloid slant.

- Varicose veins or hernia or uterine/rectal prolapse.

HMS is diagnosed in the presence of two major criteria, or one major and two minor criteria, or four minor criteria. Two minor criteria will suffice where there is an unequivocally affected first-degree relative.

Produced with written permission from the
Hypermobility Syndrome Association

TABLE A1: Types of EDS			
Type	**Clinical features**	**Inheritance**	**Basic defect**
Classical (formerly EDS I and II gravis and mitis type)	Major: Skin hyperextensibility; widened thin scars; joint hypermobility. Minor: Smooth velvety skin; molluscoid pseudotumours; complications of loose joints; muscle hypotonia; easy bruising; manifestations of tissue extensibility (hernia, cervical insufficiency, etc.); positive family history.	Autosomal dominant	Abnormality of the pro alpha 1 (V) or pro alpha 2 (V) chain of the type V collagen encoded by COL5A1 and COL5A2 genes (in some but not all families).
Hypermobility (formerly EDS III hypermobile type)	Major: Generalised joint hypermobility; skin hyperextensibility and smooth or velvety. Minor: Recurrent joint dislocations; chronic limb and joint pains; positive family history.	Autosomal dominant	Unknown.
Vascular (formerly EDS IV arterial or ecchymotic type)	Major: Arterial/intestinal/uterine fragility or rupture; easy bruising; characteristic facial appearance. Minor: Hypermobility of small joints; tendon and muscle rupture; club feet; varicose veins; positive family history; sudden death in close relative.	Autosomal dominant	Structural defects in the proa 1 (III) chain of collagen type III, encoded by the COL3A1 gene.

Kyphoscoliosis (formerly EDS VI ocular or scoliosis type)	Major: Generalised joint laxity; severe muscle hypotonia in infancy; scoliosis present at birth and progressive; fragility of the sclera of the eye. Minor: Tissue fragility; easy bruising; arterial rupture; Marfanoid body shape; microcomea; skeletal osteopenia on X-ray; positive family history of affected siblings.	Autosomal recessive	Deficiency of lysyl hydroxylase, a collagen modifying enzyme.
Arthrochalasia (formerly included in EDS VII)	Major: Severe generalised joint hypermobility with dislocations; congenital bilateral hip dislocation. Minor: Skin hyperextensibility; tissue fragility and scarring: easy bruising; muscle hypotonia; kyphoscoliosis; skeletal osteopenia on X-ray; positive family history.	Autosomal dominant	Deficiencies of the proa(I) or proa 2(I) chains of collagen type due to skipping of exon 6 in the COL1A1 or COL1A2 gene.
Dermatospraxis (formerly included in EDS VII)	Major: Severe skin fragility; sagging, redundant skin. Minor: Soft, doughy skin texture, easy bruising; premature rupture of foetal membranes; hernias.	Autosomal dominant	Deficiency of procollagen 1 N-terminal peptidase in collagen.

*Source: www.ehlers–danlos.org/index.php?option=com_*
content&task=view&id=4&Itemid=5. With kind permission of EDS-UK
(consent obtained).

Sample forms

Physiotherapy/other medical practitioner: sample patient contract

I, _____, will try to:

- self-manage standard symptoms and pain using the appropriate resources (including medication) in between physiotherapy sessions
- avoid unnecessarily texting and emailing my physio unless there is an out-of-context emergency or acute incident resulting in a new or different trauma (e.g. ending up in hospital)
- respect my physio's right to privacy and time out from my case including vacations/weekends when he/she is otherwise unavailable to me
- in an emergency, seek advice from other medical professionals/present to A&E, as appropriate, within the context of the situation
- negotiate with my physio the type of psychological/emotional support that he/she is comfortably and clinically able to offer me at an appropriate time to her/him
- look at my other resource banks/alternative support bases to avoid unnecessarily fatiguing my physio but not seek other physiotherapy unless my physio is away and I am in crisis.

I, Physio, will try to:

- avoid introducing my patient to particularly new/risky movement patterns that are likely to incur flare-ups or acute symptoms when either she or I are going to be unavailable for support (e.g. vacation times)

- support my patient as I continue to challenge psychological and physical patterns that are likely to be either raw for her, or new movement patterns that are likely to cause temporary chaos

- support my patient towards greater independence of self-management (in line with what my patient is going to try to do) and avoid feeling guilty if my patient ends up in pain or crisis when I am unavailable to her

- tell my patient when it is not appropriate for her to contact me (e.g. vacation) and to remind her about email overload, if required again, and reset boundaries.

Signed _____ (Patient)   Date _____

Signed _____ (Physiotherapist) Date _____

HMS physiotherapy subjective

A. Patient DOB: _____

Acute summary	Musculoskeletal	Sleep/fatigue
POTS/asthma	Psychology	Pain
Exercise	Bladder	Digestive
Gynaecology	Psychology	Support

EDSIII physiotherapy subjective graph

Date: _____

A. Patient DOB: _____

Scale measurement

0 = no pain, no symptoms; 10 = severe symptoms and pain; NA = not available

Comment:

Spasm	0	1	2	3	4	5	6	7	8	9	10	N/A
Neck pain	0	1	2	3	4	5	6	7	8	9	10	N/A
Headaches	0	1	2	3	4	5	6	7	8	9	10	N/A
Neurological	0	1	2	3	4	5	6	7	8	9	10	N/A
Thoracic spine	0	1	2	3	4	5	6	7	8	9	10	N/A
Lumbar spine	0	1	2	3	4	5	6	7	8	9	10	N/A
Hip/groin	0	1	2	3	4	5	6	7	8	9	10	N/A
Knee(s)	0	1	2	3	4	5	6	7	8	9	10	N/A
Sleep	0	1	2	3	4	5	6	7	8	9	10	N/A
Fatigue	0	1	2	3	4	5	6	7	8	9	10	N/A
Bladder	0	1	2	3	4	5	6	7	8	9	10	N/A
Asthma	0	1	2	3	4	5	6	7	8	9	10	N/A
POTS	0	1	2	3	4	5	6	7	8	9	10	N/A
IBS	0	1	2	3	4	5	6	7	8	9	10	N/A
Gynae/endo	0	1	2	3	4	5	6	7	8	9	10	N/A
Sport	0	1	2	3	4	5	6	7	8	9	10	N/A
Mood	0	1	2	3	4	5	6	7	8	9	10	N/A
Psychology/other	0	1	2	3	4	5	6	7	8	9	10	N/A
_____	0	1	2	3	4	5	6	7	8	9	10	N/A
_____	0	1	2	3	4	5	6	7	8	9	10	N/A

Physiotherapy update: confidential physio 'SWOT' analysis

Strengths	Weaknesses
Opportunities	Threats

Goal-setting

Write down today's date and goals that you would like to achieve in the next six months. Do not worry about how you will achieve the goals.

Name _____ Date _____

Why did you write what you wrote?

What was special about the goals you chose?

What will your action plan be?

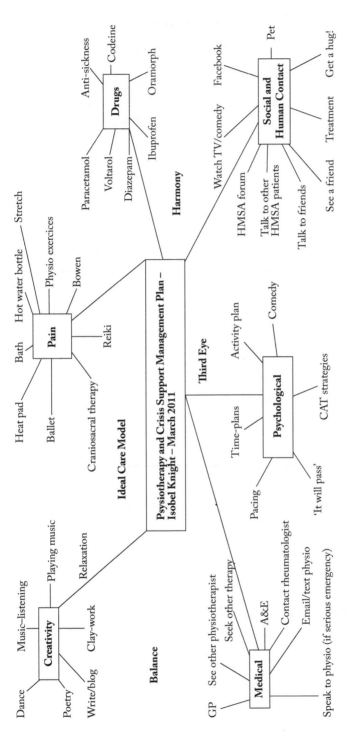

Physiotherapy and Crisis Support Management Plan –
Isobel Knight – March 2011

Ideal Care Model

Pain
- Heat pad
- Bath
- Hot water bottle — Stretch
- Physio exercices
- Bowen
- Ballet
- Reiki
- Craniosacral therapy

Drugs
- Paracetamol
- Anti-sickness
- Codeine
- Oramorph
- Ibuprofen
- Voltarol
- Diazepam

Harmony

Social and Human Contact
- Watch TV/comedy
- Facebook
- Pet
- HMSA forum
- Talk to other HMSA patients
- Talk to friends
- See a friend
- Treatment
- Get a hug!

Creativity
- Dance
- Music–listening
- Playing music
- Poetry
- Relaxation
- Write/blog
- Clay-work

Balance

Third Eye

Psychological
- Activity plan
- Comedy
- Time-plans
- Pacing
- CAT strategies
- 'It will pass'

Medical
- GP
- See other physiotherapist
- Seek other therapy
- A&E
- Contact rheumatologist
- Email/text physio
- Speak to physio (if serious emergency)

* agreement with physio about when this is appropriate. If physio is away, then seeing other therapies, A&E, as required.
Demand protection! – if depressed/other psychological emergency – Samaritan, A&E, friends!!!

Useful contacts

CONTACTING THE AUTHOR
Isobel Knight
Email: bowtherapy@gmail.com
www.bowenworks.org
http://danceinjuryrecovery.blogspot.co.uk
https://twitter.com/IsobelKnight2
http://uk.linkedin.com/pub/isobel-knight/38/3a7/a6b

EDSIII CENTRES OF EXPERTISE FOR TREATMENT
Glasgow
Professor William Ferrell
Centre for Rheumatic Diseases
Glasgow Royal Infirmary
Glasgow G31 2ER

Royal National Orthopaedic Hospital (RNOH)
Royal National Orthopaedic Hospital NHS Trust
Stanmore
Middlesex HA7 4LP
Tel: 0208 909 5521

University College Hospital (for adults)
Professor Rodney Grahame/Dr Hana Kazkaz
The Hypermobility Clinic
Department of Rheumatology
University College Hospital
3rd Floor
250 Euston Road
London NW1 2BU

Also useful:
Hospital of St John and St Elizabeth (private hospital with hypermobility rehab clinic; Rosemary Keer and Dr Jane Simmonds practise here)
60 Grove End Road
St John's Wood
London NW8 9NH
Tel: 020 7806 4000
Email: info@hje.org.uk

BOWEN TECHNIQUE
The Bowen Association
PO Box 210
Boston PE21 1DD
Tel: 01205 319100
0700 BOWTECH (0700 269 8324) (national rates apply)
Email: office@bowen-technique.co.uk

Bowtech Pty Ltd (Bowen therapy)
PO Box 733
Hamilton,
Victoria, 3300
Australia
Tel: +61 (0) 3 5572 3000
Fax: +61 (0) 3 5572 3144
Email: bowtech@h140.aone.net.au

BOWEN THERAPISTS
Isobel Knight (London)
Email: bowtherapy@gmail.com
www.bowenworks.org

John Wilks (also Bowen instructor)
Email: cyma@btinternet.com
www.cyma.org.uk

COUNSELLING AND PSYCHOTHERAPY
British Association for Counselling and Psychotherapy
BACP House,
15 St John's Business Park,
Lutterworth,
Leicestershire LE17 4HB
Tel: 01455 883300 (general enquiries)
Email: bacp@bacp.co.uk
www.bacp.co.uk

EHLERS-DANLOS
Ehlers-Danlos Support Group (UK)
PO Box 748
Borehamwood WD6 9HU
Tel: 020 8736 5604
www.ehlers-danlos.org

ENDOMETRIOSIS
Endometriosis UK (registered charity number 1035810)
Provides support and information to women with endometriosis.
Suites 1&2
46 Manchester Street
London, W1U 7LS
Tel (free helpline): 0808 808 2227
www.endometriosis-uk.org

FELDENKRAIS
Feldenkrais Guild
The Guild does not maintain a central postal address; but if you require a postal address, please write to:
Scott Clark
13 Camellia House,
Idonia Street
London SE8 4LZ
Tel: 07000 785 506
Email: enq@feldenkrais.co.uk
www.feldenkrais.co.uk

Feldenkrais teacher
Maggy Burrowes (London-based)
Email: info@vocaldynamix.com
www.vocaldynamix.com/index.html

HYPERMOBILITY SYNDROME
Hypermobility Syndrome Association (HMSA)
49 Orchard Crescent
Oreston
Plymouth PL9 7NF
Tel: 0845 345 4465
www.hypermobility.org

OCCUPATIONAL HEALTH
College of Occupational Therapists
106–114 Borough High Street
Southwark
London SE1 1LB
Tel: 020 7357 6480
www.cot.co.uk/homepage

PHYSIOTHERAPISTS
Rosemary Keer
Central London Physiotherapy Clinic
106 Harley Street
London W1G 7JE
(See also Hospital of St John and St Elizabeth)

PHYSIOTHERAPY
Chartered Society of Physiotherapy
14 Bedford Row
London WC1R 4ED
Tel: 020 7306 6666
www.csp.org.uk

PILATES
Pilates Foundation
Pilates Foundation Administrator
PO Box 58235
London N1 5UY
Tel: 020 7033 0078
www.pilatesfoundation.com/newsite2/index.php

Pilates teacher trainer/Pilates teacher:
Jessica Moolenaar
jessica@mindfulpilates.co.uk
www.mindfulpilates.co.uk

PSYCHOLOGY
The British Psychological Society
St Andrews House
48 Princess Road East
Leicester LE1 7DR
Tel: 0116 254 9568
Email: enquiries@bps.org.uk

SPEECH AND LANGUAGE THERAPY
Royal College of Speech and Language Therapists
2 White Hart Yard
London SE1 1NX
Tel: 020 7378 1200
www.rcslt.org

WEBSITE RESOURCES ON THE TOPIC OF BIRTH
www.wonderfulbirth.com
www.fatherstobe.org
www.violence.de
www.conscious-embodiment.co.uk
www.beba.org
www.wombecology.com
www.birthworks.org/site/primal-health-research.html
www.birthinternational.com
www.cyma.org.uk
www.birthpsychology.com

WRITER'S RETREATS (WONDERFUL PLACE TO WRITE OR REST)
Retreats for you
The Court
Sheepwash
Beaworthy
Devon EX21 5NE
Tel: 01409 231252
www.retreatsforyou.co.uk

References

Adams, N. (1997) *The Psychophysiology of Low Back Pain*. Edinburgh: Churchill Livingstone.

Alexandre, N. M., Nordin, M., Hiebert, R. and Campello, M. (2002) 'Predictors of compliance with short-term treatment among patients with back pain.' *Revista Panamericana de Salud Pública 12*, 2, 86–94.

Ang, D., Kesavulu, R., Lydon, J., Lane, K. and Bigatti, S. (ND) 'Exercise-based motivational interviewing for female patients with fibromyalgia: a case series.' *Clinical Rheumatology 26*, 11, 1843–1849.

Azpiroz, F., Dapoigny, M., Pace, F., Muller-Lissner, S. *et al.* (2000) 'Nongastrointestinal disorders in the irritable bowel syndrome.' *Digestion 62*, 1, 66–72.

Baker, S. M., Marshak, H. H., Rice, G. T. and Zimmerman, G. J. (2001) 'Patient participation in physical therapy goal setting.' *Physical Therapy 81*, 5, 1118–1126.

Ballweg, M. L. (2003) *Endometriosis: The Complete Reference for Taking Charge of your Health*. Chicago: McGraw-Hill.

Banks, S. and Kerns, R. (1996) 'Explaining high rates of depression in chronic pain.' *Psychological Bulletin 119*, 1, 95–110.

Baptistella Ferão, M. and Traebert, J. (2008) 'Prevalence of temporomandibular dysfunction in patients with cervical pain under physiotherapy treatment.' *Fisioter Movement 21*, 4, 63–70.

Bartley, J. (2011) 'Breathing and temporomandibular joint disease.' *Journal of Bodywork and Movement Therapies 15*, 291–297.

Bassett, S. and Petrie, K. (1999) 'The effect of treatment goals on patient compliance with physiotherapy exercise programmes.' *Physiotherapy 85*, 3, 130–137.

Becker, R. (1985) *The Body Electric*. New York: Morrow.

Beighton, P., Grahame, R. and Bird, H. (2012) *Hypermobility of Joints* (4th edn). Berlin: Springer.

Bembry, J. and Ericson, C. (1999) 'Therapeutic termination with the early adolescent who has experienced multiple losses.' *Child and Adolescent Social Work Journal 16*, 3, 177–189.

Bennett, R. (2002) 'Growth hormone in musculoskeletal pain states.' *Current Rheumatology Reports 6*, 266–273.

Bennum, I. (1988) 'Systems Theory and Family Therapy.' In E. Street and W. Dryden (eds) *Family Therapy in Britain*. Milton Keynes: Open University Press.

Berne, K. (2002) *Chronic Fatigue Syndrome, Fibromyalgia and Other Invisible Illnesses: The Comprehensive Guide*. Alameda, CA: Hunter House Publishers.

Bird, H. (2004) 'Rheumatological aspects of dance.' *Rheumatology 31*, 1, 12–13.

Bird. H. (2007) 'Joint hypermobility.' *Musculoskeletal Care 5*, 1, 4–19.

Bohora, S. (2010) 'Joint hypermobility syndrome and dysautonomia: expanding spectrum of disease presentation and manifestation.' *Indian Pacing Electrophysiology Journal 10*, 4, 158–161.

Boudreau, S., Farina, D. and Falla, D. (2010) 'The role of motor learning and neuroplasticity in designing rehabilitation approaches for musculoskeletal pain disorders.' *Manual Therapy 15*, 5, 410–414.

Boudreau, S., Romaniello, A., Wang, K., Svensson, P., Sessle, B. J. and Arendt-Nielsen, L. (2007) 'The effects of intra-oral pain on motor cortex neuroplasticity associated with short-term novel tongue-protrusion training in humans. *Pain 132*, 1–2, 169–178.

Bravo, J., Sanhueza, G. and Hakim, A. (2010) 'Neuromuscular Physiology in Joint Hypermobility'. In A. Hakim, R. Keer and R. Grahame (eds) *Hypermobility, Fibromyalgia and Chronic Pain*. Edinburgh: Churchill Livingstone.

Brawner, C., Keteyian, S. and Saval, M. (2010) 'Adaptations to Cardiorespiratory Exercise Training.' In American College of Sports Medicine (ed.) *ACSM's Resource Manual for Guidelines for Exercise Testing and Prescription* (6th edn). London: Lippincott Williams and Wilkins.

Bryden, L. (2010) 'The Cervical Spine and Jaw: Temporomandibular Joint – Physiotherapy Management.' In A. Hakim, R. Keer and R. Grahame (eds) *Hypermobility, Fibromyalgia and Chronic Pain.* Edinburgh: Churchill Livingstone.

Bulbena, A., Aguillo, A., Pailhez, G., Martin-Santos, R. *et al.* (2004) 'Is joint hypermobility related to anxiety in a non-clinical population also?' *Psychosomatics 45,* 5, 432–437.

Bulbena, A., Gago, J., Pailhez, G., Sperry, L., Fullana, M. A. and Vilarroya, O. (2011) 'Joint hypermobility syndrome is a risk factor trait for anxiety disorders: a 15-year follow-up cohort study.' *General Hospital Psychiatry 33,* 362–370.

Campbell-McBride, N. (2010) *Gut and Psychology Syndrome.* Cambridge: Medinform Publishing.

Cardozo, L. (2011) 'Systematic review of overactive bladder therapy in females.' *Canadian Urological Association Journal,* October 5, 5 Suppl. 2: S139–S142.

Carter, C. S. (2003) 'Developmental consequences of oxytocin.' *Physiology and Behavior 79,* 383–397.

Chamberlain, D. (1998) *The Life of your Newborn Baby.* Berkeley, CA: North Atlantic Books.

Chang, H. (2008) *Autoethnography as Method.* Walnut Creek, CA: Left Coast Press.

Child, A. H. (1986) 'Joint hypermobility syndrome: inherited disorder of collagen synthesis.' *Journal of Rheumatology 13,* 239–243.

Cooper, K., Smith, B. H. and Hancock, E. (2008) 'Patient-centredness in physiotherapy from the perspective of the chronic back pain patient.' *Physiotherapy 94,* 244–252.

Coppack, R. J., Kristensen, J. and Karageorghis, C. I. (2012) 'Use of a goal setting intervention to increase adherence to low back pain rehabilitation: a randomized controlled trial.' *Clinical Rehabilitation 26,* 11, 962–3.

Cuccia, A. and Caradonna, C. (2009) 'The relationship between the stomatognathic system and body posture.' *Clinics* (São Paulo) *64,* 1, 61–66.

Damasio, A. (2000) *The Feeling of What Happens: Body, Emotion, and the Making of Consciousness.* London: Vintage Books.

Daniel, C. (2010) 'Pain Management and Cognitive Behavioural Therapy.' In A. Hakim, R. Keer and R. Grahame (eds) *Hypermobility, Fibromyalgia and Chronic Pain.* Edinburgh: Churchill Livingstone.

Davenport, H. S. (2012) 'Principles of Functional Rehabilitation' (lecture notes). University of Hertfordshire, Hatfield, UK.

Denman, C. (2001) 'Cognitive analytical therapy.' *Advances in Psychiatric Treatment 7,* 243–256.

Dietz, V., A. Gollhofer, M. Kleiber and M. Trippel (1992) 'Regulation of bipedal stance.' *Experimental Brain Research 89,* 1, 229–231.

Eccles, J., Beacher, F., Gray, M., Jones, C. *et al.* (2012) 'Brain structure and joint hypermobility: relevance to the expression of psychiatric symptoms.' *British Journal of Psychiatry 200,* 508–509.

Ercolani, M., Galvani, M., Franchini, C., Baracchini, F. and Chattat, R. (2008) 'Benign joint hypermobility syndrome: psychological features and psychopathological symptoms in a sample pain-free at evaluation.' *Perceptual and Motor Skills 107,* 246–256.

Falla, D., Jull, G. and Hodges, P. (2004) 'Feed forward activity of the cervical flexor muscles during voluntary arm movements is delayed in chronic neck pain.' *Experimental Brain Research 157,* 1, 43–48.

Falla, D. L., Jull, G., Russell, T., Vicenzino, B. and Hodges, P. (2007) 'Effect of neck exercise on sitting posture in patients with chronic neck pain.' *Physical Therapy 87,* 408–417.

Farmer, A. and Aziz, Q. (2010) 'Bowel Dysfunction in Joint Hypermobility Syndrome and Fibromyalgia.' In A. Hakim, R. Keer and R. Grahame (eds) *Hypermobility, Fibromyalgia and Chronic Pain.* Edinburgh: Churchill Livingstone.

Fass, R., Fullerton, S., Tung, S. and Mayer, E. (2000) 'Sleep disturbances in clinic patients with functional bowel disorders.' *The American Journal of Gastroenterology 95,* 5, 1196–2000.

Ferrell, W. and Ferrell, P. (2010) 'Proprioceptive Dysfunction in JHS and its Management.' In A. Hakim, R. Keer and R. Grahame (eds) *Hypermobility, Fibromyalgia and Chronic Pain.* Edinburgh: Churchill Livingstone.

Ferrell, W., Tennant, N., Baxendale, R., Kusel, M. and Sturrock, R. (2007) 'Muscular reflex function in the joint hypermobility syndrome.' *Arthritis Care and Research 57,* 7, 1329–1333.

Ferrell, W., Tennant, N., Sturrock, R. D., Ashton, L. *et al.* (2004) 'Amelioration of symptoms by enhancement of proprioception in patients with joint hypermobility syndrome.' *Arthritis and Rheumatology 50*, 3323–3328.

Fishbain, D., Cutler, R., Rosomoff, H. and Rosomoff, R. (1997) 'Chronic pain-associated depression: antecedent or consequence of chronic pain? A review.' *Clinical Journal of Pain 13*, 2, 116–137.

Fisher, K. and Hardie, R. J. (2002) 'Goal attainment scaling in evaluating a multidisciplinary pain management programme.' *Clinical Rehabilitation 16*, 871–877.

Fitt, S. (1996) *Dance Kinesiology* (2nd edn). New York: Schirmer.

Flanagan, M. (2010) *The Downside of Upright Posture*. Minneapolis: Two Harbors Press.

Flor, H., Kerns, R. D. and Turk, D. C. (1987) 'The role of spouse reinforcement, perceived pain, and activity levels of chronic pain patients.' *Journal of Psychosomatic Research 31*, 251–259.

Follonier Castella, L., Buscemi, L., Godbout, C., Meister, J-J. and Hinz, B. (2010) 'A new lock-step mechanism of matrix remodelling based on subcellular contractile events.' *Journal of Cell Science 123*, 1751–1760.

Foster, K., McAllister, M. and O'Brien, L. (2005) 'Coming to autoethnography: a mental health nurse's experience.' *International Journal of Qualitative Methods 4*, 4, 2–13.

Foster, M. (2004) *Somatic Patterning*. Longmont, CO: EMS Press.

Franklin, E. (1996) *Dynamic Alignment through Imagery*. Champaign, IL: Human Kinetics.

Fredriksen, K., Rhodes, J., Reddy, R. and Way, N. (2004) 'Sleepless in Chicago: tracking the effects of adolescent sleep loss during the middle school years.' *Child Development 75*, 1, 84–95.

Friedman, P. and Eisen, G. (1980) *The Pilates Method of Physical and Mental Conditioning*. New York: Penguin Press.

Gawthrop, F., Mould, R., Sperritt, A. and Neale F. (2007) 'Ehlers Danlos syndrome.' *British Medical Journal 335*, 448–450.

Gazit, Y., Menahem Nahir, A., Grahame, R. and Giris, J. (2003) 'Dysautonomia in the joint hypermobility syndrome.' *The American Journal of Medicine 115*, 1, 33–40.

Gellhorn, E. (1967) *Principles of Autonomic-Somatic Integrations*. Minneapolis: University of Minnesota Press.

Gluckman, P. D., Hanson, M. A., Cooper, C. and Thomburg, K. L. (2008) 'Effect of in utero and early-life conditions on adult health and disease.' *The New England Journal of Medicine 359*, 61–73.

Golier, J., Yehuda, R., Bierer, L., Mitropoulou, V. *et al.* (2003) 'The relationship of borderline personality disorder to posttraumatic stress disorder and traumatic events.' *American Journal of Psychiatry 160*, 11, 2018–2024.

Graef, F. and Kruel, L. (2006) 'Heart rate and perceived exertion at aquatic environment: differences in relation to land environment and applications for exercise prescription – a review. *Revista Brasileira de Medicina do Esporte 12*, 4, 198e–204e.

Grahame, R. (2009) 'Hypermobility: an important but often neglected area within rheumatology.' *Hypermobility Syndrome Association News*, Spring, 4–5.

Grahame, R. (2010) 'What Is the Joint Hypermobility Syndrome – JHS from Cradle to Grave.' In A. Hakim, R. Keer and R. Grahame (eds) *Hypermobility, Fibromyalgia and Chronic Pain*. Edinburgh: Churchill Livingstone.

Grahame, R. and Bird, H. (2001) 'British consultant rheumatologist's perceptions about the hypermobility syndrome.' *Rheumatology 40*, 559–562.

Grahame, R. and Keer, R. (2010) 'Pregnancy and the Pelvis.' In A. Hakim, R. Keer and R. Grahame (eds) *Hypermobility, Fibromyalgia and Chronic Pain*. Edinburgh: Churchill Livingstone.

Grbich, C. (2007) *Qualitative Data Analysis: An Introduction*. London: Sage Publications Ltd.

Greenwood, N. L., Duffell, L. D., Alexander, C. M. and McGregor, A. H. (2011) 'Electromygraphic activity of pelvic and lower limb muscles during postural tasks in people with benign joint hypermobility syndrome and non hypermobile people. A pilot study. *Manual Therapy 16*, 623–628.

Grubb, B.P. (2008) 'Postural tachycardia syndrome – clinician update.' American Heart Association, http://circ.ahajournals.org/content/117/21/2814.full, accessed 26 July 2010.

Guimberteau, J-C. (2010) *Muscle Attitudes*. DVD.

Guimberteau, J-C., Bakhach, J., Panconi, B. and Rouzaud, S. (2007) 'A fresh look at vascularized flexor tendon transfers: concept, technical aspects and results.' *Journal of Plastic, Reconstructive and Aesthetic Surgery 60*, 7, 793–810.

Gurley-Green, S. (2001) 'Living with hypermobility syndrome.' *British Journal of Rheumatology 40*, 487–489.

Hakim, A. and Grahame, R. (2003) 'Joint hypermobility.' *Best Practice and Research Clinical Rheumatology 17*, 6, 989–1004.

Hakim, A., Grahame, R., Norris, P. and Hopper, C. (2005) 'Local anaesthetic failure in joint hypermobility syndrome.' *Journal of the Royal Society of Medicine 98*, 2, 84–85.

Hakim, A., Keer, R. and Grahame, R. (2010) *Hypermobility, Fibromyalgia and Chronic Pain*. Edinburgh: Churchill Livingstone.

Hakim, A. and Grahame, R. (2004) 'Non-musculoskeletal symptoms in joint hypermobility syndrome: indirect evidence for autonomic dysfunction.' *Rheumatology 43*, 1194–1195.

Hakim, A. (2012) 'Results of (HMSA) patient experiences survey: perspectives on care and treatment outcomes.' *HMSA Newsletter*, November, p.25. In the *Daily Telegraph* 25 June 2012.

Hall, M. G., Ferrell, W. R., Sturrock, R. D., Hamblen, D. L. and Baxendale, R. H. (1995) 'The effect of the hypermobility syndrome on knee joint proprioception.' *Rheumatology 34*, 2, 121–125.

Hamilton-Fairley, D. (2004) *Lecture Notes: Obstetrics and Gynaecology*. Oxford: Blackwell Publishing.

Hameroff, S., Rasmussen, S. and Mansson, B. (1988) 'Molecular Automata in Microtubules: Basic Computational Logic of the Living State?' In C. Langton (ed.) *Artificial Life, SFI Studies in the Sciences of Complexity* (Vol. VI). Redwood City, CA: Addison-Wesley.

Hanna, T. (1988) *Somatics*. Cambridge, MA: Da Capo Press.

Hankinson, E. A. (2012) 'Nutrition Model to Reduce Inflammation in Musculoskeletal and Joint Diseases.' In R. Schleip, T. W. Findley, L. Chaitow and P. Huijing (eds) *Fascia: The Tensional Network of the Human Body. The Science and Clinical Applications in Manual and Movement Therapy*. Edinburgh; New York: Churchill Livingstone/Elsevier.

Harding, V. (2003) 'Joint Hypermobility and Chronic Pain: Possible Linking Mechanisms and Management Highlighted by a Cognitive-behavioural Approach.' In R. Keer and G. Grahame (eds) *Hypermobility Syndrome – Diagnosis and Management for Physiotherapists*. Philadelphia, PA: Elsevier.

Hardy, L., Jones, G. and Gould, D. (1996) *Understanding Psychological Preparation for Sport*. Chichester: Wiley and Sons.

Haw, C., Hawton, K., Houston, H. and Townsend, E. (2001) 'Psychiatric and personality disorders in deliberate self-harm patients.' *The British Journal of Psychiatry 178*, 48–54.

Heffez, D. S., Ross, R. E., Shade-Zeldow, Y., Kostas, K. *et al.* (2004) 'Clinical evidence for cervical myelopathy due to Chiari malformation and spinal stenosis in a non-randomized group of patients with the diagnosis of fibromyalgia.' *European Spine Journal 13*, 6, 516–523.

Hemmings, B. and Povey, L. (2002) 'Views of chartered physiotherapists on the psychological content of their practice: a preliminary study in the United Kingdom.' *British Journal of Sports Medicine 36*, 61–64.

Henderson, L. and Wood, R. (2000) *Explaining Endometriosis*. Crow Nest, NSW: Allen and Unwin.

Hendler, N. (1984) 'Depression caused by chronic pain.' *Journal of Clinical Psychiatry 45*, 3, 30–38.

Hinz, B. and Phan, S. H. (2007) 'The myofibroblast – one function, multiple origins.' *The Americal Journal of Pathology 170*, 1807–1816.

Ho, M-W. and Knight, D. (1998) 'The acupuncture system and the liquid crystalline collagen fibres of the connective tissues.' *American Journal of Complementary Medicine 26*, 3–4, 251–263.

Holt, N. (2003) 'Representation, legitimation and autoethnography – an autoethnographic writing story.' *International Journal of Qualitative Methods 2*, 1, 18–27.

Hunsley, J., Aubry, T., Verstervelt, C. and Vito, D. (1999) 'Comparing therapist and client perspectives on reasons for psychotherapy termination.' *Psychotherapy: Theory, Research, Practice, Training 36*, 4, 380–388.

Hunter, A. (2011) 'Tearing up the rule book.' *Royal College of Speech and Language Therapists Bulletin/May*, pp.20–21.

Hypermobility Syndrome Association (2011) 'New rare disease UK report.' *Hypermobility Syndrome Association Newsletter*, Spring, p.13.

Jack, K., McLean, S. M., Moffett, J. K. and Gardiner, E. (2010) 'Barriers to treatment adherence in physiotherapy outpatient clinics: a systematic review.' *Manual Therapy 15*, 3, 220–228.

Janov, A. (1990) *The Primal Scream*. London: Abacus.

Jentoft, S., Kvalvick, A. and Mengshoel, A. (2001) 'Effects of pool-based and land-based aerobic exercise on women with fibromyalgia/chronic widespread muscle pain.' *Arthritis Care & Research 45*, 42–47.

Jones, K., Deodhar, P., Lorentzen, A., Bennett, R. M. and Deodhar, A. A. (2007) 'Growth hormone perturbations in fibromyalgia: a review.' *Seminars in Arthritis and Rheumatism 36*, 6, 357–379.

Juhan, D. (2002) *Job's Body: A Handbook for Bodywork*. New York: Station Hill Press.

Jull, G. A., O'Leary, S. P. and Falla, D. L. (2008) 'Clinical assessment of the deep neck flexor muscles: the craniocervical test.' *Journal of Manipulative Physiological Therapeutics 31*, 525–533.

Kanjwal, K., Karabin, B., Kanjwal, Y. and Grubb, B. (2009) 'Postpartum postural orthostatic tachycardia syndrome in a patient with the joint hypermobility syndrome.' *Cardiology Research and Practice*, doi:10.4061/2009/187543.

Katon, W. and Sullivan, M. (1990) 'Depression and chronic medical illness.' *Journal of Clinical Psychiatry 51*, 6, 3–11.

Kavuncu, V., Sahin, S., Kamanli, A., Karan, A. and Aksoy, C. (2006) 'The role of systemic hypermobility and condylar hypermobility in temporomandibular joint dysfunction syndrome.' *Rheumatology International 26*, 257–260.

Keays, S. L., Bullock-Saxton, J. E., Newcombe, P. and Bullock, M. I. (2006) 'The effectiveness of a pre-operative home-based physiotherapy programme for chronic anterior cruciate ligament deficiency.' *Physiotherapy Research International 11*, 4, 204–218.

Keefe, F. J. and Van Horn, Y. (1993) 'Cognitive behavioral treatment of rheumatoid arthritis pain: understanding and enhancing maintenance of treatment gains.' *Arthritis & Rheumatism 6*, 4, 213–222.

Keefer, L., Stepanksi, E., Ranjbaran, Z., Benson, L. and Keshavarzian, A. (2006) 'An initial report of sleep disturbance in inactive inflammatory bowel disease.' *Journal of Clinical Sleep Medicine 2*, 4, 409–416.

Keer, R. (2003) 'Physiotherapy Assessment of the Hypermobile Adult.' In R. Keer and G. Grahame (eds) *Hypermobility Syndrome: Diagnosis and Management for Physiotherapists*. Philadelphia, PA: Elsevier.

Keer, R. (2010) 'The Cervical Spine and Jaw: a) The Cervical Spine.' In A. Hakim, R. Keer and R. Grahame (eds) *Hypermobility, Fibromyalgia and Chronic Pain*. Edinburgh: Churchill Livingstone.

Keer, R. and Butler, K. (2010) 'Physiotherapy and Occupational Therapy in the Hypermobile Adult.' In A. Hakim, R. Keer and R. Grahame (eds) *Hypermobility, Fibromyalgia and Chronic Pain*. Edinburgh: Churchill Livingstone.

Keer, R. and Grahame G. (eds) (2003) *Hypermobility Syndrome: Diagnosis and Management for Physiotherapists*. Philadelphia, PA: Elsevier.

Keer, R. and Simmonds, J. (2011) 'Joint protection and physical rehabilitation of the adult with hypermobility syndrome.' *Current Opinion in Rheumatology 23*, 131–136.

Kennedy, J. and Gazvani, S. (2000) *The Investigation and Management of Endometriosis*. London: RCOG.

Kerr, A., Macmillan, C. E., Uttley, W. S. and Lugmani, R. A. (2000) 'Physiotherapy for children with hypermobility syndrome.' *Physiotherapy 86*, 313–317.

Keuthen, N., Deckersbach, T., Wilhelm, S., Engelhard, I. *et al.* (2001) 'The skin picking impact scale (SPIS).' *Psychosomatics 42*, 5, 397–403.

Kirby, A. and Davies, R. (2007) 'Developmental coordination disorder and joint hypermobility syndrome – overlapping disorders? Implications for research and clinical practice.' *Child Care Health Development 33*, 5, 513–519.

Kirby, A., Davies, R. and Bryant, A. (2005) 'Hypermobility syndrome and developmental coordination disorder: similarities and features.' *International Journal of Therapy and Rehabilitation 12*, 10, 431–437.

Kiresuk, T. J., Smith, A. and Cardillo, J. E. (eds) (1994) *Goal Attainment Scaling: Applications, Theory and Measurement*. Hillsdale, NJ: Lawrence Erlbaum Associates.

Klonsky, D., Oltmanns, T. and Turkheimer, E. (2003) 'Deliberate self-harm in a nonclinical population: prevalence and psychological correlates.' *American Journal of Psychiatry 160*, 8, 1501–1508.

Knezevic, M., Guillermo, M., Vicente, M., Francisco, G. *et al.* (2008) 'Physical rehabilitation treatment of the temporomandibular pain dysfunction syndrome.' *Facta Universitatis 15*, 3, 113–118.

Knight, I. (2006) *The History of My Skin: An Autobiography*. Unpublished.

Knight, I. (2009) *Skin Collection*. London: Chipmunka Publishing.

Knight, I. (2011) *A Guide to Living with Hypermobility Syndrome: Bending without Breaking*. London: Singing Dragon Press.

Kram, R. and Dawson, T. J. (1998) 'Energetics and biomechanics of locomotion of red kangaroos.' *Comparative Biochemistry and Physiology B120*, 41–49.

Kurth, L. and Haussmann, R. (2011) 'Perinatal pitocin as an early ADHD biomarker: neurodevelopmental risk.' *Journal of Attention Disorders 15*, 5, 423–431.

Laibow, R. (1991) 'Circumcision: relationship attachment impairment.' NOCIRC International Symposium on Circumcision, San Francisco, April 1991, 14.

Latthe, P., Hills, R. and Khan, K. (2006) 'Factors predisposing women to chronic pelvic pain.' *British Medical Journal 322*, 7544, 749–755.

Levin, S. and Martin, D-C. (2012) 'Biotensegrity. The Mechanics of Fascia.' In R. Schleip, T. W. Findley, L. Chaitow and P. Huijing (eds) *Fascia: the Tensional Network of the Human Body: The Science and Clinical Applications in Manual and Movement Therapy.* Edinburgh; New York: Churchill Livingstone/Elsevier.

Levine, P. (1997) *Waking the Tiger: Healing Trauma.* Berkeley, CA: North Atlantic Books.

Levinkind, M. (2008) 'Consideration of whole body posture in relation to dental development.' Oral Health Report, Vol. I, 2008, *British Dental Journal Supplement.*

Levy, H.P. (2012) 'Ehlers-Danlos Syndrome, Hypermobility Type.' In Pagon, R.A., Bird, T.D., Dolan, C.R., Stephens, K. and Adam, M.P. (eds). *Gene Reviews™* [Internet] Seattle, WA: University of Washington. Available from www.ncbi.nlm.nih.gov/books/NBK1279, accessed on 12 February 2013.

Lew, H., Otis, J., Tun, C., Kerns, R., Clark, M. and Citfu, D. (2009) 'Prevalence of chronic pain, posttraumatic stress disorder and persistent post concursive symptoms in veterans.' *Journal of Research Development 46*, 6, 697–702.

Li, Y., Foster, W., Deasy, B. M., Chan, Y. *et al.* (2004) 'Transforming growth factor-β1 induces the differentiation of myogenic cells into fibrotic cells in injured skeletal muscle.' *The American Journal of Pathology 164*, 3, 1007–1019.

Locke, E. A. and Latham, G. P. (2002) 'Building a practically useful theory of goal setting and task motivation: a 35-year odyssey.' *American Psychologist 57*, 9, 705–717.

Locker, D. (1997) 'Living with Chronic Illness.' In G. Scambler (ed.) *Sociology as Applied to Medicine.* London: W. B. Saunders Company Ltd.

Magee, D. J. (2008) *Orthopedic Physical Assessment* (5th edn). St Louis, MO: Saunders.

Maillard, S. and Murray, K. (2003) *Hypermobility Syndrome in Children,* In R. Keer and G. Grahame (eds) *Hypermobility Syndrome: Diagnosis and Management for Phsyiotherapists.* Philadelphia, PA: Elsevier.

Maitland, G. D. (ed.) (1986) *Spinal Manipulation* (5th edn). Butterworths: London.

Mallik, A. K., Ferrell, W. R., McDonald, A. and Sturrock, R. D. (1994) 'Impaired proprioceptive acuity at the proximal interphalangeal joint in patients with the hypermobility syndrome.' *British Journal of Rheumatolgy 33*, 7, 631–637.

Mannerkorpi, K. and Daly, M. (2003) 'Physical exercise in fibromyalgia and related syndromes.' *Clinical Rheumatology 17*, 4, 629–647.

Manning, J., Korda, A., Benness, C. and Solomon, M. (2003) 'The association of obstructive defecation, lower urinary tract dysfunction and the benign joint hypermobility syndrome: a case-control study.' *International Urogynaecology Journal 14*, 128–132.

Marlatt, G. A. and Gordon, J. R. (1980) 'Determinants of Relapse: Implications for the Maintenance of Behaviour Change.' In P. O. Davidson and S. M. Davidson (eds) *Behavioral Medicine: Changing Health Lifestyles.* New York: Brunner/Mazel.

Martin-Santos, R., Bulbena, A. and Crippa, J. (2010) 'Anxiety Disorders, their Relationship to Hypermobility and their Management.' In A. Hakim, R. Keer and R. Grahame (eds) *Hypermobility Fibromyalgia and Chronic Pain.* Edinburgh: Churchill Livingstone.

Martin-Santos, R., Bulbena, A., Porta, M., Gago, J., Molina, L. and Duro, J. (1998) 'Association between joint hypermobility syndrome and panic disorder.' *American Journal of Psychiatry 155*, 11, 1578–1583.

Masi, A. T., Nair, K., Andoinian, B. J., Prus, M. P. *et al.* (2011) 'Integrative structural biomechanical concepts of ankylosing spondylitis.' *Arthritis,* doi:10.1155/2011/205904.

Maslow, A. (1970) *Motivation and Personality.* New York: Harper and Row Publishers.

McCormack, M., Briggs, J., Hakim, A. and Grahame, R. (2004) 'Joint laxity and the benign joint hypermobility syndrome in student and professional ballet dancers.' *Journal of Rheumatology 31*, 1, 173–178.

McIntosh, L., Mallett, V., Frahm, J., Richardson, D. and Evans, I. (1995) 'Gynaecologic disorders in women with Ehlers-Danlos syndrome.' *Journal of the Society for Gynaecologic Investigation 2*, 3, 559–564.

McLeod, J. (1998) *An Introduction to Counselling* (2nd edn). Buckingham: Open University Press.

Mears, J. (1996) *Coping with Endometriosis*. London: Shelton Press.

Medina-Mirapeix, F., Escolar-Reina, P., Gascon-Conovas, J., Montialla-Herrador, J. and Collins, S. (2009) 'Personal characteristics influencing patients' adherence to home exercise during chronic pain: a qualitative study.' *Journal of Rehabilitative Medicine 41*, 347–352.

Middleditch, A. (2010) 'Physiotherapy and Occupational Therapy in the Hypermobile Adolescent.' In A. Hakim, R. Keer and R. Grahame (eds) *Hypermobility, Fibromyalgia and Chronic Pain*. Edinburgh: Churchill Livingstone.

Mills, D. and Vernon, M. (1999) *Endometriosis: A Key to Healing through Nutrition*. Shaftesbury, Dorset: Element.

Montpetit, L. (2012) *Breaking Free from Persistent Fatigue*. London: Singing Dragon Press.

Morgan, A., Pearson, S., Davies, S., Gooi, H. and Bird, H. (2007) 'Asthma and airways collapse in two heritable disorders of connective tissue.' *Annals of the Rheumatic Diseases 66*, 10, 1369–1373.

Mujika, I. and Padilla, S. (2000) 'Detraining: loss of training-induced physiological and performance adaptations. Part II: Long term insufficient training stimulus.' *Sports Medicine 30*, 3, 145–154.

Muller, D. and Schleip, R. (2012) 'Suggestions for a Fascia-oriented Training Approach in Sports and Movement Therapies.' In R. Schleip, T. W. Findley, L. Chaitow and P. Huijing (eds) *Fascia: The Tensional Network of the Human Body. The Science and Clinical Applications in Manual and Movement Therapy*. Edinburgh; New York: Churchill Livingstone/Elsevier.

Murray, K. (2006) 'Hypermobility disorders in children and adolescents.' *Clinical Rheumatology 20*, 2, 329–351.

Myers, T. (2001) *Anatomy Trains*. London: Churchill Livingstone.

Myers, T. and Frederick, C. (2012) 'Stretching and Fascia.' In R. Schleip, T. W. Findley, L. Chaitow and P. Huijing (eds) *Fascia: The Tensional Network of the Human Body. The Science and Clinical Applications in Manual and Movement Therapy*. Edinburgh; New York: Churchill Livingstone/Elsevier.

Nager, C. W. and Albo, M. E. (2004) 'Testing in women with lower urinary tract dysfunction.' *Clinical Obstetrics and Gynecology 47*, 1, 53–69.

Naylor, I. (2012) 'Dupuyten's Disease and Other Fibrocontractive Disorders.' In R. Schleip, T. W. Findley, L. Chaitow and P. Huijing (eds) *Fascia: The Tensional Network of the Human Body. The Science and Clinical Applications in Manual and Movement Therapy*. Edinburgh; New York: Churchill Livingstone/Elsevier.

Nicolakis, P., Erdogmus, B., Kopf, A., Ebenbichler, G. *et al.* (2001) 'Effectiveness of exercise therapy in patients with internal derangement of the temporomandibular joint.' *Journal of Oral Rehabilitation 28*, 1158–1164.

Niere, K. R. and Torney, S. K. (2004) 'Clinicians' perceptions of minor cervical instability.' *Manual Therapy 9*, 3, 144–150.

Odent, M. (1986) *Primal Health*. London: Century Hutchinson.

Oliver, K. and Cronan, T. (2002) 'Predictors of exercise behaviors among fibromyalgia patients.' *Preventative Medicine 35*, 4, 383–389.

Oschman, J. (2003) *Energy Medicine in Therapeutics and Human Performance*. Edinburgh: Butterworth Heinemann.

Oschman, J. (2012) 'Fascia as a Body-wide Communication System.' In R. Schleip, T. W. Findley, L. Chaitow and P. Huijing (eds) *Fascia: The Tensional Network of the Human Body. The Science and Clinical Applications in Manual and Movement Therapy*. Edinburgh; New York: Churchill Livingstone/Elsevier.

Oschman, J. and Oschman, N. (1995) 'Somatic recall. Part 1 – Soft tissue memory.' *Massage Therapy Journal 34*, 3, 36–45; 111–116.

Panjabi, M. M. (1992) 'The stabilizing system of the spine. Part II. Neutral zone and instability hypothesis.' *Journal of Spinal Disorders 5*, 390–397.

Panjabi, M. M., Cholewicki, J., Nibu, K., Grauer, J., Babt, L. B. and Dvorak, J. (1998) 'Critical load of the human cervical spine: an in vitro experimental study.' *Clinical Biomechanics 13*, 1, 11–17.

Parker, H., Dumat, W. and Booker, C. K. (2000) 'The Pain Management Programme.' In C. J. Main and C. C. Spanswick (eds) *Pain Management: An Interdisciplinary Approach*. Edinburgh: Churchill Livingstone.

Paris, J. (2005) 'Borderline personality disorder.' *Canadian Medical Association Journal 172*, 12, 1579–1583.

Peck, C. and Love, A. (1986) 'Chronic Pain.' In N. J. King and A. Remengi (eds) *Healthcare: A Behavioural Approach*. Sydney: Grune and Stratton.

Pilates, J. and Miller, W. (1998) *A Pilates Primer: The Millennium Edition*. Incline Village: Presentation Dynamics Inc.

Porges, S. (2001) 'The polyvagal theory: phylogenetic substrates of a social nervous system.' *International Journal of Psychophysiology 42*, 123–146.

Potter, M., Gordon, S. and Hamer, P. (2003a). 'The difficult patient in private practice physiotherapy: a qualitative study.' *Australian Journal of Physiotherapy 49*, 53–61.

Potter, M., Gordon, S. and Hamer, P. (2003b) 'The physiotherapy experience in private practice: the patients' perspective.' *Australian Journal of Physiotherapy 49*, 195–202.

Powell, D. W., Mifflin, R. C., Valentich, J. D., Crowe, S. E., Saada, J. I. and West, A. B. (1999) 'Myofibroblasts. II. Intestinal subepithelial myofibroblasts.' *American Journal of Physiology – Cell Physiology 277*, 2, 183–201.

Preference Collaborative Review Group (2008) 'Patients' preferences within randomized trials: systemic review and patient level meta-analysis.' *British Medical Journal 337*, a1864.

Price, C., Hoggart, B., Olukoga, O., Williams, A. and Bottle, A. (2012) National Pain Audit – Final Report (2010–2012). (Obtained with kind permission from The British Pain Society).

Pritchard, A. (2009) *Ways of Learning*. Abingdon: Routledge.

Proctor, M. and Farquhar, C. (2006) 'Diagnosis and management of dysmenorrhoea.' *British Medical Journal 332*, 7550, 1134–1138.

Rahman, A. and Holman, A. (2010) 'Pharmacotherapy in Fibromyalgia.' In A. Hakim, R. Keer and R. Grahame (eds) *Hypermobility Fibromyalgia and Chronic Pain*. Edinburgh: Churchill Livingstone.

Raj, S. (2006) 'The postural tachycardia syndrome (POTS): pathophysiology, diagnosis and management.' *Indian Pacing and Electrophysiology Journal 6*, 2, 84–99.

Raven, P. B., Welch-O'Connor, R. M. and Shi, X. (1998) 'Cardiovascular function following reduced aerobic activity.' *Medicine and Science in Sport and Exercise 30*, 7, 1041–1052.

Reinagel, M. (2007) *The Inflammation-free Diet Plan*. London: McGraw-Hill.

Rejeski, W. J., Brawley, L. R., Ettinger, W., Morgan, T. and Thompson, C. (1997) 'Compliance to exercise therapy in older participants with knee osteoarthritis: implications for treating disability.' *Medicine and Science in Sport and Exercise 29*, 8, 977–985.

Remvig, L. (2007) 'General joint hypermobility and tissue stiffness: a review.' 1st International Fascia Research Congress, Boston, October.

Remvig, L., Schleip, R., Kristensen, J. H., Krogsgaard, M. and Juul-Kristensen, B. (2007) 'Do patients with Ehlers-Danlos syndrome and/or hypermobility syndrome have reduced number of contractile cells in fascia?' 1st International Fascia Research Congress, Boston, October.

Richards, R. (2008) 'Writing the othered self: autoethnography and the problem of objectification in writing about illness and disability.' *Qualitative Health Research 18*, 12, 1717–1728.

Romano, J. and Turner, J. (1985) 'Chronic pain and depression – does the evidence support a relationship?' *Psychological Bulletin 97*, 1, 18–34.

Rombaut, L., Malfait, F., Cools, A., De Paepe, A. and Calders, P. (2010) 'Musculoskeletal complaints, physical activity and health-related quality of life among patients with the Ehlers-Danlos syndrome hypermobility type.' *Rehabilitation 32*, 16, 1339–1345.

Rooks, D. (2008) 'Talking to patients with fibromyalgia about physical activity and exercise.' *Current Opinion in Rheumatology 20*, 2, 208–212.

Rooks, D., Silverman, C. and Kantrowitz, F. (2002) 'The effects of progressive strength training and aerobic exercise on muscle strength and cardiovascular fitness in women with fibromyalgia: a pilot study.' *Arthritis Care and Research 47*, 1, 22–28.

Rothschild, B. (2000) *The Body Remembers*. New York: W. W. Norton and Company.

Roy-Byrne, P., Smith, W., Goldberg, J., Afari, N. and Buchwald, D. (2004) 'Posttraumatic stress disorder among patients with chronic fatigue.' *Psychological Medicine 34*, 2, 363–368.

Russek, L. (1999) 'Hypermobility syndrome.' *Physical Therapy 79*, 6, 591–599.

Sacks, O. (2011) *Musicophilia*. Croydon: Picador.

Sahin, N., Baskent, A., Cakmak, A., Salli, A., Ugurlu, H. and Berker, E. (2008) 'Evaluation of knee proprioception and effects of proprioception exercise in patients with benign joint hypermobility syndrome.' *Rheumatology International 28*, 10, 995–1000.

Sahrmann, S. A. (2002) *Diagnosis and Treatment of Movement Impairment Syndromes*. St Louis: Mosby.

Sahrmann, S. A. and Associates (2011) *Movement System Impairment Syndromes of the Extremities, Cervical and Thoracic Spines*. St Louis, MO: Elsevier Mosby.

Sakaguchi, K., Mehta, N. R., Abdallah, E., Forgione, A. *et al.* (2007) 'Examination of the relationship between mandibular position and body posture.' *The Journal of Craniomandibular Practice 25*, 4, 237–249.

Sanes, J. N. and Donoghue, J. P. (2000) 'Plasticity and primary motor cortex.' *Annual Review of Neuroscience 23*, 393–415.

Sansone, R., Pole, M., Dakroub, H. and Butler, M. (2006) 'Childhood trauma, borderline personality symptomology, and psychophysiological and pain disorders in adulthood.' *Psychosomatics 47*, 2, 158–162.

Sansone, R., Whitecar, P., Meir, B. and Murry, A. (2001) 'The prevalence of borderline personality among primary care patients with chronic pain.' *General Hospital Psychiatry 23*, 193–197.

Sawicki, G. S., Lewis, C. L. and Ferris, D. P. (2009) 'It pays to have a spring in your step.' *Exercise Sports Science Review. 37*, 3, 130–138.

Scambler, G. (ed.) (1997) *Sociology as Applied to Medicine*. London: W. B. Saunders Company Ltd.

Schleip, R. (2003) 'Fascial plasticity – a new neurobiological explanation.' *Journal of Bodywork and Movement Therapies 7*, 1, 11–19 and 7, 2, 104–116.

Schleip, R. (2009) Webinar presentation.

Schleip, R. and Klingler, W. (2007) 'Fascial strain hardening correlates with matrix hydration changes.' 1st International Fascia Research Congress, Boston, October.

Schleip, R., Findley, T. W., Chaitow, L. and Huijing, P. (eds) (2012) *Fascia: The Tensional Network of the Human Body. The Science and Clinical Applications in Manual and Movement Therapy*. Edinburgh; New York: Churchill Livingstone/Elsevier.

Scobbie, L., Wyke, S. and Dixon, D. (2009) 'Setting and applying psychological theory to setting rehabilitation goals.' *Clinical Rehabilitation 23*, 4, 321–333.

Shaikh, M., Hakim, A. and Shenker, N. (2010) 'The Physiology of Pain.' In A. Hakim, R. Keer and R. Grahame (eds) *Hypermobility, Fibromyalgia and Chronic Pain*. Edinburgh: Churchill Livingstone.

Sharp, T. (2004) 'The prevalence of posttraumatic stress disorder in chronic pain patients.' *Current Pain Headache Report 8*, 2, 111–115.

Sharp, T. and Harvey, A. (2001) 'Chronic pain and posttraumatic stress disorder: mutual maintenance.' *Clinical Psychological Review 6*, 857–877.

Shaver, J., Lentz, M., Landis, C., Heitkemper, M., Buchwald, D. and Woods, N. (1997) 'Sleep, psychological distress, and stress arousal in women with fibromyalgia.' *Research in Nursing and Health 20*, 3, 247–257.

Shilling, C. (1993) *The Body and Social Theory*. London: Sage Publications Ltd.

Siler, B. (2000) *The Pilates Body*. London: Penguin.

Simmonds, J. (2003) 'Rehabilitation, Fitness, Sport and Performance for Individuals with Joint Hypermobility.' In R. Keer and G. Grahame (eds) *Hypermobility Syndrome: Diagnosis and Management for Physiotherapists*. Philadelphia, PA: Elsevier.

Simmonds, J. (2010) 'Principles of Rehabilitation and Considerations for Sport, Performance and Fitness.' In A. Hakim, R. Keer and R. Grahame (eds) *Hypermobility Fibromyalgia and Chronic Pain*. Edinburgh: Churchill Livingstone.

Simmonds, J. (2012) 'Hypermobility and the Hypermobility Syndrome' In R. Schleip, T. W. Findley, L. Chaitow and P. Huijing (eds) *Fascia: The Tensional Network of the Human Body. The Science and Clinical Applications in Manual and Movement Therapy*. Edinburgh; New York: Churchill Livingstone/Elsevier.

Simmonds, J. and Keer, R. (2007) 'Hypermobility and the hypermobility syndrome.' *Manual Therapy 12*, 4, 298–309.

Simmonds, J. and Keer, R. (2008) 'Hypermobility and the hypermobility syndrome, part 2. Assessment and management of hypermobility syndrome: illustrated via case studies.' *Manual Therapy 13*, 2, E1–E11.

Simpson, M. (2006) 'Benign joint hypermobility syndrome: evaluation, diagnosis and management.' *Journal of American Osteopath Association 106*, 9, 531–536.

Smekal, D., Velebova, K., Hanakova, D. and Lepsikova, M. (2008) 'The effectiveness of specific physiotherapy in the treatment of temporomandibular diseases.' *Acta Universitalis Palackianae Olomucensis. Gymnnica 38*, 2, 45–53.

Spanswick, C. C. and Parker, H. (2000) 'Clinical Content of Interdisciplinary Pain Management Programmes.' In C. J. Main and C. C. Spanswick (eds) *Pain Management: An Interdisciplinary Approach.* Edinburgh: Churchill Livingstone.

Stenström, C. H., Arge, B. and Sundbom, A. (1997) 'Home exercise and compliance in inflammatory rheumatic diseases – a prospective clinical trial.' *Journal of Rheumatology 24*, 3, 470–476.

Tinkle, B. (2008) *Issues and Management of Joint Hypermobility.* Greensfork, Indiana: Left Paw Press.

Tinkle, B. (2010) *Joint Hypermobility Handbook.* Greens Fork, IN: Left Paw Press.

Tinkle, B. T., Bird, H. A., Graham, R., Lavallee, M., Levy, H. P. and Sillence, D. (2009) 'The lack of clinical distinction between the hypermobility type of Ehlers-Danlos syndrome and the joint hypermobility syndrome (a.k.a. hypermobility syndrome).' *American Journal of Medical Genetics 149A*, 11, 2368–2370.

Tomasek, J., Gabbiani, G., Hinz, B., Chaponnier, C. and Brown, R. A. (2002) 'Myofibroblasts and mechano-regulation of connective tissue remodelling.' *Nature Reviews 3*, 5, 349–363.

Tsao, H., Galea, M. P. and Hodges, P. W. (2008) 'Reorganization of the motor cortex is associated with postural control deficits in recurrent low back pain.' *Brain 131*, 8, 2161–2171.

Turvey, M. T. (2007) 'Action and perception at the level of synergies.' *Human Movement Science 26*, 657–697.

Tyc, F., Boyadjian, A. and Devanne, H. (2005) 'Motor cortex plasticity induced by extensive training revealed by transcranial magnetic stimulation in human.' *European Journal of Neuroscience 21*, 1, 259–266.

Van der Kolk, B. (1994) 'The body keeps the score: memory and the evolving psychobiology of posttraumatic stress.' *Harvard Review of Psychiatry 1*, 5, 253–265.

Vaughan, M. B., Howard, E. W. and Tomasek, J. J. (2000) 'Transforming growth factor-β1 promotes the morphological and functional differentiation of the myofibroblast.' *Experimental Cell Research 257*, 180–189.

Voermans, N. C., Altenburg, T. M., Hamel, B. C., de Haan, A. and van Engelen, B. G. (2007) 'Reduced quantitative muscle function in tenascin-X deficient Ehlers-Danlos patients.' *Neuromuscular Disorders 17*, 8, 597–602.

Warner, L. and McNeill, M. E. (1987) 'Mental imagery and its potential for physical therapy.' *Physical Therapy 68*, 4, 516–520.

Wilks, J. (2007) *The Bowen Technique: The Inside Story.* Corton Denham: CYMA.

Williams, B. and Poijula, S. (2002) *The PTSD Workbook.* Oakland, CA: New Harbinger Publications.

Williamson, D., Robinson, M.E. and Melamed, B. (1997) 'Pain behaviour, spouse responsiveness, and marital satisfaction in patients with rheumatoid arthritis.' *Behaviour Modification 21*, 97–118.

Wipff, P-J., Rifkin, D. B., Meister, J-J. and Hinz, B. (2007) 'Myofibroblast contraction activates latent TGF-β1 from the extracellular matrix.' *Journal of Cell Biology 179*, 6, 1311–1323.

Wolfson, A. and Carskadon, M. (1998) 'Sleep schedules and daytime functioning in adolescents.' *Child Development 69*, 4, 875–887.

Zarate, N., Farmer, A., Grahame, R., Mohammed, S. *et al.* (2010) 'Unexplained gastrointestinal symptoms and joint hypermobility: is connective tissue the missing link?' *Neurogastroenterology and Motility 22*, 3, 252–262.

Zittel Conklin, C. and Westen, D. (2005) 'Borderline personality disorder in clinical practice.' *American Journal of Psychiatry 162*, 5, 867–875.

Further reading

Ellis, C. and Bochner, A. P. (2000) 'Autoethnography, Personal Narrative, Reflexivity: Researcher as Subject.' In N. Denzin and Y. Lincoln (eds) *The Handbook of Qualitative Research* (2nd edn). Thousand Oaks, CA: Sage.

Gunderson, J. (1993) 'The phemonological and conceptual interface between borderline personality disorder and PTSD.' *The American Journal of Psychiatry 150*, 1, 19–27.

Koenigsberg, H., Harvey, P., Mitropoulou, V., Schmeidler, J. *et al.* (2002) 'Characterizing affective instability in borderline personality disorder.' *American Journal of Psychiatry 159*, 5, 784–788.

Mohammed, S., Lunniss, P., Zarate, N., Farmer, A. *et al.* (2010) 'Joint hypermobility and rectal evacuatory dysfunction: an aetiological link in abnormal connective tissue?' *Neurogastroenterology and Motility 10*, 1085–e283.

Nicholas, M., Molloy, A., Tonkin, L. and Beeston, L. (2005) *Manage your Pain*. London: Souvenir Press.

Rose, S., Cottencin, O., Chouraki, V., Wattier, J. *et al.* (2009) 'Study on personality and psychiatric disorder in fibromyalgia.' *La Presse Médicale 38*, 5, 695–700.

Skegg, K., Nada-Raja, S., Dickson, N., Paul, C. and Williams, S. (2003) 'Sexual orientation and self-harm in men and women.' *American Journal of Psychiatry 160*, 3, 541–546.

Tragesser, S., Bruns, D. and Disorbio, J. (2010) 'Borderline personality disorder features and pain: the mediating role of negative affect in a pain patient sample.' *Clinical Journal of Pain 26*, 4, 348–353.

Tsao, H., Galea, M. P. and Hodges, P. W. (2010) 'Driving plasticity in the motor cortex in recurrent low back pain.' *European Journal of Pain 14*, 8, 832–839.

List of contributors

I am exceptionally fortunate to have contributions from the following very experienced medical team, including Professor Howard Bird, Dr Alan Hakim, Rosemary Keer, Dr Andrew Lucas, Dr Jane Simmonds and John Wilks, as well as contributions from Feldenkrais teacher Maggy Burrowes and Pilates Instructor Jessica Moolenaar. Here are their biographies:

Professor Howard Bird MA MD FRCP

Howard Bird has been Emeritus Professor of Pharmacological Rheumatology at the University of Leeds since his retirement in 2010 from the posts of Academic Sub-Dean and Honorary Consultant Rheumatologist. As a clinician, for some 25 years he was responsible for the Leeds rheumatology clinic devoted to Inherited Abnormalities of Connective Tissue. His MD thesis was entitled 'Joint Hypermobility' and he has published numerous books, chapters and original scientific 'papers', in this and in other fields.

In 2011 he was appointed Visiting Professor at University College London in conjunction with their newly established MSc in Performing Arts Medicine. He has held clinics for musicians and dancers for some 20 years and now teaches and researches in Performing Arts Medicine and in joint flexibility at University College, Laban Conservatoire for Dance and the Royal College of Music.

Dr Alan Hakim MA FRCP

Dr Hakim studied and trained as a junior doctor in Cambridge before specialist training in Rheumatology at University College Hospital and undertaking research as an Arthritis Research Campaign Fellow at St Thomas' Hospital, London. It was during his research that Dr Hakim met Professor Grahame and was introduced to the world of hypermobility. Having been a consultant for 12 years, Dr Hakim enjoys a variety of roles as a clinician, researcher, author and health care manager, working across London and nationally within clinical leadership and clinical commissioning in England.

Dr Hakim is a Consultant Physician and Rheumatologist at Whipps Cross University Hospital, Barts Health NHS Trust, London, and at the Hypermobility Unit, Hospital of St John and St Elizabeth in London. He is an Honorary Senior Lecturer in Experimental Medicine and Rheumatology at Queen Mary University in London and Chief Medical Officer and Trustee of the Hypermobility Syndrome Association, UK.

Rosemary Keer

Rosemary Keer is a chartered physiotherapist with many years of unrivalled experience of treating patients with joint hypermobility syndrome and EDS. She has worked closely with Professor Grahame developing a successful approach to managing the difficult symptoms of this complaint and lectures nationally and internationally to spread the word. Rosemary is the lead editor along with Professor Grahame of the much acclaimed text for physiotherapists on hypermobility syndrome and its treatment (*Hypermobility Syndrome: Diagnosis and Management for Physiotherapists*, 2003), as well as a more recent book with Professor Grahame and Dr Hakim which updates and expands our knowledge of the syndrome (*Hypermobility, Fibromyalgia and Chronic Pain*, 2010). Rosemary splits her time between working at the Hospital of St John and St Elizabeth and in her own clinic on Harley Street. She is also an advisor to the Hypermobility Syndrome Association (HMSA).

Dr Andrew J. Lucas BSc (Hons) MSc MSc D.Psych C.Psychol C.Sci AFBPsP

Dr Lucas is a Consultant Health Psychologist specialising in musculo-skeletal chronic pain management and holds degrees in Psychology (BSc Hons), Health Psychology (MSc) and Pain Management (MSc). His doctoral thesis was awarded from City University London for original research on chronic pain-related disability and pain self-efficacy. He is a chartered health psychologist, chartered scientist and associate fellow of the British Psychological Society. Health psychologists specialise in physical health management and are employed in the clinical setting in such fields as cardiac rehabilitation, oncology, HIV and AIDS, and chronic pain management. Chronic illness needs long-term management rather than cure, and the approach is to help patients develop self-management strategies and new coping skills. Dr Lucas has worked at the Royal National Orthopaedic Hospital (RNOH), Stanmore since 1999. The RNOH has delivered in patient pain management programmes (PMP) for over 20 years. He is consultant lead psychologist and head of the Clinical Health Psychology department.

Andrew Lucas's research interests are primarily concerned with explaining chronic pain-related disability; for example, he has investigated the role of family and health-related beliefs. Consistent with other research, no clear relationship has been found between pathology and disability. A patient with minor pathology may be very disabled and vice versa, and so other non-medical factors must play a role in contributing to chronic pain-related disability; his research explores the contribution of these 'other factors'.

Dr Jane Simmonds FHEA MCSP MMACP

Jane Simmonds is a principal lecturer, physiotherapy research lead and post-graduate programme leader at the University of Hertfordshire. Originally from Western Australia, she has worked in a wide range of sport, clinical and educational settings in Australia and the UK. Jane is a clinical specialist in Ehlers-Danlos syndrome (hypermobility type) and hypermobility syndrome at the Hypermobility Unit in central London. She completed a professional doctorate in 2010 entitled 'Advancing Practice in Hypermobility and Osteoporosis' and regularly contributes and reviews research and clinical papers at conferences and for peer-reviewed publications.

John Wilks MA FRSA RCST BTAA

John has been practising the Bowen technique and craniosacral therapy full time since 1995, and works at clinics in the south-west of England. He is a former chairman of the Bowen Association of the UK, the Craniosacral Therapy Association of the UK and the Cranial Forum. He is the author of three books, including *Understanding the Bowen Technique* and *Understanding Craniosacral Therapy*, both published by First Stone Publishing, and has produced two DVDs on the Bowen technique.

In 2005 he set up a two-year practitioner training for midwives in craniosacral therapy at Poole Hospital NHS Trust, the first of its kind to be accredited with the Royal College of Midwives. In 2009 he was listed in *Tatler*'s guide to the 250 best private doctors in the UK.

Maggy Burrowes

Maggy became interested in the work of Dr. Moshe Feldenkrais after many years studying movement, particularly Tai Chi Yang Style, and Martha Graham-based dance. She graduated from the first British Feldenkrais Professional Training Programme in 1990, and is still involved in the UK training programmes as an experienced practitioner, giving individual lessons to trainee practitioners in London and Sussex. Maggy has many years' experience teaching Feldenkrais, and Feldenkrais-based voice work, both privately, and in colleges, universities and adult education centres in the UK and abroad.

She has been singing professionally in the popular music field since 1983, and teaching voice and singing to a wide variety of students, including professional and trainee actors, since 1988.

Since qualifying as a Feldenkrais teacher, Maggy's ongoing project has been to develop a comprehensive awareness-based voice and singing teaching system, using the Feldenkrais approach. To this end she has explored many modern vocal teaching methods, focusing particularly on the work of Jo Estill, a highly-respected pioneer in the field of voice training, and Alison Bagnall, an Australian Feldenkrais practitioner and speech therapist. The VocalDynamix course is the culmination of her years of study, and her many years' experience of vocal exploration, experimentation and personal development.

Jessica Moolenaar

Jessica had a successful career as a performer in Contemporary Dance in the Netherlands for a decade, until injuries forced her to retire and re-train as a Pilates teacher. She undertook an MSc in Advanced Professional Practice in the school of Integrated Health of the University of Westminster to satisfy her curiosity in the context and underpinnings of her own Pilates practice. Her knowledge and interest in movement, dance, complementary and alternative health and movement practices, and the sciences underpinning them, continues to inform her Pilates practice to the general public as well as to Pilates teacher training students and professionals and movement practitioners of all levels. She also teaches dedicated remedial Pilates to injured dance students. She has been a member of and accredited Teacher Training Provider with the Pilates Foundation since 2001 and is currently serving as a committee member of the Professional Standards Committee. Jessica teaches fluid and effortless movement incorporating a mindfulness approach in order to instil better movement habits without losing sight of the whole person and their functional needs. She is particularly interested in working with clients with neurological conditions, scoliosis, hypermobility syndrome, chronic pain syndromes and trauma.

Subject Index

Author Index